THE
ABANDONMENT
RECOVERY
WORKBOOK

Also by Susan Anderson

Black Swan: Twelve Lessons of Abandonment Recovery

The Journey from Abandonment to Healing: Surviving through and Recovering from the Five Stages That Accompany the Loss of Love

Taming Your Outer Child: Overcoming Self-Sabotage and Healing from Abandonment

THE ABANDONMENT RECOVERY WORKBOOK

Guidance through the 5 Stages of Healing from Abandonment, Heartbreak, and Loss

SUSAN ANDERSON

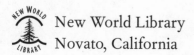
New World Library
Novato, California

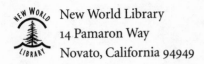 New World Library
14 Pamaron Way
Novato, California 94949

Text design by Tona Pearce Myers

Library of Congress Cataloging-in-Publication Data is available.

First New World Library printing, August 2016
ISBN 978-1-60868-427-4
Ebook ISBN 978-1-60868-428-1
Printed in Canada on 100% postconsumer-waste recycled paper

 New World Library is proud to be a Gold Certified Environmentally Responsible Publisher.
Publisher certification awarded by Green Press Initiative.
www.greenpressinitiative.org

10   9   8   7   6   5   4   3   2   1

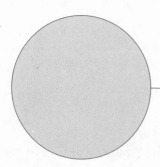

A Note to Readers

Although this book helps people get in touch with their feelings and take positive steps in their lives, it is not a substitute for professional mental health services. If you feel you are at risk or are experiencing serious psychiatric problems, it is important to seek psychiatric intervention. Those interested in enhancing the abandonment recovery process are encouraged to seek additional help from sponsors, psychotherapists, support groups, and other professional mental health services.

In all of the case studies cited here, the names are fictitious and identifying details have been changed to protect the privacy of individuals involved. The testimonies came from clients, members of support groups, and people submitting their personal stories to www.abandonment.net. Many people were eager to contribute to the legacy of abandonment recovery and gave me permission to publish their names. I demurred, understanding that they might not feel as comfortable sharing personal information after more time passes and their heartbreak is further behind them.

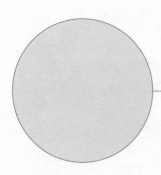

Contents

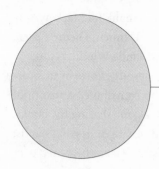

Acknowledgments

The impetus for writing this book came from the personal stories I received at my website, www.abandonment.net. They were sent by abandonment survivors from all over the world and all walks of life. Their outpouring of pain and personal truth has contributed to the growing legacy of abandonment and recovery.

Compiling the influx of anecdotal data was clearly too much for me to accomplish alone. Two psychotherapists came forward, Celeste Carlin and Donna Carson. They had dealt with the issue of abandonment in all its forms for decades. They helped me bear witness to the extraordinary legacy of childhood abandonment and how it can create vulnerability to heartache in adult relationships. They witnessed the relief people expressed about finding a listening place where others wanted to hear their stories—and even use them to help—and about finally having the pain of abandonment validated.

Celeste and Donna tallied hundreds of requests from people who wanted a more personal connection to the healing process as well as instructions for setting up abandonment support groups. They urged me to write a book to take abandonment recovery to the next level. To help me get started, Donna wrote a foreword for a proposed workbook, and Celeste wrote Akeru-to-Go exercises. Without their encouragement, moral support, and direct help, this book would not have been written.

I want to express my gratitude to abandonment survivors who wrote to me from as far away as Tasmania, Thailand, the Sudan, Singapore, Maui, Canada, South Africa, Ecuador, and Japan, as well as clients and members of the abandonment workshops I ran in Manhattan and Huntington, New York; and at Esalen Institute, Kripalu Center for Yoga and Health, New York Open Center, Breitenbush Hot Springs, and elsewhere around the country. The testimonies offered by abandonment survivors greatly enhanced the research and clinical data I had amassed over the years, and are woven into this workbook.

I am grateful to Paul, whose love, steadfastness, and support are valuable beyond description; my son, Adam, and my daughter, Erika, for providing my life's purpose, direction, and pride; my father, Dexter Griffith, for striking the balance between creativity and self-discipline; my mother, Barbara Griffith, for being the wind beneath my wings; my sister, Marcia Gerardi, and my brothers, Dexter and Robert Griffith, for their constant love and connection; Mark Gerardi, Karen Griffith, Randy Davis

Griffith, Michele Tanner, Jessica Gerardi, Kristi Griffith, Dylan Griffith, Bryan Griffith, Jesse Mark Cohen, Alexander Cohen, and Laura Cohen for their support and love. I want to thank Jill Mackey, Amy Wapner, Carole Ann Price, Pat Malone, Gina Hoffman, Pat Dennis, Anthony Damien, Diedre Olsen, Edith Drucker, Fran Friedman, Deborah Greenwood, Florence McManus, and Linda Whol.

I am indebted to Robert Gossette, Ph.D., for his discerning mind and generous efforts in mentoring the research for this book; Peter Yelton, my friend and personal guru, who contributed a wealth of conceptual material along with love and inspiration; Richard Robertiello, M.D., for sharing his books, articles, and personal guidance, Susan Golomb for believing in my work and placing it in good hands; Jason Gardner, Kim Corbin, Kristen Cashman, Tona Pearce Myers, and Christine Zika, who pored over the manuscript with loving care; Michele Monteforte for beautiful website graphic art and design; Laura Goodman, L.C.S.W., for her devotion to the abandonment community at abandonment.net; Tyler Jordan for keeping the site running smoothly; Edward Kannel, Hannelore Hahn, and IWWG for writing encouragement; and T.K., Rigo, Sheila, and the gang at my favorite waterside café—T.K.'s Galley—for putting up with my writing paraphernalia.

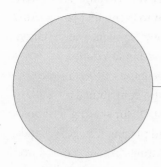

Foreword

This book is meant to be held when you need it and put away when you must. It can lie sleeping on your shelf and then be embraced quickly as you feel necessary.

It has been designed this way because abandonment does not follow a calendar year, but flows along its own silent course, creating an undercurrent of invisible triggers, making it hard to predict when and where the painful reminders might intrude. It is not only Valentine's Day, New Year's Eve, or the first day of spring that evoke painful memories but a shared song or a familiar scent. Sometimes just bumping into a mutual friend can send your whole day into a swirl.

There can be no right or wrong way to experience abandonment. There is only your way, your pace, your daily needs, your destiny to follow. It doesn't matter if it is the first time you've picked up this book or the twentieth, whether it lay on the shelf for a month or whether you determinedly read every word of every page, driven by the possibility for healing. There is enough food for thought, discovery, and healing to sustain you and help you grow.

This book offers many options for living life more fully. You may want to start an abandonment support group. You may want to go online to abandonment.net in the middle of the night to share your situation and feelings. You may choose to read, write, or reflect as a way of centering yourself. Each time you move toward embracing your hurt, each time you reach out for solace or direction, this book is there to guide and support you.

There is no time pressure of a daybook or performance pressure of a written journal. Abandonment has too much stress of its own to impose any additional burdens. Open to any page and it greets you with a salutation, a praise, a nugget of valuable information, an option to change and grow. Or if you wish, start from the beginning and follow incremental steps toward transforming your life and increasing your capacity for love.

—Donna Carson, L.C.S.W.

What Is Abandonment?

A loss of love, a feeling of disconnection, being left behind…

Abandonment. Just the mention of the word is like dropping a pebble into a still pond. Tiny waves of emotion rise up from the deep, disturbing the calm surface of life.

Abandonment conjures up children left at birth, fathers packing their suitcases and moving out, mothers dying and leaving their whole family bereft of nurturance, and lovers betraying one another's hearts. But abandonment breaks our hearts in subtle ways, too, as when we are not recognized for our accomplishments, dismissed by a friend, or not invited to a party.

This book is dedicated to abandonment survivors seeking to heal the universal wound of abandonment.

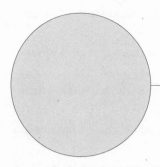

What Is Abandonment.net?

This workbook is interactive. It works in conjunction with a website whose address is abandonment.net.

Abandonment.net is exactly that—an abandonment net, a supportive base available for anyone experiencing loss, disconnection, or uncertainty about themselves or a relationship. You can log on anytime, day or night. Move from the isolation of your home to a supportive online listening space.

Abandonment survivors and therapists from all over the world reach out to us. We read what you share with interest and empathy. We respond to connect with you, express our gratitude, and provide you with updated information about how to find workshops and other materials on abandonment recovery.

We offer a wealth of resources at abandonment.net. You might begin by clicking on ABANDONMENT HELP. Then click on the question mark in the middle of the Help Center pinwheel to compare your situation to others'.

Or click on the PERSONAL STORIES button to tell us about your situation. Add your voice to the collection of wisdom from thousands of others who struggle with abandonment issues. When you share your feelings and situations, they are kept strictly confidential.

If you're interested in joining or setting up an abandonment support group, you'll find directions in Appendix A of this book, or you can click on ABANDONMENT GROUPS. You can contact us for additional support.

Maybe it's not you going through heartbreak, but you're a family member or friend. If so, you can find out how to help by clicking HELPING A FRIEND?

Mental health professionals can click on HELPING A CLIENT? to access the Professional Page, which also includes a link to find out about professional abandonment training.

Imaginary Support Group

In writing this workbook, I created a prototypic group of abandonment survivors so that I could imagine how each exercise and program might relate to their needs.

Who was included in my imaginary group?

A woman in her early twenties who feels destined to loneliness because she's afraid to risk closeness and is too vulnerable to put herself out there in the singles' world.

A man who keeps sabotaging his relationships due to anxious, insecure feelings that crop up from his previous losses and disconnections.

A woman in her fifties who's been dumped after thirty years of marriage and who has lost her financial security, her identity as a woman, and her sense of future.

A man in his twenties who others find attractive but who feels demoralized because he has just lost the love of his life and wants to die.

A woman in her thirties who's been in and out of relationships and is beginning to wonder if it's her. Does she have unresolved abandonment issues creating patterns and blocking her from finding love?

A woman in her forties going through the ending of a long, agonizing affair.

A married professional woman who is Korean, who wants to resolve *han*—a word in her native language that means "bruised spirit."

A man aged forty who is happily married and seeks to resolve depression, which he believes goes back to when he was ten and his father had left the family.

A man in his sixties who's just been abandoned by his beloved wife of forty years for whose love he toiled in his business, made untold sacrifices, did everything he could to provide for her and the family—a gentle man, who never acted selfishly or took advantage of male dominance and yet was left by his wife, who walked out the door telling him she no longer had feelings for him and now is madly in love with someone else and going through her second youth.

A woman in her thirties who's been left by her lover of seven years and who's had to relocate, but who does not have an empathic friend on whom to lay her burdens and who doesn't feel comfortable asking for help from the new acquaintances in her life.

A woman in her forties whose husband is having an affair, but he's trying to resolve his feelings so that he can return to their marriage, all of which leaves her dangling on a string.

A man in his thirties who broke up with his girlfriend and then found out that she's moved on and hooked up with someone else; he now feels unexpectedly devastated.

A man in his twenties whose partner left him for someone else and his pain is unbearable.

I also thought about someone who would not be able to access a support group. I imagined this book reaching out to a woman in prison in her thirties who wants to free herself of the incessant self-abusive dialogue going on in her head. She seeks to ease the eternal unhappiness of having to say good-bye to her children, children she continues to love from within her cell with an aching sense of helplessness that borders on torture.

In keeping these various scenarios in mind, I was able to consolidate the urgencies, challenges, and needs of several thousand people who have told me their abandonment stories.

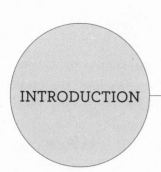

INTRODUCTION

Where the Healing Begins

I'm going to introduce myself and provide you with an overview of the process of recovery.

I am a psychotherapist trained in family, group, and individual psychotherapy techniques, but I acquired my most useful training while going through my own personal abandonment. As you read this introduction, I hope you gain a sense of knowing me—because I'm going to share from personal experience—and also a sense of perspective as I guide you through the five universal stages of abandonment and beyond. Learning the steps to take after surviving a great loss is a hopeful process. You discover your ability to benefit by the experience rather than be diminished by it.

Many of you are going through heartbreak, getting separated or divorced, or feel isolated and alone. Many of you are grieving over someone close to you who has died. Some seek recovery from childhood wounds that impinge on the quality of your current life. But our journey will take us beyond the specifics of your loss, all the way to the underlying source of the fear and despair—abandonment—the crux of the human condition.

Abandonment is a universal wound. It's what makes heartbreak so painful and what's behind the turmoil and uncertainty of divorce. It's why separation arouses such intense anxiety and why losing a friend, a job, a lover, causes our self-esteem to plummet. Abandonment is what complicates our grief when someone dies: we feel left behind. Abandonment stirs up feelings of not being worthy, not belonging, not being in control of our lives. Abandonment's wound lies deep and invisible, making it hard to let go. That's abandonment—always acting beneath the surface, spilling primal fear into moments of disconnection, disappointment, and loss. It generates feelings of insecurity and self-doubt when we attempt to love again.

This book is dedicated to healing the wound of abandonment through a step-by-step process of personal recovery. The goal is to find greater life and love than before.

Power of Example

The journey we'll take together begins with my own story.

There I was, a specialist in abandonment, helping people overcome heartbreak and loss for over twenty years, and I suddenly found myself going through my own profound abandonment. The love of my life told me one night, out of the blue, that he didn't love me anymore and wanted to leave. It came as a complete shock. We had been madly in love, deeply connected through our mutual love of nature, art, music, and so many immeasurable things. We'd led vital, interdependent lives, enhanced each other's growth, traveled the world together, built a family, a home, and celebrated life together for nearly twenty years. And now this.

Feeling as if a knife had been thrust through my heart, I struggled to cope with the same torturous pain I'd specialized in helping my clients cope with for over twenty years.

As a professional, I had already gleaned all of the available information on the subject from the existing psychology and self-help literature and found it to be sparse and simplistic when it came to abandonment. Heartbreak had been trivialized. Conventional wisdom consisted almost entirely of platitudes that were nearly impossible to apply, especially when going through the intense emotional crisis of abandonment.

Love yourself.
Find happiness from within.
You don't need a man (or woman) to make you happy.
Celebrate your pain.
Let go and move forward.

If it were easy to recover from such a deep personal injury, surely we'd all be going on with our lives. The walking wounded with chronic uncertainty and damaged self-esteem would spontaneously recover. I have never met people more motivated to *move forward* and *let go* than those surviving abandonment. But they need more than placebo advice. Faced with the real burden of recovery from so damaging a wound, people need realistic steps that are well researched, clinically tested, and really work. That is what this book is designed to provide.

Being left by someone you love creates such intense anxiety and despair that many people turn to sedatives like alcohol, pills, or illicit drugs.[1] Some commit or try to commit suicide.[2]

Others commit or try to commit homicide. We hear about this all the time. Someone's ex, heartbroken and unable to deal with the rejection, goes off on a rampage to choke her former spouse or to set fire to the social club where his old girlfriend and her new boyfriend are together or to shoot her in her wedding dress as she's about to marry someone else.

While these not-so-rare murders and suicides receive media attention, the powerful abandonment rage underlying these actions is rarely alluded to. Yet it is there, an unspoken reminder of everyone's vulnerability. We understand only too well how difficult it is to contain the seething, burning anger of rejection and feel deeply disturbed to see someone else lose control and destroy lives.[3]

In the course of this book, I will give heartbreak the serious treatment it deserves, investigating the source of its overpowering feelings. Together, we'll explore ways to prevent rage from inflicting such devastating consequences on self and others. We'll also learn about the lingering grief of abandonment—why it is so difficult to let go when someone leaves you.

What does a therapist do when faced with a personal crisis of gargantuan proportions in her own area of expertise? Having found nothing in the literature that spoke to the center of my pain, I decided to write my own. I began this effort by writing an allegory about a little girl who goes for a walk with her father deep into the woods…

…He walks her across a log in the water and puts her high upon a rock jutting out in the stream. "You stay here while I go pick us some huckleberries for lunch," he says.

"Don't go far, Daddy," begs the little girl.

"I won't," he promises. He makes his way back across the log and into the forest as the little girl studies the back of his red shirt to keep track of him. He is momentarily hidden, first behind this tree and then behind that one. Suddenly there is no sight of red at all.

Perched atop the giant rock, the little girl begins calling to her daddy, hoping he is right nearby only teasing her. "Daddy, I'm here," she calls. "Daddy, where are you?" But after a while she can't hold back her terror. She screams into the forest with all her might. The forest remains silent.

As night falls, the little girl is frozen with fright on the cold, hard rock…

She has been abandoned.*

When I first wrote this story, it had no resolution—the image of the child on the rock remained a literary still-life intended to represent the desolation and terror we all feel when left by someone we love. It expressed the depths of my own pain.

As most people discover when going through the pain that accompanies a loss of love, just surviving each day becomes a full-time job. Life is suddenly devoted to pain management.[4] From years of clinical work helping people through abandonment, I knew the best way to ensure my own emotional survival was to get into the moment and stay there as long as possible.

I'd need to practice the art of mindfulness—become a Buddhist in my everyday life.[5] This meant going places and doing things that stimulated my senses—using my senses of hearing, sight, and touch and breathing in a deliberate, conscious new way to attend more closely to the moment.

The moment is nature's refuge from pain. Getting into the moment brings you out of your head where all of your painful thoughts reside and into the sensations that are present in your immediate environment. By concentrating your attention on what you are experiencing now on a sensory level, you momentarily take leave of your fearful thoughts about your future or your sorrowful thoughts about your loss. You substitute the sensations of the moment for the obsessively painful chatter going on in

---

*   Excerpted from my book *Black Swan* (1999).

your head. In present-tense mode, there is only now. Opening your senses to the sounds and smells and sights of the moment allows you to co-exist with your feelings without having to suppress them. As you learn how to use the moment, you learn how to experience life more intensely, gaining self-nurturance, self-generosity, and emotional self-reliance.

"Aren't you supposed to embrace your pain?" people have asked me "—to stay with it in order to work it through?"

When someone you love leaves you, getting through the pain is a matter of survival. Your primary task during the initial crisis is emotional rescue. Owing to the circumstances of abandonment, you are usually left to do this alone. You are in disconnect mode. Separation anxiety is coursing through your every waking moment. You are struggling to survive at a time when your life feels over, when everything you care about is suddenly gone. Getting into the moment helps you discover your ability as a separate human being to withstand the pain and anxiety of being left. You discover that you can stand on your own two feet and live and function in spite of being bombarded by unwanted emotion. In the moment, you can find relief without attempting to deny the reality that confronts you or suppress the feelings. In my case, I knew that to manage the emotional crisis and gain strength from it, the best thing I could do was to get into the moment and stay there as much as possible.

Getting into the moment is how we learn one of life's greatest lessons: that we can survive as a separate human being—as long as we take it one moment at a time. Grief work is about accepting the pain of loss. In the moment, rather than try to resist the emotion that envelops us, we learn to accept its reality and remain fully intact in spite of the overwhelming panic, rage, and despondency we experience. Using our sensory organs to tune in to the sights and sounds of the here and now, we can stop fretting about what will happen tomorrow.

Attending to now gets you out of your head, instantly lifting you above your fears about the future and your sorrow about the past. You go from disconnect mode to reconnect mode: you reconnect to life in a profound new way—in the moment.

In the midst of the devastation of abandonment, getting into the moment is an exercise that takes determination, discipline, and grit. But it is worth the effort. The moment offers an oasis of safety and calm. We'll explore a specific exercise for getting into the moment in chapter 3.

During my own abandonment crisis, I found it difficult to stay in the moment for more than a few seconds at a time. My mind kept pulling me back into my despair, panic, grief, and hurt. But I persevered at this exercise the same way I coached my clients to do over the years. Each time I succeeded at getting into the moment, I gained another notch in my ability to rely on my own personal resources. Gaining self-reliance was not much of a consolation in light of my overwhelming sorrow, but I knew that the exercise's intent was not to console me; it was to survive the pain. Gaining personal strength was a side effect.

So, the morning after my beloved life partner of twenty years moved out, I took the world's most deliberately conscious walk, concentrating intently on seeing and noticing everything possible with my eyes, skin, ears—all to get into the moment. Walking downhill toward the harbor, I kept lapsing into nightmarish thoughts about my new situation, then catching myself and focusing all of my energy on getting back into the moment.

The pain stood on either side of the moment. When I'd think about the past—how just yesterday he'd been in my life—I'd feel overwhelming grief. When I thought about my future—the prospect of being alone—I faced the terrifying abyss of the unknown.

Would I succumb to this fear and pain? Would I die alone?

The moment has no future and no past. It is about now. It contains the sensations of life, which include the birds high in the treetops and the car engines down on the highway, all happening in the present. The split second of the moment cuts a path between past and future and offers a safety zone, an oasis to return to in time of need.

When we are racked in emotional pain, getting into the moment requires real effort and know-how. The most efficient way to get into the moment is to isolate one of the sensory organs and use it in a deliberate, systematic way to tune in to what's going on within and around you. For many of my clients, workshop attendees, as well as myself, our sense of hearing helps us most quickly gain entry into the moment.

So as I made my way toward the harbor, whenever the pain hit, I stopped walking and shut my eyes to tune out everything but the background noises. I'd concentrate with all my might until my ears could detect the faint buzzing of insects in the grass and the rustling of leaves in the bushes. Listening intently to these sounds brought me momentarily above the depths of despair. Then, to intensify this present-tense oasis, I'd gradually reopen my eyes to attend to a few carefully selected sights, such as the lace pattern of sunlight sprinkling through the tree branches. Using the moment's respite, I remained in tune with the sensations of the here and now as long as I could, which would usually last all of about four seconds. Then I'd dissolve into fear and despair once again.

Reaching the harbor in this stop-and-start manner, an astounding spectacle awaited me. A black swan. I was stunned. This was not a black cormorant or a charcoal-gray Canada goose. This was a black swan with a beautiful long neck and bright-red beak gliding in and among a flock of white swans. This spectacular sight was enough to distract me from my pain, at least for a moment.

I never knew such a creature existed. How could this be? Where had he come from?

I couldn't help but be moved by the timing of such an event. I decided to interpret the arrival of the black swan as a gift, a windfall, an opportunity—for what I wasn't yet sure.

My swan certainly wasn't home in these waters; he was strange to the region—to the country—and obviously isolated. I identified my own situation with his.

Every morning I took my stop-start staccato walk down to the harbor, counting my breaths along the way or intently listening to the background sounds—all to seek momentary refuge in the moment. And when I'd arrive at the harbor, I was always heartened to see my swan still there. As I photographed him, I observed how he loved to glide far out into the harbor, as far away from the other swans as he could get, as if to exaggerate his aloneness. I knew there was a lesson in this for me, but I wasn't yet sure exactly how to apply it.

I kept steady watch on his behavior. As I learned more about him, I started to write about the black swan in my allegory about the child on the rock. I knew the swan beheld wisdom that could help her, but it meant I'd have to first get her down from the rock. As a therapist, I knew I couldn't leave the little girl up there in a helpless, passive position. She'd have to climb down and find her way out of the forest before she would be in an active enough position to take hold of the opportunity that was to come to her by way of the mystical black swan. I could hardly wait to see what was going to transpire between them. Over many months, my allegory transformed from a simple vignette to the *Iliad* and the *Odyssey* of the heart. There were to be a succession of twelve lessons between the black swan and the little girl as she made her way along the path of healing.

There is something ironic about healing. Even though it is a *natural* process, people going through a devastating experience like abandonment, loss, or disappointment often go against it. They do the very opposite of what will help them.

That's why it so often takes a long time for the emotional turmoil to go away—and why we get stuck in our anxiety and pain. We fight the process, and this emotional protest can cause some of us to invert our sense of loss into rage, numbness, or depression. Abandonment recovery shows us how to give up our relentless protest and work *with*, rather than *against* the feelings.

The swan had slowly emerged in my mind as a figure of mystical proportions on whom I managed to project untapped wisdom coming from somewhere within my higher self.

He seemed to hold the key that unlocked the code of recovery. I observed my mysterious mentor closely over many months and wrote him into my evolving epic. The majestic black swan slowly unraveled the sequence of steps involved in healing the primal wound of abandonment. Through his lessons, he helped the little girl absorb them one by one. In revealing the Twelve Lessons of Emotional and Spiritual Healing, he guided my own path of recovery.

THE TWELVE SWAN LESSONS

1. Centering
2. Cleansing
3. Attending
4. Separating
5. Beholding
6. Accepting
7. Increasing Love
8. Letting Go
9. Reaching Out
10. Integrating and Owning
11. Transcending
12. Connecting

As the little girl followed the steps of recovery, she performed a physical gesture for each lesson. These are the universal gestures I have observed people use, even when they're not conscious of it, as they come to terms with a great loss. Since the primal pain of abandonment is often wordless, much of our healing is through these gestures. For example, as you will see in the next chapter, when the little girl learned to find her peaceful center within—the beginning point of healing—she placed her hands across her chest. I have seen countless people perform this gesture when attempting to center themselves during a stressful moment.

As we make our way through the chapters, we will review each of the Swan Lessons along with the twelve gestures that accompany them. I have shared these gestures during my workshops and support groups, and I have acted as a conductor, leading a movement choir of people in performing the twelve gestures in front of an audience, accompanied by music.[6] We stretch the gestures out, exaggerate each one, and then bring them back to the same simple gestures we all practice in everyday life. One gesture flows into the next, creating a flowing signature of healing that is unique to each person.

It is important for readers to realize that the little girl was able to benefit by the black swan's guidance because she climbed down from her rock and actively participated in each of the twelve lessons. I hope you take example from this as you make your way through the Swan Lessons by becoming active in your own recovery. Reading is a passive activity, writing is active. Jotting down your thoughts and feelings on paper helps draw you directly into the process. This book provides a way for you to take action—not only with the lessons but with the other healing balms presented throughout. Participate in your own recovery. Rather than just reading or imagining what the exercises are like, you will gain most by *doing* them.[7]

Take a little break from reading this book and think about an experience in life that left you feeling as if you had been put up on the rock. Describe.

How old were you? _____ How did you feel?

Obviously, you've survived this. What strengths helped you climb down from the rock and find your way out of the forest?

Is this strength present in you today? Name this strength.

You can practice each of the twelve Swan Lessons and other recovery exercises by writing your responses here, in the boxes provided, or you can expand on them in your own journals and notebooks. You can bring the Qs into your abandonment support groups and use them as the basis for powerful group discussions.*

---

* See Appendix A for instructions for setting up abandonment support groups. Abandonment.net offers more help. Contact us.

Exploring S.W.I.R.L.

I spent the next year discovering, writing about, and incorporating into my life each of the Swan Lessons, as well as sharing them with my clients. I performed the lessons every day, using the gestures that go with them, and over time I began to feel stronger and more confident than I'd ever felt before. One morning about a year after my breakup, I set out for my usual walk around the harbor, unaware that I was about to have an epiphany. I was aware only that I was happy and in love, grateful for where my life was. When I reached the harbor, I felt a tingling sensation as it occurred to me that the dark cloud of grief, no longer above me, suddenly seemed far behind me. Observing its shape and dimensions from a distance, I was able to see for the first time that abandonment has its own kind of grief—a powerful grief universal to human beings. I could see where its natural folds lay—that it broke down into five universal stages: Shattering, Withdrawal, Internalizing, Rage, and Lifting.

Each of the stages affects a different aspect of human functioning and calls forth a different emotional response. They overlap one another as part of one inexorable process of grief and recovery.

I was awestruck at the cyclonic nature of this all-encompassing cloud that had enveloped me for so long. This had been a profoundly difficult life process I had been through and that I helped my clients through over the years. Now that I was on professional as well as personal terms with this process, I had the vantage point of having been inside the universal pain and experienced for myself what it took to survive it.

Here is a brief overview of the stages of abandonment grief, each of which is discussed fully in the chapters to come. I show you how the twelve lessons of healing fit the five stages as we make our way—stage by stage, lesson by lesson—through this journey beyond heartbreak to connection.

The Five Stages of Abandonment

Shattering: The painful tear in your attachment, a stab wound to the heart. The sudden disconnection sends you into panic, devastation, shock, and bewilderment. You feel symbiotically attached to your lost love—as if you couldn't survive alone. You're in crisis and feel as if you'd been severed from your Siamese twin and you were in the recovery room in pain and alone. You try to keep remnants of your fractured self together, but your whole sense of reality feels destroyed. One minute you succumb to the overwhelming despair, suicidal feelings, and sorrow. The next, you see glimmers of hope.

Withdrawal: Love withdrawal is just like heroin withdrawal—each involves intense yearning for the object of desire, and this craving is mediated by opioids within your body.[8] You feel a painful aching, longing, needing a love fix and can't get one. You feel strung out. Your mind incessantly waits for your lost love to call or return. You're plagued with separation anxiety—an expectant, urgent feeling of heightened vulnerability. Physical components of withdrawal from love are the same as they are for withdrawal from heroin. You're in withdrawal from your endogenous opiates[9] as well as suffused with fight-or-flight stress hormones. Your withdrawal symptoms include wasting, weight loss, wakefulness.

Internalizing: You begin to turn your rage over being rejected against yourself, which accounts for the intense depression that accompanies abandonment.[10] You idealize your lost love at your own expense, indicting yourself for losing the most important person in your life. You internalize the rejection, interpreting the dismissal as evidence of your alleged personal unworthiness. Internalizing is the most critical stage, when your wound can become infected, scarring your self-image.[11] You inculcate a narcissistic injury.[12] Your self-doubt has the power to implant an invisible drain deep within the self that insidiously leaches self-esteem from within. You have grave doubts about your ability to hold someone's love and blame yourself for the loss. Old feelings of insecurity merge into your new wound, creating lingering insecurity. Without recovery, this feeling can interfere in future relationships.

Rage: You attempt to reverse the rejection, expressing rage over being left. You are restless to get your life back in order and riddled with low frustration tolerance, your anger spurting out of control.[13] You resent being thrust into aloneness against your will.[14] You regress into fantasies of revenge and retaliation. Your aggressive energy is like a pressure cooker. You boil over easily, sometimes spewing anger onto innocent bystanders (like your friends when they fail to understand what you're going through). Many of you who have difficulty with assertiveness tend to invert your rage into an agitated depression.

Lifting: Life begins to distract you, lifting you back into it. You experience intervals of peace and confidence. Abandonment's lessons are learned, and you get ready to love again. Without recovery, some of you make the mistake of lifting above your feelings, losing touch with your emotional center, becoming more isolated than before.[15]

You swirl through the stages within an hour, a day, a year, cycles in cycles, and you emerge out the end of its funnel-shaped cloud a changed person. As you learn how to handle the feelings at each stage of this overwhelming process, this transformation lifts you to greater life and love.

The S.W.I.R.L. Process provides a framework by which to organize your overwhelming experience. Since recovery is greatly enhanced by your active participation, once again, I offer an opportunity to relate your own situation to each of these stages.

Bear in mind that the stages are not discrete time packets but rather one continuous process. We tend to go back and forth among them, sometimes experiencing two or more at once; and just as we think we're through, something happens that seems to thrust us right back to the beginning.

THE FIVE STAGES OF ABANDONMENT

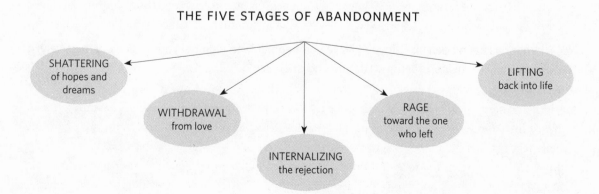

SHATTERING of hopes and dreams

WITHDRAWAL from love

INTERNALIZING the rejection

RAGE toward the one who left

LIFTING back into life

Actually, it only feels that way. Each time you swirl through the stages, you come out with greater awareness, strength, and capacity for love than before. This book will help you use the cyclonic feelings of each stage to make profound personal changes and transform your life. You need to remain determined to turn abandonment—one of life's most painful experiences—into an opportunity for profound personal growth.

We have all been through the S.W.I.R.L. Process at one time or another as we flow through the disconnections and disappointments of everyday life. Briefly review the stages to answer the following questions. Remember, we will cover each of the stages in greater depth as we continue our journey.

What has the S.W.I.R.L. Process been like for you?

Shattering: What has Shattering been like? How have you handled the feelings?

Withdrawal: Describe any Withdrawal symptoms you have experienced. How have you handled the yearning and longing?

Internalizing: What has your experience been like going through the Internalizing process? Has heartbreak hurt your self-esteem? How?

Rage: What has Rage been like for you? Have you been able to channel your Rage constructively, or has it bottlenecked inside, creating agitation and depression?

Lifting: Describe your experience with Lifting. What experiences help you lift above the pain, even if momentarily?

We each have our own way of dealing with these stages, our own signature. Everyone's swirl is unique. Here is an example from a group I ran several years ago.

> "I seem to swirl backward," says Keaton. "It's the story of my life—even on good days I manage to put my socks on inside out, so why shouldn't I expect to swirl in reverse too?"
>
> Members of the group laughed, having come to enjoy Keaton's unique take on life.
>
> "When my girlfriend and I first broke up," he continues, "I began with the last stage, Lifting [stage 5]—thinking my life would be better than ever, feeling relieved that our hassles were over. But then I found myself going through Rage [stage 4] because I was aggravated that things weren't going as good for me as I planned. And then I began Internalizing [stage 3] the whole mess, taking it personally that she no longer wanted me and began to beat myself up for being stupid enough to let her go. Then I went into severe Withdrawal [stage 2] from missing all the good things about being together, and this put me right back to the beginning into Shattering [stage 1]—which got me cycling backward."

Our own unique style of swirling through the stages is based on patterns we developed from having survived previous losses, heartbreaks, and disconnections during childhood and adolescence. It's also affected by our temperament and personality, and our susceptibility to feeling rejected. Incidentally, rejection sensitivity runs rather high among abandonment survivors, as you might well have noticed.

The many people who have shared their stories with me have used the term *swirl* in many different ways, describing how they've been "Swirling all of their lives," "Sucked into the swirl," or "Drowning in swirl," to quote a few.*

How does the concept of *swirl* apply to your current life situation?

---

*   To submit your personal story, contact us at abandonment.net.

Does it apply to previous times of loss in your life? How?

Which stage of swirl do you feel you tend to get stuck in the most?

How has this concept been useful to you?

 Mini-Swirls

Most therapists understand that the underlying abandonment wound can be easily accessed in their client's most mundane events of everyday life. For survivors of childhood abandonment, as well as those who are going through a heartbreak, the abandonment nerve twinges if, in the course of a normal day, they feel criticized, excluded, misunderstood, overlooked, taken for granted, belittled, disrespected, or made to wait.

With our vulnerability heightened, almost anything can cause us to begin swirling. It can be very subtle. Feeling left out, ignored by a friend, or failing to get recognition at work can set swirl in motion. On a bad day, losing your keys can send you swirling. Most of us realize we're overreacting, but we tend to fault ourselves rather than recognizing the universal process beneath our taut nerves and tender feelings.

You might even go into a mild swirl if, for example, a member of your abandonment support group fails to show up one night. You, along with the other group members, experience the absence of that person as a slight letdown, a disconnection (a mild Shattering). You feel a slight anticipation—waiting for him to arrive, wishing, wondering why he's not there (Withdrawal). Then you feel slightly rejected, a little dismissed, that the group just wasn't important enough to him (Internalizing). You may not even be conscious of the mild self-doubt and self-deprecation that set in. You think to yourself, "I guess the group is more important to me than to him. We're not special or interesting enough." Then you feel a twinge of annoyance over the fact that he didn't bother to let one of us know, or couldn't hold to his commitment (Rage). And finally, even before these subliminal thoughts reach your awareness, you lift into the group discussion as it starts to get under way (Lifting). You went through swirl on such a subtle level you weren't even conscious of it. But the vulnerability was there, tingeing the moment with a little more self-doubt and disappointment than usual.

Take a moment to reflect on your own unique style of the mini-swirl. Can you think of a recent instance that caused one?

Were you conscious of overreacting at the time?

What was this mini-swirl like for you? Can you identify any of its stages, however subtle? If so, which stage was most difficult?

How do you handle mini-swirls?

How would you like to handle the next one?

AKERU: WHAT IS AKERU?

Akeru is the name I've given to a program that turns the pain of an ending into the beginning of positive change. Akeru is a Japanese word with many meanings: to end, to begin, to pierce, to start, to expire, to unwrap, to turn over, to close, and to open. It's a perfect word to describe the cycle of renewal and healing involved in abandonment recovery. Akeru also refers to the empty space created when someone leaves, allowing you to see a painful loss as an opportunity to fill a void with something new and positive.

Akeru is an innovation. Until now, abandonment has been a most difficult wound to heal. People immured in its anxiety and despair have been seeking all kinds of remedies to quell the internal disquiet. Yoga, meditation, and relaxation techniques have had an indirect impact in that they provide sustenance to the whole person. In fact, abandonment survivors have found great relief by gaining access to a place of peace and calm within. Akeru provides a way to bring this meditative and creative energy directly to the source of the abandonment wound. Akeru works with rather than against the energy involved in the pain. It taps into the powerful human drive toward attachment to create new life and connection.

Akeru recognizes abandonment as a rebirth.

Throughout the book, I guide you through each of the five Akeru exercises. There is one for each stage of the S.W.I.R.L. Process.

For Shattering, the Akeru exercise is called *Staying in the Moment.*

For Withdrawal, the exercise involves creating a *Big You / Little You Dialogue.*

For Internalizing, there is a visualization exercise called *Building a Dream House.*

For Rage, you discover a powerful self-awareness tool called *Outer Child.*

For Lifting, the exercise involves *Increasing Your Capacity for Love* and connection.

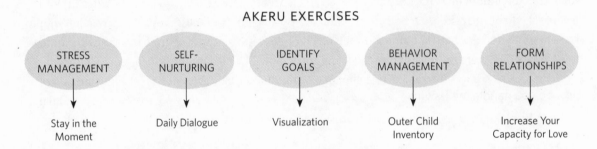

AKERU EXERCISES

STRESS MANAGEMENT	SELF-NURTURING	IDENTIFY GOALS	BEHAVIOR MANAGEMENT	FORM RELATIONSHIPS
Stay in the Moment	Daily Dialogue	Visualization	Outer Child Inventory	Increase Your Capacity for Love

We explore the stages and exercises one at a time, coming up for air along the way to give you an opportunity to apply what you are learning. In addition to Akeru and the Swan Lessons, you'll find many recovery shortcuts, including Truth Nuggets, Action Bullets, and Back to the Future, as well as the opportunity to respond to many Qs (questions) and IQs (inventory questionnaires). You'll learn how to join or set up abandonment support groups and have an opportunity to go online to abandonment.net to connect to a listening space designed for you and others going through heartbreak, loss, and disconnection.* You'll also learn about Community Projects—how to reach out to members of your community who need your special attention or support.

All of the different-sized and -shaped healing balms of this program add up to one goal: recovery from the universal wound of abandonment. Our goal is to celebrate the life around us at all times and increase our capacity for love.

---

*   For instructions to set up abandonment support groups, see Appendix A. Or go to abandonment.net for more help.

1 Centering

When I was going through Shattering, I was astounded by the intensity of my feelings. I had been at the other end of this pain for years, helping my clients cope with the panic, hopelessness, and despair of abandonment. In the midst of their initial throes of grief, it was always difficult to convince them that the devastation was temporary. Now I had trouble convincing myself.

Hopelessness is a powerful feeling belonging to the Shattering stage, but it is a feeling, not a fact. It passes, giving way to a brighter outlook. When you're in its grips, though, your sense of dead and panic feel real, warping your sense of reality with visions of *always* and *never*.

"I'll always feel broken and alone. I'll never love again."

I'm going to take you through the feelings of the Shattering stage. We'll explore what makes them so intense and what to do about them. We'll discuss the shame, fear, and sense of doom of this initial stage and take you through the first step in the healing process.

Shattering is the first stage of abandonment—when your love is torn and your security's ripped away. You are suddenly in disconnect mode. Your heart pounds and stomach turns upside down. Severing a relationship creates real trauma.[1] It sends you into shock, disbelief, bewilderment. You feel unable to face the reality of your life. You're alienated from your feelings, literally disconnected from self. Nothing seems real except the pain.

"When Julian left me," said Sandra, "he took all of my hopes and dreams with him. My future suddenly went up in smoke. I didn't want to live without him. I was shattered."

Shattering fractures the lens of reality. We experience visions of our lost love in every blue car that drives by or think we hear her voice coming from somewhere in the crowd.[2] We overreact to every love song on the radio and agonize over every lost caress.[3]

Shattering also occurs in ripples. The emotional volcano of a breakup produces aftershocks and reverberations that affect the landscape of our future. If we know how to handle the feelings, this change can be for the better. The everyday trials and tribulations of life trigger emotional memories of earlier losses, flooding our current crisis with old familiar feelings of helplessness and insecurity.[4] The tools of abandonment recovery allow us to administer to these primal needs and feelings, enabling us to finally heal from our oldest wounds.

Many people have probably been through Shattering but have yet to resolve the leftover tears and broken dreams. They experience patterns of abandonment, set in motion by the aftershocks of a previous loss. Bits and particles of a shattered self, from previous losses, continually work their way up from the wound to the surface. They block the healthy flow of your relationships and your life. The next few chapters help you work the splinters through—from your Shatterings past and present.

 ## Swirling through Shattering

If you're going through a loss of love, you tend to swirl from Shattering through the rest of the stages and then come back again to Shattering to revisit the realization that the bottom has dropped out of your world. You revisit Shattering each time you have contact with your ex, go through a Saturday night alone, or deal with another holiday and suddenly feel desperate for that special connection you no longer have. Many people attempt to medicate their pain with alcohol, drugs, sleep, food, sex, shopping—anything to dull the sensations, quell the anxiety, ease the hurt.[5]

Whether you're reading this book to heal from a recent heartbreak or because you're experiencing waves of insecurity from previous losses, the feelings of Shattering are potentially valuable. As you learn how to harness their energy, you turn adversity into triumph.

In the meantime, it's important during Shattering to accept the *possibility* that the following facts are true.[6]

Check the items you agree with.

- ❑ The intense feelings of Shattering are temporary.
- ❑ The intensity is natural and universal to human beings.
- ❑ In fact, there is a biochemical basis for feeling so wounded and afraid.
- ❑ Childhood losses remain imprinted in my brain and are being reignited by my current experience of abandonment.
- ❑ These deeply personal feelings are the tools with which I will construct my healing.
- ❑ By staying in the moment I will learn to manage my pain.

❏ Progressing through recovery, I will eventually come to view Shattering as a gift, an opportunity for a fuller self to emerge, a chance for a whole new life to start, an awakening.

❏ By facing my personal truths and maintaining a vision for a better future, I will learn to increase my capacity for love and connection.

I know that to invite *possibility* into your life requires a leap of faith. Even as you feel yourself falling into an abyss, faith in your capacity for healing helps you grow wings on the way down.[7] Eventually you lift to greater life and love than before.

This book is designed to help you take that leap of faith in yourself and the power that is within all of us to heal the deepest of wounds.

Take yourself by the hand and entertain the Power of Possibility. Consider the testimonies of others who have stood where you stand.

"If you'd told me that I'd find love again," says Sam, "I'd have punched you out. In fact people did try calming me down. 'You'll see, it'll be all right,' they'd say, 'you'll find somebody.' But I believed my life was over and I was infuriated that nobody believed me! Yet here I am today proving them right. I'm in a new relationship—the best I ever had."

"I was absolutely convinced that I was going to die of my wounds," reports Phyllis. "Being betrayed by the love of my life was a wound too great to heal. It was unbearable agony—like being burned alive very slowly over a barbecue pit—with my best friend and greatest love stoking the flames. Back then I couldn't possibly glimpse the fact that I was going to wind up with a whole new job, new career, new life, new me."

Take a moment to entertain the possibility that your abandonment is going to help your life in a profound way. Writing down your thoughts reinforces the impact of possibility.

What would entertaining the Power of Possibility mean in your life?

One of the things that therapists know too well is that most people do not acknowledge the depths of their pain. They don't give themselves the opportunity to validate the strength it takes to go on. So many of us are in survival mode. To stop and truly celebrate our strength and courage is to begin living our lives more consciously, with recognition of life's greatness—as well as our own greatness to meet its challenges.

Q

How have you persevered through this difficult time? Give yourself credit for doing so.

> People frequently ask: "Why can't I control the pain or at least make it calm down?"
>
> I explain: If you've lost your significant other, you've sustained a real wound—a wound that must be taken care of. Like it is with any other serious injury, you can't just switch off the pain. Strangely, most of us think we should be able to.

"All of this crying and desperation! It makes me feel weak," says Jean, "as if it proves my abandoner right to have dumped me."

When we find that we can't regulate the intensity, we feel ashamed for succumbing to the emotional excess.

Why Do I Feel the Way I Do?

Understanding the biological level of heartbreak is an empowering tool for negotiating its treacherous waters. Let's begin by discussing the amygdala.

The amygdala is the seat of emotional memory. We are going to learn a lot about the amygdala, because it plays a lead role in your abandonment experience.

Your amygdala is an almond-shaped structure set deep within the mammalian brain (or "limbic system,"[8] as some call it). The amygdala plays a central role in the way you emotionally respond to any threatening situation. It functions as your body's central alarm, scanning your environment for signs of imminent danger, warning and empowering you with powerful stress hormones with which to protect yourself. The danger it perceives can be a stampeding herd of buffalo, an explosion in a nearby building, or the threat of your primary relationship breaking apart.

Imprinted in your amygdala are memories of how you responded to fearful events accumulated since childhood—events that conditioned you to respond automatically to future events. Its emotional memory is believed to contain traces of your birth experience as well.[9] The amygdala reacts to abandonment as a threat. We experience this reaction as fear.[10] Our first fear is abandonment—being left with no one to ensure our survival. Witness the infant who cries in terror when his mother's face disappears from his bedside.

Anything reminiscent of previous events is able to set off the amygdala's alarm and propel you into a state of neurobiological emergency. When the threat is an armed enemy, your body goes into the fight-or-flight response, physically preparing you to endure a battle. When the threat is loss of a relationship, your body reacts the same way, but you interpret the surge of neurohormones and other physiological signs of self-defense as "going to pieces."

The amygdala is like an overprotective watchdog during abandonment. It perceives losing your emotional attachment as a direct threat to your life and acts swiftly to alert your autonomic nervous system to go into red alert. Because heartbreak is an ongoing crisis, your ever-watchful amygdala keeps you in an action-ready state, as if you were sustaining an ongoing siege of violence.

Why Does It React That Way?

This small organ in your brain was conditioned to respond to abandonment when you were a small child forming attachments to your parents.[11] Things were different then. As a child you couldn't have survived without someone taking care of you. Your amygdala is not equipped to know the difference between then and now. When you go through an adult breakup, it responds as if you were still a small child whose very existence is threatened, and it dispatches the self-defense artillery of your mammalian brain. The pounding of your heart and queasiness are signs of your body's defense mechanisms kicking in—your autonomic nervous system going into full sway. *Autonomic* means "automatic." You automatically go into survival mode, which, quoting from the annals of medical humor, include the Four Fs of Survival: *fighting*, *fleeing*, *freezing*, and *sexual reproduction*.

Shattering is the trauma stage of the S.W.I.R.L. Process; the unbearable vulnerability you feel is one of its primary symptoms. Abandonment constitutes a *sustained* emotional crisis.[12] It's not like a train crash that happens once and then you set out to recover. The stress of abandonment is sustained day after day as the ramifications of your loss mount. Each new jolt of the reality that your relationship is threatened sends your amygdala into increasingly high alert. It deploys repeated volleys of stress hormones to keep you on edge and battle ready for the long haul.

Another of the amygdala's significant functions is that it triggers emotional memories from the past—memories that are often detached from the events that caused them.[13] This floods you with old, unwelcome feelings that seem all out of proportion to the actual event.[14]

It helps to become in tune with the power of the mind-body connection so that you understand why you feel out of control. Indeed, automatic responses are taking over.

IQ   Mind-Body Checklist

Check the symptoms that apply to you.

FOURTEEN SCIENTIFIC TIDBITS[15]

❑ I can't sleep because the steady secretions of stress hormones create a sustained nocturnal vigil.

❑ I can't eat because my digestive energy is shunted to major muscle groups for battle strength.

❑ Alternately, I am ravenously hungry because glucocorticoid stress hormones[16] build up in my bloodstream and stimulate appetite to help sustain nutrients for ongoing self-defense.

❑ My eyes feel weak; I experience changes in depth perception because my pupils dilate to pinpoint my enemy at a distance.

❏ I have a tendency to sigh because respiration becomes shallow to enable me to detect sounds of danger above the sound of my own breathing.

❏ I am preoccupied with old losses, rejections, and heartbreaks because my amygdala sent a relay to other brain stations to sort through related memory banks of earlier experiences to provide life-saving information.[17]

❏ I jump at the slightest noise; I can hear his car on faraway streets because the cochlear receptors in my inner ears increase their capacity to detect faraway sounds to aid in self-protection.

❏ I feel enraged; I want to lash out because my amygdala activated a self-defense response and I am in the *fight* phase of the Four Fs of Survival.

❏ I can't move forward, can't make decisions, feel stunned, dazed, immobilized because I'm in the *freeze* phase of the Four Fs of Survival.

❏ I feel a frequent urge to masturbate because I am in the fourth phase of the Four Fs of Survival.

❏ I have a strained, possibly higher pitched voice because my vocal cords tighten to emit distinctive sounds of fright to signal my allies that danger is present.

❏ I have a high pulse rate and high blood pressure because more oxygen and blood nutrients are needed to fuel my battle performance.

❏ I run to the bathroom because my body is voiding its waste products to make me lighter on my feet to better fight my enemy or sprint away from him.

❏ I flinch easily because stress hormones surge to increase my response time, allowing me to dart out of the way of a hurled rock.

Most of these effects dissipate as you come out of the Shattering crisis, but some can last longer or become chronic. For instance, you might wake up with separation anxiety each morning or feel shock waves of despair during certain moments in your day for an ongoing period.

Q

Take a moment to consider your current mind-body state. Write a phrase or sentence that describes some of your current feelings and how they seem to manifest in your body.

How do these feelings interfere in your life?

Name a strength you use to cope with them.

Shame and Self-Blame

Many people have trouble accepting the intense fear and despair involved in loss. Faulting yourself for feeling miserable only makes the crisis worse because it creates shame—a destructive emotion.[18] Shame is a major component of heartbreak, especially if you feel rejected. Losing someone's love can feel demoralizing and plunge you into self-doubt, causing you to feel unworthy, defective even. It is humiliating to feel that you've been thrown away by someone you love.

Shame is an insidious and destructive emotion. Unless you challenge its assumptions, it can go underground and become an internal saboteur, bent on using your most vulnerable feelings against you.

The antidote to shame is self-acceptance.

To assess your current level of shame, explore these questions.

Are you able to accept the automatic (autonomic) nature of your response to your loss or do you fault yourself because your emotions are too out of control?

Describe what aspects of your current situation cause you to feel humiliated, guilty, or ashamed.

Do you blame yourself for your breakup? Does self-blame engender feelings of unworthiness or inadequacy?

Give yourself a message of self-acceptance for withstanding such difficult feelings.

What strengths do you use to prevent heartbreak from damaging your sense of self-worth?

Accepting the Pain of Loss

Learning to accept the pain of loss helps reduce shame. This is a critical step in healing. Until people learn this acceptance, they remain in protest. Protesting your current circumstances is an unrealistic attempt to ward off having to face your reality.[19] Rather than divest your energy in defending yourself against rejection, faulting yourself, beating yourself up, or trying to fight the grief, take a moment to accept the simple fact that your turmoil is about loss. What you are feeling is the pain of losing someone's love. Indeed this is painful, and you have every right to feel devastating loss. Accepting the universal basis of this pain helps you inch toward accepting the reality of the loss and progress through the inevitable process of grief.

> When I mention the word "acceptance," some abandonment survivors, impatient for relief ask: "Acceptance. Is that all there is to do? Just grin and bear it?"
>
> I answer: Acceptance is only a first step. It centers you in reality. It reduces shame, because you realize that your pain is legitimate. It helps end the protest and restore calm. It prepares you to use the emotional turbulence of abandonment to gain inner strength. This is why we'll continue to work on acceptance throughout our journey.

Take a moment to reassure yourself that you are truly not in a life-or-death battle. Tell yourself that no matter how dire it feels, you do not need to be in self-defense mode. The emotional crisis you're experiencing feels out of control because your overzealous amygdala—in its primitive, imprecise way—is reacting as if you were fighting for your life.

In fact, your survival is not threatened. You may wonder, however, how you are supposed to convince your mammalian brain of this. Actually, we engage in this type of communication all the time. One of the functions of our higher brain—the cerebral cortex—is to talk sense to our emotional brain. In this manner, human beings have calmed themselves down over the centuries.

Whereas your mammalian brain's asset is its ability to make snap judgments—to act automatically without taking the time to think first—your cerebral mind's strength is its ability to provide you with more detailed information with which to better evaluate the situation, but it takes longer to process the information.[20] You realize after you've jumped ten feet that the loud noise wasn't a bomb after all, but a thunderclap. The fast-moving object that caused you to flinch wasn't a predator, but a tree branch. The loss of your relationship that has your life in a swirl isn't the end of the world after all, but the loss of an attachment to one person.

Providing precise cognitive information is one of the ways your cerebral cortex distinguishes you from the rest of the animal kingdom. Your cortex is critical in providing the rational, calming reassurance you need during Shattering. Maybe your amygdala can't tell you that your life is not over, that indeed you're able to be on your own, but your cognitive mind can. Leading from your higher brain, you are able to find a rational voice, one that brings your emotional crisis under cerebral control time and time again during the crisis of Shattering. Use the emotional turbulence of Shattering to discover your inner strength. Let your cognitive brain commend you for that strength—a permanent acquisition that will serve your life ongoing.

Take a moment to check the items that, in spite of your amygdala's state of emergency, your cognitive mind can now accept as true.

- ❏ I am an able-bodied adult.
- ❏ I can stand on my own two feet.
- ❏ I can survive on my own.
- ❏ I can turn my life in a positive direction.

Most of us envy people who seem self-assured. Now, thanks to your abandonment, you get to exercise your own capacity to become self-assured. Using your higher brain to calm yourself during this crisis is exactly how you learn to develop this enviable quality. Reassure yourself that you are indeed capable of taking care of yourself, that being in disconnect mode is temporary. Remind yourself that the emotional excess is just your mammalian brain's way of trying to overprotect you. While you may appreciate your amygdala's effort to wage an all-out life-or-death battle on your behalf, you don't need that much protection. You can survive this crisis as an adult. Calmly, patiently talk to yourself until your cognitive reasoning has effectively taken back the reins from your mammalian brain's tenacious grip on your nervous system. Each time the crisis becomes unbearable, guide yourself to solid ground.

Dear Emotional Brain,

Although I appreciate your attempts to defend me from what you believe is a threat to my life, I want to reassure you that…

Facing Fear

As you learn to take your emotional self in hand, it becomes more and more difficult for your amygdala to hijack your grief process. Now it is your ever-evolving adult self taking back control. Yet even the most self-assured of us still harbor doubts about the future when surviving abandonment, because we are human. It is scary to face the fact that, admittedly, your future remains unknown. Having learned to strengthen your rational, adult self, your next task is to use your calming wisdom to face your fears.

The fears that accompany loss are like batteries that eventually run out of juice but feel very real while they still have any charge. Some of them have a short life; others seem more like Energizer Bunnies.

Commonly expressed fears include the following:

My life will never be the same.
I will die lonely.
I will never love again.
The pain will get worse and I won't be able to withstand it.
What if I die of heartbreak?

Stating your fears helps you face them.

Name a few of your own fears:

It also helps to share your fears with a good friend—someone who is a good listener and won't try to "fix" it. It may be difficult, though, to find someone who can bear to listen to your dire circumstances without wanting to talk you out of your feelings. Friends and family often tend to give simplistic advice, dismissing the gravity of your situation, because they can see what you can't while in the midst of your crisis—that your fears are feelings, not facts. They also may want to deny the pain because abandonment—everyone's worst nightmare—hits them too close to home. Tell your friends or family that you need someone to just sit with you during your pain, listen without giving advice, and be on hand to support your struggle.

The most important thing I gained from sharing my fears with a friend was…

The most helpful thing a friend said to me was…

The most nonempathetic thing a friend said to me was…

If you're going through abandonment, now is a good time to consider professional counseling. Your emotional self is more accessible than at any other time to benefit from the process. Professionals are trained to listen and provide feedback without overidentifying with your situation, dismissing your feelings, or losing patience with you. They provide guidance to help you weather the storm, and they support the insight you are gaining from the experience.

It's important to reach out to others so that you can discover that your fears are universal, that you are not alone in being alone.[21] Reaching out to friends, joining support groups, finding an e-buddy, getting into therapy, and reconnecting with family members all provide human comfort during the crisis.*

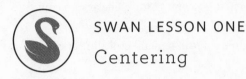

SWAN LESSON ONE
Centering

In the story about the little girl I mentioned earlier, I had written a new section in which she climbed down from the rock and emerged from the forest. She was alone, grief stricken, and in shock. It was time to initiate a meeting between her and the majestic swan to see what might unfold.

The little girl watches the black swan glide through the water. To her amazement he approaches her at the shoreline. Her grief is so great, she cannot speak, but the swan is able to hear her silently spoken feelings.

"Go inside, Amanda," says the swan, "so you can find your listening place."

"It hurts," cries the little girl within herself.

"Yes, inside is where your feelings are," he says. "You must go through your feelings all the way to the very center of them to find your listening space so that you can hear what I have to say."

"Daddy, Mommy, where are you? Please come and take me home!" cries the little girl inside.

"Go to the very center where you exist all by yourself. Your parents are not here with you now. In this moment you are alone, as we are all alone," says the swan. "In the very center exists your surviving self. Can you find it?"

"I'm afraid," weeps the little girl silently in her heart. "It's awful. I'm all alone."

"You must find your way to the very center of the awfulness. In the very center lives an aloneness that is so real, it isn't awful anymore. It is where your peaceful self resides. It is an aloneness we all share. Go inside and find it."

The little girl closes her eyes and crosses her hands over her chest.

"Can you find it all the way in the very center?"

The little girl presses her hands harder against her chest and nods her head yes.

"Alone is where your healing self resides," says the swan. "When you are all the way inside, aloneness isn't awful anymore, is it? It just is. Aloneness is reality, yours as well as mine. It is a sacred place, an alone place just for you," says the swan. "It will be your special place to come to each time we meet."

---

*   For instructions to set up abandonment support groups, see Appendix A. Log on to abandonment.net to reach out to us.

As the little girl learned to find her center, she commenced the emotional and spiritual process of healing from the deep wound of abandonment.

It is important for readers to notice as we make our way through the twelve lessons that the little girl is able to benefit from the swan's guidance because she actively practices each lesson. As she practices this first lesson—centering—she crosses her hands over her chest, a simple gesture I have seen countless people perform as they center themselves during times of turmoil.

Take a break from reading and think about the earliest time you can remember feeling at peace and entirely calm within yourself.

Q

How old were you? _____

Where were you? Who were you with? Were you alone?

What were the special circumstances of this peaceful memory?

Describe the peaceful experience.

Now close your eyes and go inside. Place your hands over your chest to help you center in. See if you can find this feeling again. Can you find peacefulness within? Does it feel familiar? Or is it new? Describe.

How can centering help you cope with your Shattering experience?

As you make your way to that peaceful place inside, you might come across uncomfortable feelings—fear, doubt, or sorrow. Rather than fight the pain, imagine that you are cutting a path right through it, all the way to the very center of the turmoil to a sacred, protected place inside. In this center, there is no past or present, no fear or sorrow—only your awareness of being alive now.

What uncomfortable feelings must you make your way through to feel peaceful and free inside?

Can you get to the very center where you experience a protected internal place?

What is it like?

Finding your peaceful inner center is easier when life is going smoothly. When you're going through the initial stages of abandonment, it can feel as if the very center of yourself had been shattered, making it quite a challenge to discover the peace that resides deep within yourself. Don't give up. Begin by imagining what an ideal internal space would feel like.

Describe your ideal internal space.

What strengths help you find your center?

Consider the testimonies of those who have entered this beginning point of the healing process.

"I had a real instinct for feeling inner peace as a child and found it easy to meditate when I grew up," says Bob. "But when Sarah left me, I felt so broken up inside that my sense of self was scattered to the four winds. What used to come naturally now took all my effort. I was too anxious to locate any inner peace at first. But I knew it was there somewhere and that I just had to find a way to create it again. I discovered that counting my breaths helped me center in. And there it was, an oasis inside—an oasis I could return to when my nerves got on edge, no matter how much effort it took."

"Inside my center is a place where I can accept my aloneness without feeling afraid," says Jon. "I feel okay being alone in there—alone and yet connected to the universe at the same time."

"My new center is a refuge," says Jackie. "I go constantly to this new place inside myself to get away from all the fear and confusion."

Describe what feelings and thoughts come to you while centering.

Back to the Future

Centering sets the stage for working through the powerful feelings of fear, hopelessness, and shame of the Shattering stage. What follows is an exercise I call Back to the Future, which builds on your ability to tune in to your inner resources by tapping into the problem-solving properties of your imagination. Imagination is one of the most underused commodities of the human mind, especially as it relates to problem solving.

Through thirty years of clinical practice treating people suffering from heartbreak and then going through it myself, I've found that traditional methods aren't able to get at the source of the intense anxiety and despair of this type of wound. Reciting affirmations in the mirror or just going to therapy isn't enough to reach the underlying insecurity and sadness of abandonment. The fear is too primal, the self-doubt too deep. The only human resources strong enough to heal the powerful feelings of abandonment are your awareness and your imagination. Awareness is what helped you find your center, and imagination helped you create peacefulness and hope within it.

Back to the Future doesn't rely on traditional inroads into your psyche. By gaining entry through your imagination, it disarms your internal gatekeepers—those psychological gremlins who work unconsciously to maintain the status quo in your life. Back to the Future is not about maintaining your old patterns; it's about changing them.

Back to the Future is a life-changing technique that helps you overcome your deeply entrenched patterns of self-sabotage and achieve your true potential. It provides a shortcut to recovery, but it does not work by magic. It involves taking action. First, you imagine your life as it might look in the future after having removed all of the obstacles within your power. Then you exercise your problem-solving skills by determining your best course of action. Next you exercise your will by following through with action.

The exercise involves three levels: visualization, problem solving, and action. The visualization part is actually an encapsulated version of another exercise, one you will learn about in chapter 8 when we explore Building Your Dream House.

To explain how Back to the Future works, let's use karate as a metaphor. When karate masters prepare to break a cinder block with their bare hands, they visualize not the cinder block but the space beyond the cinder block to break through it. Likewise, Back to the Future uses your imagination to focus on the space beyond your own blocks and yields the same powerful results. To visualize the possibility of the future is to focus your energy on the solution rather than the problem.[22]

I'm going to ask you to create a hypothetical scenario—an idyllic scene that takes place about two years in the future when it's conceivable to imagine that your current problems are already behind you. Two years gives your imagination plenty of time to make the changes necessary to set your life where you want it.

Then, I'm going to ask you to stretch your imagination all the way toward figuring out what you might have done to have resolved your problems. Figuring out how you hypothetically solved your problems involves working backward from the future.

Let's Try It

Begin by getting into a relaxing position. Close your eyes and find your peaceful inner center. Imagine the following scene taking place at some time in the future. Again, two years is a feasible period in which to accomplish just about any change. Imagine that you are sitting in a beautiful room, on an extremely comfortable chair, gazing at a pleasurable view. Place yourself fully in this scene. As you sit, envision feeling completely at peace and happy in the future, because all of your current problems are resolved. Maybe you have acquired all of the love and fulfillment you ever desired. Maybe you've resolved personal issues that have long interfered in your success. You've moved whatever has been blocking you out of the way, and you feel fulfilled and successful because of the accomplishment.

Describe the chair, room, view, and feelings of your futuristic scene.

If this were purely a visualization exercise, we would continue with this pleasurable scene. But we are going to use this idealistic place as a springboard from which to do some rigorous problem solving. In the next task, I'm going to ask you to work backward from this future scene to figure out what steps you might have taken to get there.[23] I pose some questions to help you with this hypothetical conundrum.

In contemplating the scene, describe what changed in your life that enabled you to feel this happy and fulfilled two years from now.

Name some of your current problems that you had to move out of the way.

Can you identify the main obstacle you had to overcome to achieve this fulfillment?

How might you have removed this obstacle? (This question takes some head-scratching, scalp-scrunching mental exertion.)

Yes, that last question involves some effort. For those of you who found the answer easily, it probably means that you didn't give it enough thought. If you really knew how to remove the obstacle blocking your life, you would have already removed it!

Here is an abbreviated version I borrowed from Stephen, a member of an abandonment support group, to give you a better idea how this works.

My future scene?	"I'm more at peace with myself, feel successful, content to be alone."
What improvements, what changed?	"I stopped obsessing about my ex, used the energy to get a new job."
What problems are behind me?	"My neediness and insecurity."
What obstacle was in the way?	"Lack of confidence."
How did you remove it?	"I started believing in myself."

Before we celebrate Stephen's final answer, let's consider the fact that a big problem remains: How is Stephen supposed to start believing in himself? Doesn't this sound like another one of those easier-said-than-done solutions that just keeps going in circles?

Tackling this conundrum is a real brainteaser. Persevere, stay with me, and together we'll get it done. To take Back to the Future to the next level, you need to ask yourself, "What did I do differently on a behavioral level that helped me remove the obstacle?" Or another way of putting it, "What would a fly on the wall observe me doing differently as I took the necessary steps to make this change?" In Stephen's case, he asked, "What specific steps did I take to begin to believe in myself?"

His answer: "Between now and two years from now, I started going to interviews and networking to find a better job."

Let's try it. Answer by referring to your previous responses.

Name a specific action you might have taken to remove this obstacle.

If you find yourself struggling to come up with an action, go Back to the Future and imagine the scene again in which you feel happy and at peace, with all of your problems behind you. Use that pleasurable scene to refresh your imaginative powers. Stay focused on the chair, room, view, and contentment. Imagine feeling extremely good about yourself in the future for having removed the obstacle to your success. Imagine that it was your own determination, commitment, and follow-through that propelled you forward. Then see yourself in action. Imagine yourself taking little steps to overcome the obstacle. From this position, with your imagination focused on the space beyond your problems, it is easier to come up with a single action you might have taken in making this progress. You don't need to come up with a whole action plan, or the "perfect" action. Any single action, however small a step, that heads in the direction of your desired goal will do.

To complete the Action Vow that follows, think of a tiny step you can take today that will inch you in the direction of your goals. Make a personal vow to take this first tiny step within twenty-four hours. Make sure your Action Vow is small and doable so that you'll be sure to follow through. Here is Stephen's Action Vow:

"Within twenty-four hours I will go online and download Monday's employment section."

Action Vow: Within the next twenty-four hours, I will _____ .

Back to the Future channels your actions productively, even when you're not conscious of moving forward. Conjuring up a positive futuristic image sends psychological energy to the space beyond your obstacles. This bypasses your greatest doubts, breaks through your own mental blocks, and taps into your power to change. It gets your imagination to work on problem solving and offers new perspective on the underlying issues that have been in your way all along, how to resolve them, and what first steps to take.

Back to the Future is a powerful change vehicle, but don't take my word for it. Begin using it on a daily basis, taking a tiny step every day in the direction of your desired goals. Within a short time you will notice your daily actions guided by an emerging higher self. Soon you become alert to new opportunities and seemingly more opportunities will come your way. You may spot relevant announcements in the newspapers or overhear a pertinent conversation while you're waiting at the bus stop. More attentive to the possibilities and options surrounding you, you will find your actions tend to flow more easily. You think more confidently and positively. Once you start taking small steps, larger behaviors begin to change spontaneously. You tend to pick up the phone to follow through rather than just thinking about picking up the phone. You start to take positive risks, expanding your range of activity. And what's more, your patterns change.

As your actions become more goal directed, you begin to notice small improvements right away, with larger structural changes taking longer—a period of months or even years.

Visualization combined with baby steps create the momentum for real change. Naturally, success takes more than performing a single exercise. Staying at the level of solution in your life requires repeated use of this exercise, frequent visits Back to the Future. That's why you will find this technique repeated throughout the book.

Consider Sarah's testimony after she tried this exercise for a few months.

"I had trouble asserting myself at work and had this really good idea for a new program, but I couldn't get the team to take me seriously. As usual, it was my own reticence holding me back. So I began doing Back to the Future every day, each time visualizing my new program as if it were

already up and running. I pictured this scene taking place about a year in the future, with my teammates cooperating with me and giving me credit. Most of my daily Action Vows had to do with asserting myself in little ways. Within a month or so, I found myself acting more confidently at work and getting more response. When I expressed my ideas, I spoke to the right people. I noticed my eye contact increasing. I also didn't let people interrupt me as much. I didn't take no for an answer when something was really important. It took a few months of visualizing and taking baby steps, but my new program started coming together. I'm in charge of it and people are helping me."

It takes a leap of faith to entertain the Power of Possibility and stick with it. It also takes great effort.

Now that you've used your imagination to work on your most resistant problems, you've performed a strenuous mental workout. You used the problem-solving muscle of your brain—equal to running ten laps around the football field. After such mental exertion, let's taper off with some easy, straightforward questions that require little effort.

Check all that apply.

❑ Am I determined to move beyond my emotional challenges and scale my prison walls of isolation, shame, and grief?
❑ Am I ready to put an end to my self-sabotage?
❑ Do I have the will to find the love I've always wanted?
❑ Can I reach my potential as a human being?
❑ Will I put in the effort?
❑ Will I work to get there?
❑ Will I persevere even when I'm discouraged?
❑ Am I ready to follow through?

Write a statement that commits your solid determination to achieve your goals. *I will…*

To reinforce your commitment, it helps to share your goals with others—trusted friends, family, e-buddies, abandonment support group members, and therapists. Working through the overwhelming feelings of heartbreak and the obstacles holding you back requires endurance and know-how. Keeping other people aware of your effort keeps you motivated and on track. According to a Chinese proverb, "The journey of a thousand miles begins with the first step."[24]

More Food for Thought

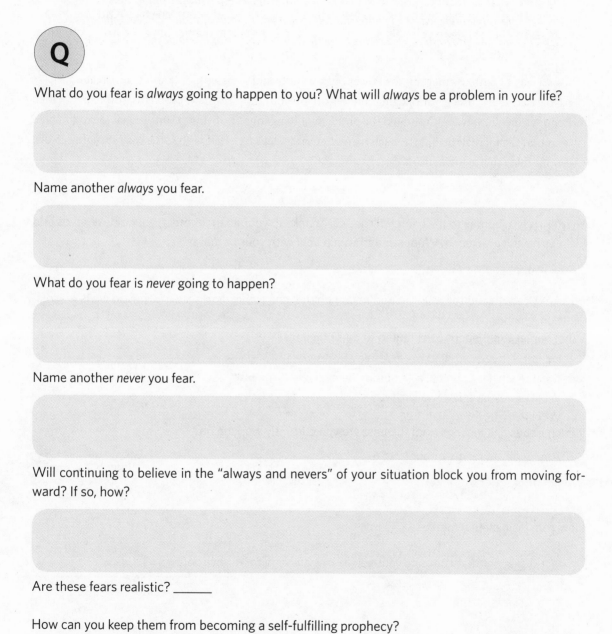

Q

What do you fear is *always* going to happen to you? What will *always* be a problem in your life?

Name another *always* you fear.

What do you fear is *never* going to happen?

Name another *never* you fear.

Will continuing to believe in the "always and nevers" of your situation block you from moving forward? If so, how?

Are these fears realistic? _____

How can you keep them from becoming a self-fulfilling prophecy?

What strengths and insights are you using?

Do you feel that being rejected by someone you love is a negative reflection on you? Write a compassionate, empathetic note to yourself, accepting the humanness and dignity of your current situation.

Dear Worthy Self,

Shattering is a journey to the center of the self. Thanks to your abandonment, your oldest needs and feelings have reawakened. What strengths help deal with your primal self?

What earlier experiences contributed to these feelings?

Which issues and feelings from the past are you currently working on?

How can this benefit your life?

Shattering means you've hit an emotional bottom. This bottom can help you transform your life. It's up to you to discover the larger purpose of your current turmoil. What is this experience calling for you to change?

How does it benefit your personal growth to develop a larger purpose for your problems?

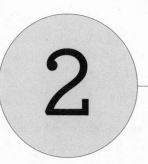

2 Cleansing

"Will I ever love again?"

People in the throes of a breakup universally express the fear that they will never love again. I was afraid of this myself for a few months after losing my life partner. In the midst of the despair and hopelessness of Shattering, we believe that losing our loved one means losing the possibility for love and connection forever. It is this fear, above all, that makes ending a relationship so anguishing. Therapists know only too well how hard it is to convince people that their lives are not over. My message in this chapter is that there are steps we can take to ensure a brighter future.

If I'd had a crystal ball during my own abandonment that promised I'd find love again, I could have endured the awful isolation more easily at the time. If I could have foretold the future and known that I was not in permanent hell, but in a transitional period heading toward even greater happiness, this knowledge would have quelled much of the fear and desolation of the Shattering stage.

Almost anything is bearable if we know it is temporary.

Now that my ordeal is behind me, how I wish I had a crystal ball for the many thousands of people who contact me during their own time of Shattering to let them see that if they are willing to perform the work of recovery, they will be able to find the love they always sought. That is the hopeful message this chapter brings.

Not everyone needs to find a relationship to be happy, but all of us need to know we could succeed at one if we wanted it.

Some people feel chronically shattered because they desperately want someone to care about but, after years of effort, can't find a relationship. Their future looms ahead of them, a frightening spectacle of loneliness. They have a sense of endless doom and a heightened vulnerability running just below the surface of their everyday lives.

"My biological clock is running out," says Beverly. *"It's too late for true happiness now. It feels as if my whole mission in life has been aborted."*

Some people going through a breakup feel especially desperate because it's happened before. They're caught up in patterns in which they keep getting abandoned over and over again. Once again, they've failed to get a relationship to last. They describe the anxiety, wakeful nights, and loss of confidence in themselves.

"Am I condemned to loneliness for the rest of my life?"

"Will I ever love again?"

It may seem too early to address these questions even before you've come to terms with a recent breakup. But most people need immediate answers to these burning questions, especially during the early throes of heartbreak when hopelessness runs at an all-time high.

The answer is that, of course, you will find connection and love again, even if it means having to discover more about yourself. Even if it means that in the midst of your desolation you have to face your feelings, face yourself, face your reality, and *change*.

This chapter allows you to counter the helplessness and despair of the Shattering stage with a vision of change. You can have a future filled with vitality and love—if you're willing to work toward it. This vision will take you beyond the hopelessness of Shattering to *cleansing*, the next step of healing. You'll learn to cleanse your abandonment wound of the self-defeating patterns that have caused love to go awry, as well as the virulent messages of rejection and unworthiness you have picked up from previous heartbreaks and losses. You'll explore your own personal love map[1] to discover why it's so hard to let go of a former love and connect to a healthy new one.

During the angst of heartbreak, most of you vow you'll never go through this again but don't know how to go about breaking your cycles of abandonment. You need to know that tools are available—new information and hands-on exercises—to help you make a healthy lasting connection to someone you love.

> Some people protest, asking: "Isn't this jumping the gun? Is it too soon to worry about finding someone else when I'm still grieving the last one?"
>
> I answer: This initial stage of Shattering is an ideal time to address the patterns that may sabotage your attempts to find love. When your defenses are shattered, you are most receptive to reconstructing new patterns.[2]

It's important to point out that not everyone's heartbreak is part of a destructive pattern.

"I never had a problem with other relationships. They ended amicably when we realized it didn't work. But now I'm heartbroken for the first time."

"What patterns? There's only been one person in my life and now he's gone."

Some of you will move from the pain of heartbreak to a period of emotional self-reliance and, if you choose, to a successful new relationship, all without a hitch. Others can fall into a pattern of reabandonment partly owing to the neurochemicals triggered by going through the trauma of abandonment, a common problem we'll be exploring fully throughout this book.

I'm going to help you discover some of your personal truths and share new information with which to inoculate yourself against future heartbreak. Once you know how to identify your cycles, you will no longer be a victim of heartbreak but a person with a mission to transform your life. We'll take an inventory of your old values and your current ideas about love to assess problem areas. Once you know where to place the fulcrum in your life, you can apply your energy where it's needed and lift your life to your desired goal, moving beyond Shattering to connection.

Lookin' for Love in All the Wrong Places

Millions of people are in a chronic form of abandonment grief. They are searching for love and can't find it. They're in a state of involuntary aloneness and don't know how to get out. Operating on hunches, I've learned to ask my isolated clients questions that may seem irrelevant to them at the time, like, "Whom do you sit next to at work?" What I've learned from my detective work as a psychotherapist is that in many cases, they have found love on numerous occasions but weren't able to recognize it. They were looking for another feeling and dodged the opportunity for a real relationship.

In addressing the thousands of personal stories people have sent to abandonment.net, I am reminded once again about how widespread this problem is—the tendency to avoid the opportunity for a real relationship based on false values and ideas. In fact, love might be staring you in the face at this very moment, but a potential mate remains emotionally invisible to you. Instead, you are pining away for someone who is unavailable, someone who left you feeling abandoned.

What Happens When Love Is Invisible?

At the beginning of a breakup, it is usually only your ex who remains emotionally visible to you. You really can't see or feel anyone else. The new suitors fall short because of who they *aren't*—they aren't your ex. They only make you miss your ex more. New potential sources of love and security seem to lack that special appeal. They remain romantically invisible because your ex dominates your attention.

While you're in acute heartbreak, it might seem irrelevant to consider whether or not at some critical point in the past, you might have overlooked a person with whom you could have developed a loving relationship—a relationship that might have nurtured your self-image, confidence, and security. It's true that we can't change the past, but at least we can learn from it.

Many of you may be resistant to considering the idea that you could have overlooked an available lover.

If That Were True, I'd Have Felt Some Sort of Attraction

We belong to a culture immersed in the romantic notion that attraction is destiny.[3] We go around looking for someone who stirs up the right chemistry.[4] Contrary to conventional wisdom, it is possible to develop chemistry toward a person you may not have felt initially attracted to. There are millions of people populating the planet whose successful, loving marriages were arranged by their parents. In these cases, intense love feelings and attachment develop after the union was formed. There are biological mechanisms in place to see that this happens.[5] Sleeping in proximity to someone promotes bonding, as does skin-to-skin contact, kissing, caressing, hugging, intimate sex, and orgasm. So do promises of fidelity, financial interdependency, and steadfast companionship. Caring together for children or pets, working in partnership toward mutual goals, and marking your milestones as a couple with rituals and celebrations—all of these deepen attachment and kindle the love bond between two people.

To suggest that people reared in Western societies are sometimes unable to recognize love even when it hits them over the head may seem preposterous.[6] Many people think they are specially equipped with radar to detect the right person—if not at first sight, at least by the second date. But a common bind for millions of lonely people is that they are attracted only to emotionally unavailable partners. Their radar homes in on those who are destined to leave them in the end. They're drawn like moths to abandonment's flame.

At this point, consider the proposition that your body and mind might contain false notions about love, about what a relationship is supposed to be, and about what kind of partner to choose.

Here are some Qs to get you thinking.

 ## LOOKING A LOVE HORSE IN THE MOUTH

Have you suspected that any of your friends are looking for love in all the wrong places? Name an example.

How did it make you feel to watch her push someone away just because he didn't stir up the right chemistry—when you suspected all along that this person might have been right for her and brought her security?

How did you feel watching your friend pursue an abandoner?

Do you think there was ever an instance in which love showed up in your own life and you weren't able to see it? Describe.

Did any of your friends recognize it, even when you couldn't?

What potential benefit does considering these insights have in your life?

A common and vexing problem keeping many of you on the outside of love is a condition of the heart that I call abandoholism. It occurs when abandonment takes on a mind of its own and becomes a compulsion.[7] You've heard of foodaholism, workaholism, shopaholism, and, of course, alcoholism. Well, here comes another addictive pattern—abandoholism.

Abandoholism is similar to the other -holisms, but instead of being addicted to a substance, you're addicted to the emotional drama of heartbreak. So you pursue unavailable partners to keep the romantic intensity going and to keep your body's love chemicals flowing.[8]

What Makes Someone an Abandoholic?

Abandoholics are people who've been hurt in the past, and the abandonment fear they acquired conditions them to equate insecurity with love. Unless they're pursuing someone they're insecure about, they don't believe they're in love. When someone comes along who wants to be with them, this suitor seems too easy to get to arouse that required level of insecurity they've come to associate with love. If they can't feel those yearning, lovesick sensations, they aren't feeling anything. So they keep pursuing unavailable partners who bring out craving, pursuing feelings.[9]

The reason I call this pattern *abandoholism* is because it's psychobiologically addictive.[10] Many people have a compulsion to be abandoned because they're addicted to the high-stakes drama of an emotionally challenging relationship—and the love chemicals that go with it.

One of the underpinnings of abandoholism is *fear of abandonment*. Feeling attracted to someone creates a fear of losing that person. Fear of being abandoned can become so intrusive that it disrupts your ability to maintain your emotional balance while pursuing a new relationship. Try as you might to hide your insecurity, it drains your confidence. You try to put your best foot forward, but your neediness and desperation show through, causing your partners to lose romantic interest. They sense your emotional suction cups aiming straight toward them and get scared away.

Another aspect of abandoholism is *fear of engulfment*. Fear of engulfment is at the opposite end of the emotional spectrum. It occurs when someone is pursuing you and now it's *you* who's pulling back. You feel engulfed by the suitor's emotional attraction toward you. When fear of engulfment kicks in, you zealously guard your autonomy at all costs and feel threatened lest your suitor take it away.

Fear of engulfment can erupt in mini-anxiety attacks. The panic is about the fear of losing yourself in becoming emotionally obligated to that person. Their needs and expectations might engulf you, causing you to abandon yourself.

Whether fear of engulfment sets in gradually or all at once, it effectively shuts you down emotionally and sexually. You want out of this relationship because you feel burdened by taking on the emotional responsibility of an available partner.

Fear of engulfment is one of the most common causes for the demise of new relationships, but it is carefully disguised in excuses like the following.

Check those that seem familiar.

❏ He just doesn't turn me on.
❏ I don't feel any chemistry.
❏ She's too nice to hold my interest.
❏ I need more of a challenge.
❏ I feel nauseous whenever she tries to get closer.

Abandoholics tend to swing back and forth between these emotional poles. Your pendulum swings between *fear of abandonment* and *fear of engulfment*. You're either pursuing hard-to-get lovers, driven by a desperate urge to bond with them, or you're feeling turned off because someone is genuinely interested in you. You're always at opposite ends of the emotional spectrum, never on mutual ground, never secure, never at peace.

Some people are so afraid of rejection that they avoid relationships altogether. This is called *abandophobism*.[11]

Abandophobics are closely related to abandoholics; in fact, they're just another variety of the same difficulty. Abandophobics act out their fear of abandonment by remaining socially isolated or by appearing to search for someone, when in fact they are pursuing people who are unattainable, all to avoid the risk of getting attached to a real prospect—someone who might abandon them sooner or later.

There's a little abandophobism in most abandoholics.

Many of you describe getting hooked on someone who dangles the possibility of a relationship in front of you but never emotionally follows through. What better way to avoid a real relationship than to pursue an eternally unavailable partner? To help you interact with these insights, here is a snap quiz.

Check off all that might possibly be true for you.

- ❏ I choose unavailable partners who keep me insecure.
- ❏ Insecurity is my favorite aphrodisiac.
- ❏ I am afraid to risk the closeness of a real relationship.
- ❏ I feel attracted only when I'm in pursuit.
- ❏ I need hot, fresh, new love to keep me always on the move for the next relationship.
- ❏ I feel engulfed when someone wants me.
- ❏ I have unrealistic expectations of my partners.
- ❏ I think I haven't found the right person.
- ❏ I wouldn't join any club who would have me as a member.
- ❏ I need an emotional challenge to sustain my interest.

How Do These Patterns Set In?

For both abandoholics and abandophobics, a negative attraction tends to be more compelling than a positive one.[12]

The syndrome of self-sabotage underlying this was most likely cast in childhood. You may have formed an insecure attachment to one or both of your parents. You struggled to get more attention from them, to get them to favor you, accept you, and treat you nicely, but they failed to provide what you craved most—unconditional love and attention. The insecurity, yearning, and neediness you felt toward your parents caused you to doubt your self-worth and put them on pedestals. Over time, you internalized this need for approval and you idealized others at your own expense. It became a pattern.

Now, as an adult, you re-create this scenario by giving your love partners too much power. By elevating them above yourself, you re-create that old familiar yearning you grew accustomed to as a child. Feeling emotionally deprived and "less-than" is what you've come to expect. It's the only scenario you can *feel*. You've come to associate these needy, lovesick, insecure feelings with being in love.

Not all people who have an abandonment compulsion came from insecure attachments.[13] Some of you had loving, caring parents but felt insecure in your relationships with peers. You felt attracted to heartthrobs in high school but didn't feel strong enough about yourself to negotiate mutual relationships with them. Adolescent relationships are notoriously fickle[14] to begin with; their emotional dynamics are painfully unstable and scarring. Many of you internalized self-doubt during this volatile time and inculcated fears that continue to haunt the future.

Why Does the Insecurity Linger?

Rejection from your past and present heartbreaks is harbored deep within the self, conditioning your amygdala (discussed in chapter 1) to "fear" that what happened in the past will happen again. Recent scientific research shows that rather than dissipate, fear tends to incubate.[15] It gains intensity over time. The internal worry "Am I worthy?" grows louder each time you go through another rejection. The mounting uncertainty compels you to look to others for something you've become too powerless to give yourself: esteem. When you seek acceptance from a withholding partner, you place yourself in a one-down position, re-creating the unequal dynamics you had with your parents or peers. You choreograph this scenario over and over, playing out a fantasy in which you try to win love and acceptance from a hard-to-get lover and remain enslaved by your own need for approval.

People develop these patterns after years of emotional conditioning. Your losses, heartbreaks, and disappointments have a cumulative effect, causing you to respond most keenly to those who treat you less-than and stir up the old familiar feelings of want, need, and desperation. Conversely, you are *un*able to feel anything when someone freely admires or appreciates you as much as you do them.

It is helpful for therapists seeking to help people overcome these entrenched patterns to provide specialized support and prepare to vigorously challenge their client's tightly held beliefs. These patterns do not give up without a fight because the roots of the problem run so deep.*

Why Do We Elevate Those Who Hurt Us?

Being left by someone you love activates fear—primal abandonment fear—set deeply into your mammalian brain. Abandoners become powerful figures to your amygdala, owing to the pain they caused by leaving you. Pain is a powerful reinforcer, conditioning you to feel aroused whenever you think about or see this person. This ongoing reactivity (known as carrying a torch) confuses you into thinking that you must still love the person and that she must be very special to hold your interest for so long. In fact, your ex may not have been special at all, but because she caused such intense pain, you confuse your lingering reactivity as proof of how irreplaceable and special she was. This may not be true at all. What you are experiencing is separation anxiety—a natural biological concomitant to breaking an attachment and adjusting to the rigors of being alone[16]—regardless of the specialness of your former partner.

Feeling insecure and idealizing those who cause pain set the stage for developing abandoholism.

Once you make your abandoner special, your life is ruled by contradictions. You confuse calmness for boredom, tension for excitement, insecurity for love.[17]

Abandoholics are in denial and extremely cunning at keeping the truth hidden from their friends, therapists, and themselves. What truth? That they appear to be looking for a relationship when in fact they are looking for emotional candy to feed their abandohol addiction.

As people learn about this concept, they find all kinds of ways to apply it.

"I've spent most of my thirties strung out on abandohol," declares Roberta, *having gained the awareness that her volatile emotional life has been the result of being attracted to abandoners.*

---

* Therapists interested in more information should go to the Professional Page at abandonment.net.

The abandonment compulsion is insidious. You didn't know it was developing. Until now, you didn't have a name for it. It's been unconscious. You didn't realize that you've transferred unresolved feelings from your parents and old high-school heartbreakers directly into your current relationships. Yet little by little you've grown addicted to the roller coaster of pursuing abandoners, having become your own worst enemy. Millions are caught up in this drama, a passion play I call "The Agony and the Ecstasy."

> The Ecstasy is the opportunity to conquer that love challenge—the thrill of seduction. The Agony is feeling rejected—the bittersweet tragedy of unrequited love.

When you meet people you think are better than you, you can't resist going after them because they are a challenge. You imbue them with power, see them as special, and then feel immediately insecure. They respond by treating you as if you were not good enough. Now you're hooked. You get conquest fever, drawn to the drama. You obsess about how to win them over. You're incessantly craving a love fix. The more your partners withhold, distance from you, and reject you, the more intense the craving. You feel ecstasy when you're trying to seduce them and agony when they're pulling away.[18]

Abandoholics have learned to associate the Agony and Ecstasy with being in love. They get propelled into the drama full throttle.

Insecurity Is an Aphrodisiac

If you are a hard-core abandoholic, you're drawn to a kind of love that is highly combustible. The hottest sex is when you're trying to seduce a hard-to-get lover. Insecurity becomes your aphrodisiac. You can't appreciate the Ecstasy without the Agony. These intoxicated states are produced when you sense emotional danger—the danger being your lover's propensity to abandon you the minute you get attached.

At the other end of the seesaw, you turn off and shut down when you happen to successfully

SCIENTIFIC TIDBIT

Being with someone who is a challenge stimulates surges of catecholamines (adrenaline, norepinephrine), which, combined with your endogenous opiates and other hormones, cause you to feel infatuated. Infatuation is a cocaine-like emotional high that intensifies your sexual feelings and medicates the rigors of intimacy. Caught up in the heat of passion (mediated by these neurochemicals), two people just getting acquainted are able to be intimate without embarrassment. To stay high, abandoholics keep seeking uncommitted partners. When someone comes along who is available, your body doesn't produce enough catecholamines to support this high. You experience this as having no chemistry and go into withdrawal from your addiction. Unless you're inebriated on love chemicals, you can't tolerate the intimacy of a real relationship. So you run.

Like a junkie desperate for a love fix, you search for another lover who arouses just the right dose of fear to get you emotionally loaded. You're in denial: When your body is attracted (addicted), it tells you you're in love. When your partner becomes available, your love-stress hormones stop flowing, and you fall out of love.

win someone's love. If your lover succumbs to your charms—heaven forbid—you suddenly feel too comfortable, too sure of him to stay interested. There's not enough challenge to sustain your sexual energy. You interpret your turn-off as his not being right for you.

Do Your Friends and Therapists Help or Hinder You?

Whether you're a hard-core love-junkie or just a garden-variety abandoholic, the most common maneuver is to tell your friends, "I know she seems ideal for me, but there isn't any chemistry" or "He's a nice guy, but I'm not attracted to him."

Your friends tend to believe in the mythology of the right chemistry and accept your excuses at face value (and so do many therapists). You've programmed them to agree with you. You get them to say, "You're right not to settle" or "You just need to find the right person." To break these patterns, you need to eject your old tapes and reprogram your friends. Be honest with yourself and realize that nobody is directing your life but *you.*

How about Following Your Gut?

Both ends of the spectrum—abandoholism and abandophobism—cause their victims to misinterpret self-help's latest directive to follow your gut. In your case, following your gut most likely got you into these patterns. Your gut got you to pursue someone who made your heart go pitter pat, not because she's the right one, but because she's likely to abandon you. And your gut got you to avoid someone else because she didn't press the right insecurity buttons.

Enrich your mind. Follow your wisdom. But until you overcome your abandonment compulsion, beware of your gut. Your earlier heartbreaks and disconnections have made it hard for you to read it correctly.

Gaining Self-Esteem by Proxy

Some people try to gain self-esteem by association, that is, by selecting a partner who has socially valued attributes that help you compensate for something you feel is lacking in yourself. Psychoanalyst and author Richard Robertiello referred to this type of choice as a *narcissistic extension.* The danger in seeking self-esteem by proxy is that your self-worth remains in someone else's hands. This leaves you in a one-down position and perpetuates your cycles of neediness and low self-esteem.

As you're working your way through the stages of abandonment, take advantage of the possibilities that are all around you for renewal, growth, and love. You need to learn more about yourself, come out of denial, cleanse your perspective of the negative-thinking tapes of the past, and transform your patterns.

IQ   THE ABANDOHOLIC CHECKLIST

Dig deep, be honest, and check all that apply.

IF I'VE BEEN LOOKING FOR LOVE IN ALL THE WRONG PLACES, COULD IT BE THAT...

❑ I'm unable to tolerate the sober dynamics of a mature relationship?

❑ I'm accustomed to being on the outside looking in—it's an emotional state I'm familiar with?

❑ I'm a perfectionist and this causes me to reject imperfect, yet realistic, candidates?

❑ I prefer the ideal relationships in my mind to realistic flesh-and-blood ones?

❑ My inner child is so lonely it smothers my lovers with too much neediness?

❑ I obsess about my ex because it is the only way I can maintain any connection with her even though it keeps me in pain?

❑ I'm emotionally clinging to the past to avoid taking a new risk?

❑ I'm not able to handle the emotional responsibility of being needed and wanted?

❑ I'm unable to make decisions, to commit?

❑ I'm afraid of someone getting too close to me for fear he will engulf me with his needs and expectations?

❑ I have a poor self-image and can't tolerate any obvious shortcomings in my partner, as if her flaws reflected directly on me?

❑ I seek unrealistically attractive partners to compensate for something I don't like about myself, trying to gain self-worth by proxy?

❑ I don't know how to appreciate a mutual relationship because without the lovesick feelings, I feel bored and empty?

If you answered yes to any of these questions, be assured that we will continue to identify the myths, false values, defense mechanisms, and patterns that keep you outside of love. In chapter 7, we explore the issue of how to love available partners. Taking incremental steps, you'll get unstuck and overcome your barriers to finding love.

Exploring Your Personal Love Map

Examining Your Values

If you're just coming out of a relationship, you're probably not yet ready to act on many of the insights you are reading about in this chapter. Even so, it helps to plant the seeds of these ideas now so that when they come up later they'll yield change. If you're not ready to think about anyone but your ex right now, consider the possibility that someday you may be in a position to accept a new person into your life. Your goal here is to inoculate yourself against future heartbreak.

Let's look at the cinder block wall that blocks you from love. It's usually put together by romantic myths left over from junior-high-school days and false values acquired from living in our material world. These values and myths are based on outside appearances and unrealistic expectations about what love is—fickle notions of who is a good catch. The glue holding your wall together comes from your primitive ego, not your adult wisdom. It is reinforced by old defense mechanisms that have become maladaptive to your task of finding a relationship. Finding a relationship means following the high road.

What Is Your Idea of a Good Catch?

Take time to examine your values as they relate to your choices in partners. More often than not, to break your cycles of abandonment, you have to change your values—values about who you consider to be or not to be a suitable catch. Changing your values means examining deeply held beliefs, questioning their merit, actively refuting their assumptions, and substituting more realistic ones.

Let's dig around a little bit into the foundation of your belief system and examine your concept of what you think is attractive and which attributes—such as financial success, personality, looks, confident air, educational achievement, and social background—you value most.

What attributes do you value about prospective partners?

Do you remember when you first learned to value these attributes? Where were you? What were the circumstances? Which friend or family member held similar values and may have influenced you?

Which of these old values tend to get you into the most trouble when choosing a potential partner?

What new values can you substitute that might ensure greater emotional stability in future relationships?

Repeat this line of questioning each time you identify another trait you've been attracted to.

As you begin to sort through your values, discarding some, replacing others, you are taking an important step in recovering from your addiction to abandohol. You may, for example, discover you have a weakness for men with big egos and that this usually causes your self-esteem to plummet and your heart to break. What to do? You can choose to abstain from this type of man. As you revamp your values and beliefs about love, you gain emotional sobriety. You come down from the love chemicals and high-stakes drama to a more sober place of wisdom. Rather than remain in the intoxicated pursuing role, you can remain emotionally temperate, developing a relationship with yourself to become self-reliant, ultimately choosing partners who can meet you halfway.[19] Stay grounded—connected to yourself for once—rather than giving all of your power away and pursuing the illusion of love.[20]

What would emotional sobriety look like in your life?

How would it affect your choices in forming new relationships?

What would its benefits be?

What strengths will help you recover from your abandonment cycles?

Solutions and Antidotes

Sometimes the new lesson you must learn has to do with learning how to recognize the dynamics of a healthy, secure relationship. For many of you, the lesson is learning how to tolerate being loved.

Check your heart's desire.

I WANT SOMEONE WHO...

- ❏ knows his own heart and mind.
- ❏ would rather work through the conflicts and barriers than abandon the relationship.
- ❏ doesn't lose interest even after the initial infatuation dies down and the falling-in-love feelings subside.
- ❏ wants to be together as much or more than I do.
- ❏ has real staying power.

Now, before you get all excited and think, "Yes! This is exactly what I want!" think again. Before convincing yourself that you are capable of handling an available mate, query yourself to see if you're as ready as you think you are. It may be necessary to come out of denial and peel away old layers of self-deceit before you can truly entertain this possibility.

Ask yourself: If this person were fully available to me and not going away, would I still have feelings for her?

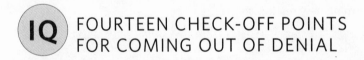

FOURTEEN CHECK-OFF POINTS FOR COMING OUT OF DENIAL

Dig deep into your soul, where your personal truth resides, and check all that apply.

WHEN SOMEONE WANTS AND NEEDS ME . . .

- ❏ I suddenly start to feel ambivalent about this extremely available person—that is, start to feel uncomfortable about some of her deficits.
- ❏ I feel stuck.
- ❏ I think I might be settling—that this person is not good enough for me, not the type I've been looking for.
- ❏ I find that my own ability to commit isn't kicking in.
- ❏ I start acting badly toward my partner to provoke him into ending it.
- ❏ I arouse my partner's insecurities by pulling away and then criticizing her for being too insecure, too needy, or too dependent on me.

❏ I suddenly think someone else is more attractive.

❏ I complain about feeling bored, confined, or pressured.

❏ I start picking at his inadequacies. On a bad day, I may become emotionally abusive.

❏ I feel envious of my single friends and wish I had my freedom back so I could meet new people.

❏ I begin to shut down emotionally, feel no passion, no sexual interest, get that proverbial headache at bedtime.

❏ I keep one foot in the relationship, one foot out and remain noncommittal.

❏ I start telling my friends that the chemistry isn't right so they can become my accomplices and dutifully recite back "You haven't met the right person yet" to help me justify my feelings of wanting to break up.

❏ I have difficulty accepting the normal ambivalence that is part and parcel of a realistic relationship.

If you checked off any of these statements, then you're like most of us. Learning to resist the emotional candy of conquest and accept the emotional sustenance of a realistic relationship requires a great deal of perspective and insight. It takes a lot of courage to admit you have a problem adjusting to the relatively tame, seemingly boring dynamics of a secure relationship. You deserve credit for being able to lift the veil of self-deceit. Denial is a dense fog that keeps the rest of the world too confused to recognize the obstacles blocking them from finding love. For you the fog is lifting. Your task is to stay grounded and focus your libidinal needs, not on hard-to-get lovers but on mutuality and trust.

> One of the tasks in forming a healthy relationship is to accept ambivalent feelings toward your partner. No one is perfect, including you. Realizing this helps us have realistic expectations, recognize ambivalence as a normal emotional response to some of our partner's traits, and celebrate one another's human qualities.

Q

When you have felt ambivalent about a partner, in what ways have you tended to act out?

What insights have you gained to seek mutual relationships?

No matter what your issues are—whether you've been ruled by fear of engulfment, have difficulty tolerating intimacy, or feel unable to take on the emotional responsibility of a real relationship, now is the time to commence real change. Although mutuality has bored you in the past and being loved turned you into a viper, after going through a painful abandonment, loneliness is even more unbearable. Loneliness holds a hidden gift. It helps you hit your emotional bottom. Falling into its dark pit motivates change. Once you learn to cleanse your wound of self-defeating behaviors, this bottom you've hit acts like a trampoline that propels you to heights of new awareness.

Abandonment recovery provides tools with which to deconstruct your invisible barriers. Your goal is to find greater life and love than before.

Cleansing Your Wound

As we have discussed, we have a tendency to idealize those whose love we long for, sometimes especially those who have deeply hurt us. One of the ways we avoid facing a loss is by psychologically tucking them into our heart where they can remain part of us. Unfortunately, we often make this mental representation more special and powerful than we make ourselves. We incorporate the abandoner so tightly that his message of rejection and unworthiness seeps into the core of our belief system, where it undermines our sense of self and interferes in the choices we make.

Shattering cracks us open to the core, exposing raw nerves and spewing contaminants. We feel everything. Our abandonment wound is open and accessible. We learned about centering in the last chapter. Our task for this chapter is to cleanse the open abandonment wound. First and foremost, we're cleansing our patterns of abandonment, sorting through and discarding the debris of false values, outdated beliefs, and negative messages left over from previous losses, disappointments, and heartbreaks. In revamping our values, we start from a new beginning.

 ### SWAN LESSON TWO
Cleansing

In the story, the little girl returned to the black swan for guidance. She had been centering and encountering feelings of terror and grief. Her need for her parents created unbearable anguish and pain. Holding them sacred created the false illusion of keeping them near, but their profound message of rejection blocked her from finding inner peace. She arrived at the water's edge, watching her beautiful swan glide toward her.

"It hurts inside," cries the little girl. "I want my daddy to come get me!"

"Your daddy is not here with you now, Amanda," says the swan. "Needing him and not having him is causing you great pain. Inside that pain, at its very center, is a special place where only you reside. Center in and cleanse it of bad feelings. Push away those who wound your feelings."

"It hurts too much! Daddy, please come back."

"You do not have to let those who cause you pain inside your sacred space," says the swan. "If someone brings bad feelings, do not share your sacred space with them. That part is there for you and you alone. Push the feelings out of your center so that you can find peace inside."

"But I don't want to push my mommy and daddy away," cries the little girl. "I only want them to come back."

"Pushing them out of your center doesn't mean pushing them out of your memory or out of your life," explains the swan. "It just means pushing them out of the space inside that is sacred. Go to this alone place in the very center of yourself and push the bad feelings away."

"I want my mommy and daddy."

"You can still love your parents and yet keep your center safe inside. Keep it a private place where only you reside."

"How?"

"It means using your imagination, Amanda. Imagine that you are pushing the people who bring bad feelings away from your center. Imagining it makes it so. Imagining creates peaceful feelings. Imagine pushing away the bad feelings."

The little girl opens her hands, palms facing outward, and begins pushing away from her chest.

"That's right, Amanda, push out those who wound you. Push away the wounders. Keep the feelings they bring out of your center. Find the space inside that is all yours and only yours and keep it safe. Let your imagination help."

Healing Gestures

As an observer of human behavior, I have seen people perform this simple "pushing gesture" with one or both hands. Their hands are slightly cupped and turned outward as they motion away from their chest. They might be describing how someone's actions have hurt them, and they use this gesture to soothe themselves. I didn't consciously register the meaning of this simple gesture, so universal to human body language, until it found its way into this, the second lesson of the black swan.

The little girl performs this gesture in an exaggerated way because she is profoundly alone and her task is enormous. Now I am able to see that this is the universal gesture people use when attempting to protect themselves from taking someone's hurtful actions to heart.

Try this simple movement yourself. Imagine that you are pushing your abandoner or others who have wounded you out of your sacred space within. Imagine that your center is a new beginning place, an emotionally serene and sober place, a place that is free from the debris of old tapes, rejection, your need for approval, and the need to make others powerful. Imagine being able to see yourself moving forward without all of the contaminating negative messages you've received over the years. Imagine leaving behind the self-defeating patterns that have kept you outside of love.

"The center I've found," says Beverly, "is actually the center of my own abandonment wound, cleansed of impurities. When I center in, I go into the center of my wound because that's where I feel life most intensely, where I love, I need, and I want—the place I know I'm alive."

Following the example of the little girl, exaggerate the cleansing gesture—one you have probably used many times without realizing it. Now deliberately push negative messages and thoughts away from your chest, as if you were cleansing your wound of the outdated values and self-defeating patterns you've accumulated over your life. No matter how attached you may still feel to someone who has wounded you, push the bad feelings out of your center so that you can find peace within.

Q

Does missing your ex cause painful feelings? Describe.

What negative messages about yourself have you picked up as a result of your abandonment?

What feelings must you work through to find freedom from the pain they bring?

Describe what it feels like when you are able to create a sacred space within—one that is free from wounded feelings and from those who created them?

What strengths enable you to push your abandoner out of your center?

What other wounders have you known? Which ones sent negative messages that have left scarring?

How did this experience affect your sense of self-worth?

What insight and strengths can you use to cleanse your inner self of negative messages and the patterns they create?

This is not the only chapter that will help you push the abandoners out of your sacred space. As we go along, you will find additional support for taking your old heartbreakers off the pedestals you've put them on, thereby cleansing yourself of their all-powerful messages about not being good enough.

 Back to the Future

Once again, the life-changing exercise Back to the Future I explained in the last chapter can propel you forward.

Imagine that it's approximately two years from now and you're sitting in your comfortable chair before your beautiful view. You're feeling at peace, fulfilled and happy because you have successfully overcome your cycle of abandonment. You feel good about yourself for having accomplished this.

Describe the pattern you've overcome in the future.

What main obstacle might you have removed to accomplish this?

How did you remove it?

What did you have to do differently on a behavioral level to make this happen?

Name the specific action you took to initiate this change.

Action Vow: Today I will _____.

More Food for Thought

Q

Describe when you've felt there was no chemistry with a person who seemed to be right in every other way.

Do you know someone who avoids available partners because they aren't ready to assume the emotional responsibility of a real relationship?

Have you ever had this problem?

Name a time when following your gut got you into romantic turmoil.

How does this awareness help?

Addiction is when you want something that you know is not good for you. Describe your own issue with this problem as it relates not to substances but to romantic partners.

Name a quality you are attracted to in a mate, one that winds up backfiring on you.

Do you feel you're making progress with these issues? How?

Name a strength for overcoming your negative attractions and emotional addictions.

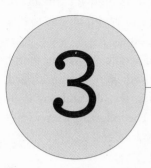

Attending to the Moment

I hope that exploring some of the patterns interfering in your relationships has given your recovery a sense of hope and direction. Taking responsibility for your side of the equation prepares you for positive change. In this chapter, we'll continue examining the origins of these patterns as we take emotional inventory of your Shattering experiences past and present. You are going to learn how to work through your feelings so that you can gain by your abandonment experience rather than be diminished by it.

Abandonment is a trauma powerful enough to produce the symptoms associated with any other type of trauma:[1] shock, disorientation, anxiety, heightened vulnerability, and lasting impact. Abandonment's wound is cumulative. It contains not only your current heartbreak but previous losses, disconnections, and disappointments as well. When your current relationship is torn, feelings from the past, stored deep within your emotional brain,[2] erupt and flow into the tear.

> *"I feel utterly helpless," says Maria. "I always prided myself on being self-sufficient, but now I can't get out of bed because I need him to come back and love me."*

Feelings of helplessness and dependency bubble up from childhood, making it feel as if you couldn't survive without your partner. You're thinking in terms of always and never, which fuels your sense of dread and panic.[3]

> *"I'll never recover from this."*

> *"I'll always be alone."*

This emotional regression is temporary, but it doesn't feel that way. In my case, it felt as though every disconnection and apprehension I'd ever experienced were coming at me in full force. I found myself gripped in the same terror I'd felt when I was three years old and my parents left me with the babysitter, and the same desolation I'd felt in the sixth grade when I didn't make the cheerleading squad.

Abandonment is a primal fear, our first fear.[4] Even those of you who grew up in idyllic childhoods within loving, intact families weren't spared this fear—the fear of being left alone with no one to care about you. The anxiety and self-doubt of abandonment continue into adulthood.

I have received thousands of personal stories* at abandonment.net from people all over the world, describing their painful and traumatic childhoods—being neglected, overlooked, ignored, or criticized. Some were left on doorsteps, shuttled back and forth between foster homes, sexually and physically abused. The love and attention needed was doled out inconsistently, if at all. The following list does not reflect the most extreme scenarios written to me, but it does represent the major areas.

 ## THE TOP THIRTY-ONE PRIMAL ABANDONMENT SCENES

Customize by checking all that apply to you and adding your own unique scenarios at the end.

CHILDHOOD PRIMAL SCENES

❑ Early abandonment of one or both parents.
❑ My mother died, father died.
❑ Custody battle—I was in the middle.
❑ Emotional, physical, sexual abuse.
❑ I witnessed family violence.
❑ Dysfunctional, chaotic, addictive family system.
❑ Divorce, family earthquake, loss of family unity.
❑ Illness of parent (cancer, alcoholism, mental illness).
❑ Birth of sibling; I lost my exclusive bond with my parents.
❑ Learning disability, lost status within family or classroom; physical disability.
❑ Parent's emotional withdrawal due to bereavement, depression, job, etc.
❑ Single-parent family; my parent was overloaded, worked full-time, or carried burdens.
❑ Both parents workaholic, self-centered, or emotionally unavailable.
❑ I went through an ugly duckling stage, parents emotionally dumped me.
❑ Parents favored another sibling.
❑ Too many babysitters, too long at day-care center or camp, too much alone time.
❑ Grandparent dies, pet dies.
❑ Parents came and went owing to business trips, marital separations, immigration problems.
❑ My brain produced too much norepinephrine.[5] (See the Scientific Tidbit on the next page).
❑ I moved a lot, always felt like the new kid on the block.

ADOLESCENT PRIMAL SCENES

❑ Felt on the outside looking in.
❑ Social discomfort, inhibition.

---

*   To submit your personal story, click on PERSONAL STORIES at the abandonment.net Help Center.

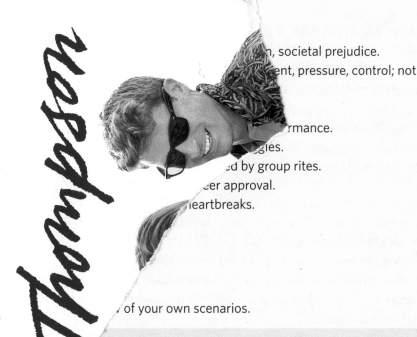

n, societal prejudice.

ent, pressure, control; not

rmance.

gles.

ed by group rites.

er approval.

eartbreaks.

of your own scenarios.

To evaluate the impact of your earlier experiences on your current emotional responses, consider that you were less able to defend yourself against loss and rejection as a child than you are now.[6] Children interpret the hurts, losses, and disappointments of life as personal failings. During adulthood, you realize that these experiences were beyond your control— not your fault—but as a child your cognitive functioning wasn't equipped to make such distinctions.[7] Children feel diminished by any disconnection or loss that makes them feel helpless to control their circumstances. Any abuse, neglect, illness, or disruption to routine causes children to doubt themselves and fear the world around them. As you enter adulthood, your heartaches get mapped onto earlier fears and losses.[8]

Fear of abandonment is cumulative. It lingers beneath the surface of life, making us vulnerable to rejection and loss later on.[9] It causes us to doubt ourselves for feeling helpless—helpless to bring our lovers back and helpless to make the pain go away.

Helplessness

As children, one of the reasons we felt diminished by losses and upsets was because we felt helpless.[10] Helplessness creates anxiety and erodes confidence in a child's fledgling sense of mastery. Many of the people writing to me about the powerlessness they feel during heartbreak describe childhood histories in which they bore witness to family violence. Most of them don't know exactly how this connects to their current despondency, but they know the old feelings of helplessness return.[11] It is known that witnessing violence is as traumatic as being the direct victim of the violence.[12] Both situations create victims because the witness feels helpless to protect the person he cares about. As a child, you needed to feel in control as much or more than you do now, and it was this abridgment—this paralyzing feeling of helplessness—that fomented the traumatic stress.[13] When children are placed in a helpless role, they learn to feel powerless, ineffectual, socially impotent, and bad about themselves. The feelings live on and come out full force during adult heartbreak, when you are once again at a loss of power, helpless to bring your life back to where it was.

Another common scenario that abandonment survivors describe is having endured sexual or physical abuse. The physical scars healed, but physical abuse hurts you even more in an emotional place. When you were hurt or attacked as a child, you felt this at its deepest level as abandonment. If the perpetrator was one of your parents, you felt he or she didn't care, didn't love you enough. You felt angry with your parent but also with yourself. You felt rejected, personally devalued, as if you weren't special enough to warrant better treatment (or better parents). You concluded you must be bad, unworthy, defective, and these basic assumptions carry through into adulthood.

When you go through an adult abandonment, your gravest self-doubts surface again and cause your self-image to plummet. Being left by someone you love feels like a form of emotional abuse. The terms *emotional murder* and *emotional rape* resonate with a lot of survivors, especially those who'd witnessed violence or been physically or sexually abused as children.

Vulnerability

It isn't just violence and abuse that increase the quotient of vulnerability in children. Anything that disrupted the emotional bond between you and your parents could have created lasting impact. Research shows the enduring effect of separations between animals and their infants. For instance, separate a rat pup from its mother for just a few weeks and observe its behavior in adulthood compared to a pup who experienced no separation. When the separated pup reaches adulthood, just look at its behaviors:

It has trouble learning new tasks, such as riding on a training wheel.
It has trouble forming new attachments.
It is more prone to depressive posturing.
Its blood levels carry high levels of glucocorticoid stress hormones.
It tends to avoid novel situations, such as being placed in a new cage or acquiring new cage mates.[14]

Thanks to the structuring of our mammalian brain, the bond between you and your primary caretaker served as a prototype for future relationships.[15] If there was alienation within your family, for example, a pattern of alienation stood a good chance of following you into your peer groups and love relationships. If you received love, support, and recognition from your parents, then in most cases you brought a sense of security into your social world, enabling you to stand up for yourself as a worthwhile individual.

The anxiety and self-doubt you accumulated from childhood disconnections bog down your attempts to get over heartbreak. All of that unfinished business resurfacing makes it harder to cope with the torrent of emotion, feel confident about your future, and face an ending.

Personality Profiles

Depending on what emotional baggage you carry, you can get stuck in one or more of the stages of abandonment. We're going to look at the effects of that stage by stage. We tend to have most difficulty working through a stage we struggled with during earlier childhood losses.

As I introduce the profiles below, you'll notice that the feelings and issues described are divvied up according to the S.W.I.R.L. Process, with a personality description for each of the five stages of abandonment. In real life, people don't fit such neat categories, so bear in mind that the descriptions are rough

> **SCIENTIFIC TIDBIT**
>
> Early separation creates dendrite damage in the hippocampus, the seahorse-shaped organ located deep within the mammalian brain, or limbic system. This affects memory as well as other brain functions, such as deregulation of glutamate, which interferes with learning, including social learning.

guides and not meant to suggest a mechanistic view of psychology[16] or that your feelings ought to fit into one of five tight little boxes. Use the descriptions to estimate the origins of some of your emotional hot spots. By determining in which of the stages you have unfinished business, you can better focus your recovery efforts. Toward the end of the chapter, we'll discuss how to work through your unresolved feelings.

 ## S.W.I.R.L. Profiles

The Shattering Personality Type: You are most likely to develop a Shattering personality profile if you went through serious or repetitious Shattering experiences in childhood, adolescence, or early adulthood, such as severe physical or sexual abuse or death of a parent. The turbulent, destructive feelings of catastrophic loss, panic, shock, fear, and helplessness tend to leach into your emotional reservoir, causing you to overreact to emotional upsets later on in life. You may have absorbed so many shattered feelings during childhood that their toxicity continues to disrupt your relationships. People with a Shattering profile tend to have a psychiatric or rehab history, have drug abuse problems,[17] or suffer chronic depression[18] or instability and extremely low self-esteem.

The Withdrawal Personality Type: If you experienced a lot of need deprivation when you were younger—perhaps your parents were alcoholic, ill, emotionally inconsistent, or otherwise unavailable—it is likely that you internalized the intense longing, craving feelings of Withdrawal. You learned to feel a chronic waiting for life, a kind of emotional emptiness—feelings that persist into adult life. Being stuck in Withdrawal can lead to dependency and co-dependency patterns in your adult relationships, in which you're too needy or too enmeshed in other people's needs. The emotional hunger gets you to self-medicate with shopping, alcohol, people, television, gambling, and other compulsive behaviors.[19]

The Internalizing Personality Type: If your parents had a tendency to be critical, dismissive, or rejecting, you may have felt you could never do anything right. Maybe you were unfavorably compared to a sibling. By Internalizing the insults and attacks, you absorbed your family's ability to make you feel small. Rejection inflicts a deep personal injury, generating insecurity, self-obsession, and the tendency to idealize others and turn your anger against yourself. These feelings fester beneath the surface, where they interfere with self-image and, later on, with forming primary relationships. People with an Internalizing profile lack the sense of entitlement and confidence to reach their true potential. They have difficulty delaying gratification;[20] their low self-worth causes them to grab for quick fixes, which sabotage their long-term goals. They eat that piece of chocolate cake because they need it now, forfeiting tomorrow's chance for having the body they desire.

> ## SCIENTIFIC TIDBIT
>
> Controlled studies have shown that rats handled during the first weeks of life secrete fewer stress hormones as adults, are less prone to avoidant or depressive behaviors, are more likely to take positive risks, and adapt more easily to novel situations than rats who were not handled.

The Rage Personality Type: If situations in your earlier life caused you to feel chronically frustrated and angry—maybe your parents were controlling, unjust, or overly punitive—you may have internalized a lot of unspent Rage, making it difficult to modulate your anger later on. Being physically violated causes children to feel rejected, guilty, unloved, undeserving, and emotionally abandoned. Inflicting physical pain or injury on a child is, on a deeper, more damaging level, another form of emotional abuse because it causes children to feel helpless, powerless, worthless. If you have a Rage profile, you have trouble staying in control of these emotions and asserting your needs appropriately at work and home. It's difficult to ask for what you want without going overboard, causing you to be either underassertive or overaggressive, expressing your anger either through passivity or impulsivity.[21] You build resentments and conflicts with people. You're prone to developing agitated depression.

The Lifting Personality Type: If you had repeated losses and disappointments in earlier life, you may have had more than the normal amount of Lifting to do. To cope, you became adept at lifting above your feelings. This may have caused some of you to develop resiliency but caused others to inadvertently detach from your emotional core.[22] As a result of overlifting, you have trouble identifying your feelings as an adult—difficulty feeling your feelings. Overlifters circumvent vulnerability by disconnecting and isolating from people. You may exhibit false self and appear emotionally remote to others. You have problems with intimacy either as a result of choosing the wrong partners or through constructing your own emotional barriers. You struggle with constancy—that is, you have difficulty sustaining love feelings toward your significant other.

Q

Which personality profiles did you identify with the most and why?

What insights and strengths help you overcome these issues?

CHILDHOOD SCENARIOS THAT CREATE EMOTIONAL BAGGAGE IN...

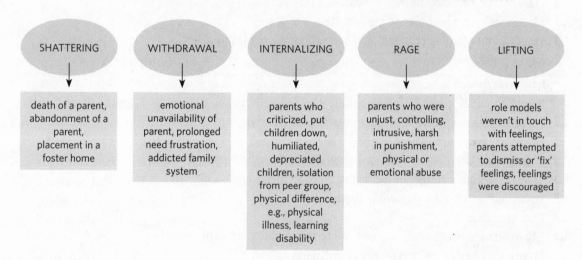

SHATTERING	WITHDRAWAL	INTERNALIZING	RAGE	LIFTING
death of a parent, abandonment of a parent, placement in a foster home	emotional unavailability of parent, prolonged need frustration, addicted family system	parents who criticized, put children down, humiliated, depreciated children, isolation from peer group, physical difference, e.g., physical illness, learning disability	parents who were unjust, controlling, intrusive, harsh in punishment, physical or emotional abuse	role models weren't in touch with feelings, parents attempted to dismiss or 'fix' feelings, feelings were discouraged

What follows is an Inventory Questionnaire to help you further identify places where you might be stuck in one or more of the stages.

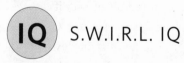 S.W.I.R.L. IQ

Check all that apply.

STUCK IN SHATTERİNG

❑ I have a pattern of depending on people who let me down.
❑ Others, especially my family, tend to scapegoat me.
❑ I have sabotaged relationships or personal successes out of fear.
❑ I constantly paint myself into corners and can't get out.

❏   I have a history of substance abuse.
❏   I am anxious or depressed a lot of the time.
❏   My life has become a roller coaster, an accident waiting to happen, an emotional disaster.
❏   I feel as if I'm missing important feelings others seem to have.
❏   I believe others see me as damaged or dysfunctional.

STUCK IN WITHDRAWAL

❏   I feel as if I'm waiting for something to happen before my life can fall into place.
❏   I have problems with food, alcohol, sex, or spending too much.
❏   I get strung out over relationships gone awry.
❏   The morning after an attempt at love, I wake up with an emotional hangover.
❏   I keep ruminating over situations and problems beyond my control.
❏   There is a big discrepancy between what I have and what I want.
❏   I am needy or overly clingy in my love relationships.
❏   I feel overpowered by others' needs.
❏   My fantasies are better than my real life.
❏   I feel an emotional emptiness, as if something were missing.
❏   I am a procrastinator.

STUCK IN INTERNALIZING

❏   I protect others even when they've treated me poorly.
❏   I have a fear of humiliation.
❏   I feel people don't really know or recognize me for who I am.
❏   I feel others are stronger or more able to cope than I am.
❏   I allow others to put me down without retort.
❏   I am inhibited.
❏   My need for perfectionism causes me to feel dissatisfied with myself.
❏   I try to stay perfect to remain above criticism.
❏   I am afraid of success because I'm afraid of competitive backlash.
❏   I am overly sensitive to rejection.
❏   I idealize others at my own expense.
❏   I am a slave for approval.
❏   I feel something holding my life back.
❏   I frequently feel slighted. I presume it to be a weakness others perceive about me.
❏   I have a constant head-trip going on in which I worry about my self-worth.
❏   I worry about how other people see me.
❏   I have experienced problems with low-grade depression.

STUCK IN RAGE

❏   I play emotional games in my love relationships.
❏   I hold out emotionally to test the other's staying power.

❏ There are dominance themes in my relationships; one side of the partnership has more control.

❏ I have a history of rebelliousness.

❏ I resist taking someone's advice, determined to do it my way, even if I know I'm being headstrong.

❏ When I feel criticized or rejected, I get vindictive urges.

❏ I vacillate between being overtolerant and overcritical.

❏ Games of one-upmanship make me anxious.

❏ I have had agitated depression.

❏ There are a lot of unresolved conflicts in my relationships.

❏ I have a tendency to brood.

❏ I hold on to a lot of resentment but act like everything is okay.

❏ My anger spurts out behind people's backs.

❏ When I underexpress or overexpress my anger, I become my own worst enemy.

> Some people recovering from abandonment have learned to identify emotional hangovers—the emotional aftershocks of the intense experience of the day before. This recognition allows you to sort out your feelings more quickly and get back on track.

STUCK IN LIFTING

❏ Others accuse me of being insincere or think of me as emotionally superficial.

❏ I sometimes feel as though others were experiencing feelings I'm not.

❏ I have trouble with intimacy.

❏ I feel numb to life.

❏ I wonder what happened to my emotions.

❏ I am always on the go, staying busy, focused on work—becoming more like a "human doing" than a human being.

❏ I shut down emotionally or sexually in the midst of a relationship.

❏ I use humor a great deal as a means of diffusing emotional situations.

❏ I suspect I have attention deficit disorder[23] or a tendency to move from one distraction to another.

WHAT PROFILE BEST DESCRIBES YOU?
Unfinished business from...

SHATTERING	WITHDRAWAL	INTERNALIZING	RAGE	LIFTING
		CREATES		
instability, self-destructiveness, psychiatric conditions	dependency, codependency, emptiness, addiction	low self-esteem, low-grade depression, poor self-image, inhibition	conflict with others, agitated depression	dys-intimacy, detachment, isolation, low emotional libido

Mining for Abandonment Gold

Getting in touch with issues and feelings arising from the cumulative wound of abandonment is like discovering a gold mine. You finally get to address your oldest, truest, and most important needs and feelings now that they have resurfaced. You may have been helpless to meet these needs as a child, but now you are a capable adult, learning the tools of recovery.

"The bad news when Sarah left me was that everything I ever went through was in my face again—my mother's death, my father's alcoholism. It all came back and I felt like hell. The good news was that I was forced to deal with myself—I mean the raw truth about what was really going on inside all this time."

The Unfinished Business Chart (page 71) can be used for continuing to mine your abandonment gold. The format allows you to collect and organize your feelings as you make your way, stage by stage, through recovery. Tracking your feelings helps you avoid picking up new emotional baggage and attend to old unfinished business at the same time.

Think about your childhood, adolescence, and adult experiences. Reflect on feelings you accumulated during each phase of your life and jot them in the chart's columns. To make the chart truly represent your personal profile, you may need to go back and review the S.W.I.R.L. Profiles and IQ. Remember, the stages overlap and real life doesn't fit into tight little boxes. The chart is designed to give you an approximate idea of where you might be stuck and where to focus your recovery.

Begin by thinking of an incident of loss or disappointment from your childhood. What feelings do you remember during the initial Shattering? Jot down the feelings in the Shattering column. Did the experience create any emotional deprivation? Did it leave you needing, wanting, waiting for reassurance that never arrived? What needs and feelings did this create? Jot down those feelings in the Withdrawal column. How did that experience affect the way you felt about yourself? Did it create self-doubt? Did it make you feel insignificant? Unspecial? Jot down those feelings in the Internalizing column. Do you remember what you did with the anger? Hold it in? Take it out on your toys? People? Yourself? Describe this in the Rage column. And finally, where did all of the feelings go? Did you stuff them? Did you give up trying to get your needs met? Become detached? Lower your expectations? Did it break your spirit? Increase your spirit? Jot down a few words in the Lifting column.

As you read across horizontally, it should give you an emotional map of the experience. You can do this for each significant emotional experience from childhood till present—and then you can look for patterns.

THE UNFINISHED BUSINESS CHART*				
SHATTERING	WITHDRAWAL	INTERNALIZING	RAGE	LIFTING

TAKING EMOTIONAL STOCK
Feelings you picked up in…

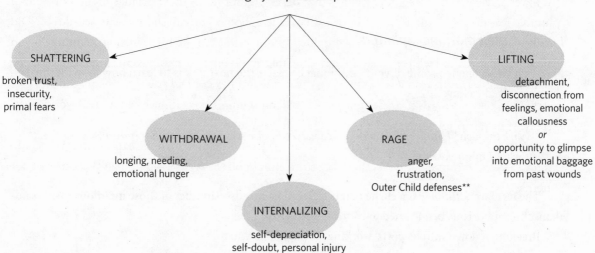

SHATTERING
broken trust,
insecurity,
primal fears

WITHDRAWAL
longing, needing,
emotional hunger

INTERNALIZING
self-depreciation,
self-doubt, personal injury

RAGE
anger,
frustration,
Outer Child defenses**

LIFTING
detachment,
disconnection from
feelings, emotional
callousness
or
opportunity to glimpse
into emotional baggage
from past wounds

---

*   You can use this chart as a handout in your abandonment support groups.

** Outer Child is discussed in depth in chapter 9.

After considering a few different experiences, take stock and consider the whole of your abandonment profile. Then examine the columns vertically. Do your feelings form an emotional theme? Which ones carry through from childhood to today?

Which loss, heartbreak, or disappointment seems to have had the greatest impact?

How can it benefit your life to resolve these long-standing feelings?

Hold on to The Unfinished Business Chart so that you can add feelings and situations to it as we continue our journey of recovery from your old wounds as well as the new.

Working through the Feelings

Pull Out the Emotional Splinters

Now that we've opened some of your emotional baggage, the next task is to learn how to work through the unresolved feelings.

> *"'Work through.' Hmmmm, should I ask? Everybody else seems to know what it means, but I don't get what I'm supposed to do."*

The term *work through* is a cliché that boggles most minds—another of those infamous easier-said-than-done aphorisms bequeathed to us from self-help.

Breaking it down into its parts, working through asks you to:

Identify a feeling. Put it into simple terms; this helps get your feelings outside of yourself and into a well-contained, safe structure. Truth Nuggets (see below) are designed to assist with this process.

Accept your feelings as part of being human. They relate to what you've gone through and do not indicate weakness on your part.

Face the reality of your feelings in the moment. The work of grief, for example, is to accept the pain of loss,[24] an enormous step accomplished not for all time but over and over again—always in the moment.

Share your feelings. Be open with a friend, discuss them with a therapist, or share them with other abandonment survivors.

> People tell me: "My feelings are such a jumble. I keep obsessing about my breakup—every word, every action, over and over. I'm driving myself and everybody else crazy. Why am I so stuck?"
>
> I explain: People surviving abandonment tend to get bogged down in the details until they learn what to do with the powerful feelings. They remain situation oriented as a way of avoiding the feelings. Remaining focused on endless details about your breakup is one of the things that wears out your friends and prolongs your pain, a tendency that lasts well into the Withdrawal stage and beyond.

The explanation for this has to do once again with your mammalian brain. Abandonment arouses your amygdala, which deploys cascades of stress hormones to surge through your mind and body. One of these, norepinephrine (NE), causes you to remain riveted on external details of the threat at hand[25]—in this case, abandonment—to help you discover clues to aid your survival. You experience this hypervigilance as being obsessed.

You don't mean to go into such detail, but you just can't seem to tell the short version, because your abandonment crisis causes the release of another stress hormone, adrenaline (a.k.a. epinephrine).[26] Adrenaline increases your impulse-to-action response, causing you to spill over the edge of your usual boundaries. Owing to these neurohormones, you automatically process what went wrong in the relationship, obsess on infinite details about your ex, and go overboard, torturing your friends with redundant concerns.

Your cognitive brain's task is to find a way to outsmart this aroused mammal's maneuvering so that your adult self can take back control.

Learning how to work with your feelings rather than ruminating about every aspect of your situation is what is going to heal you and make you strong. The following simple exercise facilitates this process.

Truth Nuggets

Truth Nuggets provide a format for safely containing your feelings while avoiding getting bogged down in the details.[27] As we continue along the path of recovery, you'll find many Truth Nuggets sprinkled throughout.

A Truth Nugget asks that you name a feeling in one simple word—for example, sad, mad, worried, disappointed, terrified, apprehensive, or happy—one that describes how you are currently feeling. Your next step is to add a brief phrase (five words or fewer) describing the situation causing the feeling.

Truth Nugget: I feel _____ because _____ .

Try one (calorie free).

Truth Nuggets have healing power because they use your cognitive brain's ability to safely interpret input from your emotional brain. Writing Truth Nuggets or speaking them out loud prevents overdramatizing and obsessing about your situation, strengthens your adult functioning, and helps you gain mastery over your life. It gets you out of the "story" and into healing.

One abandonment survivor, Jake, sent a personal story* to abandonment.net that went on for several pages. Most of us can identify with the pain he expressed in this sentence:

"When Patty left, it felt like she and her new boyfriend dropped me off in the middle of the Sahara Desert, and then took off, leaving me to die of heat and starvation."

How could Jake have put his painful feelings into a Truth Nugget? His first task would be to center in on the main feeling and identify a simple short word to describe his tumult of emotion. Then he would use a brief phrase to state the cause. His nugget might sound something like this:

I felt *hurt* because *my girlfriend betrayed me.*

As you can see, Truth Nuggets don't make interesting reading material, but they do make satisfying emotional material. They are not designed to be colorful but to help you gain strength from your ability to grasp and face your emotional reality. Once you pare your overwhelming emotions down into a simple word and attach its bite-size cause, you can swallow this reality whole. This process lifts you from the emotional soup as well as rescues you from those tediously painful details you are mired in. It encourages you to get the big picture and empowers you to focus your energy on confronting the reality you are facing.[28] You can write Truth Nuggets into your daily journal, collect them in a special place, or share them with a friend or e-buddy.

---

*   Click on PERSONAL STORIES at the abandonment.net Help Center.

SWAN LESSON THREE

Attending to the Moment

The little girl in the story learned this important step in the healing process during her third encounter with the black swan. She had been practicing the first two Swan Lessons—*centering in* and *cleansing her wound*, but then terrible fears overcame her. She beseeched her beautiful swan for help. He emphasized the importance of being able to face her reality all in one gulp. As the little girl absorbed this lesson, she took a big gasp of air and faced her reality in one sentence, feelings first.

"I'm afraid!" cries the little girl. "I don't know what's going to happen to me!"

"Go to the center of your fears, Amanda, so that you can find the oasis between past and present—the ever-flowing wellspring of now."

"I'm too afraid."

"Fear is of the future, Amanda, and we cannot do anything about the future. We have no control over it because it doesn't exist yet. There is only now. Now is where reality lives. All of your fears are about the future that is only an imagined place. You can't really know the future until you get there. Yet here is the moment, just waiting to show itself to you, and I will help you find it."

"How?"

"You already have the tools you need to find it, Amanda. They are your eyes and ears and nose and skin and heart and mind. But now you must learn to use these senses in a special new way, a way that brings you out of your fears and into the moment," says the swan.

The little girl moves closer to the swan.

"First go inside to your listening space so you can hear what I am about to say."

The little girl places her hands on her chest and burrows within.

"Find your fear and go into its very center. Can you feel your listening space?"

"I think so, yes," says the little girl.

"Now, see if you can open your ears so that you can hear the faintest sounds." The swan waits to let the sound of his own voice dissipate so that background noises can flow in.

The little girl tilts her head to listen carefully.

"Can you hear insects?" he asks, nearly whispering.

She squeezes her eyes tighter and listens. "Almost, yes."

"Can you hear anything else?"

"I can hear the waves tickling the pebbles."

As the little girl slowly tuned in to the sounds, light patterns, and skin sensations of the moment, she tilted her head—a gesture I've seen people perform when something momentarily catches their attention. As the little girl tilted her head, she consciously left her fears and entered a place of momentary calm. Once again she discovered her own strength to withstand her greatest fears—even if for a brief moment.

> People argue: "I thought you were supposed to work your feelings through, not escape from them."
>
> I explain: When you use the moment to cope with strong emotion, you're not escaping your feelings, but managing them by getting in touch with your internal strength. In learning to sustain your life as a separate person, you're neither suppressing nor denying your feelings but becoming larger than your problems by discovering your capacity to experience life in spite of painful emotion.

Here is a list of all of the things we do with uncomfortable feelings when we don't know how to handle them:

Check all you can recognize in yourself.

- ❏ I become overwhelmed by them.
- ❏ I suppress them.
- ❏ I displace them, take them out on innocent bystanders.
- ❏ I blame someone else for causing them.
- ❏ I deny them.
- ❏ I rewrite the history surrounding them in an attempt to invalidate them.
- ❏ I squelch them.
- ❏ I become situation oriented rather than face them.
- ❏ I repress them.
- ❏ I forget them.
- ❏ I ignore them.
- ❏ I project them, make them someone else's problem.
- ❏ I make them my partner's problem.
- ❏ I distract myself from them.
- ❏ I blank out, distance from them.

In contrast to these defenses, when you deal with your feelings by bringing them into the moment with you, you gain another level of self-reliance. Closely attending to the sensations in the moment allows you to co-exist with your feelings and gracefully accept their presence without being overwhelmed by them. This is what working through is all about—learning how to cope with feelings instead of overdefending yourself from them.

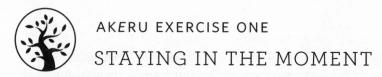

AKERU EXERCISE ONE
STAYING IN THE MOMENT

The concept of Akeru (described on page 13) helps us recognize that an ending of a relationship is truly a beginning of new life. For example, getting into the moment transforms the piercing pain of separation into an ability to gain emotional strength and experience life more intensely.

The powerful impetus to bond is ever present, but we are most aware of its pull when our relationship is ripped away. During Shattering, we feel shock, desperation, and panic because we've been cut off from everything we depended on for comfort, security, and love. The painful tear in our attachment exposes raw nerves. It is a source of intense discomfort, but we can redirect its energy to fuel our recovery.

Shattering, in effect, is an explosion of separateness. Stripped of outside support, we feel the intensity of life within and around us. It is our reawakened self that we bring into the moment with us. Getting into the moment takes advantage of our most painful emotions by working *with* its energy rather than *against* it—Akeru.

The moment is the chosen modality of healing for two reasons. First, you're powerless to control the past because it is already gone and, second, you're powerless to control the future because it hasn't yet arrived. Your power is now. You can take hold of the present. The past and future may seem very immense and overwhelming, but your reality exists now. Take a moment to think about it. Now is all there is.[29]

Feelings are now. They can best be worked through in the moment. The intense hopelessness of abandonment may feel like a life sentence, but these feelings are fueled by a negative use of your imagination. They are not reality. Any feeling can be handled when we realize it exists only for now. The moment serves as an ever-present oasis to return to during this period of stark separation.

I've used "getting into the moment" as a technique for running group therapy sessions for depressed clients in psychiatric wards. On some days, the group dynamics take a downward turn, one person's depression feeding into another's. One such day, Timothy, one of the group's more withdrawn members, tilted his chair back against the wall and remained silent while he fidgeted with the cord of the Venetian blinds. I seized on this as an opportunity to shift the group's mood. I drew attention to the fact that while the rest of us were talking about feeling stuck, Timothy was creating change for all of us. By slanting the blinds this way and that, he was changing the direction of light, creating shifting stripes of sunlight across the floor. It was amazing to see how this simple maneuver got everybody's attention. They came out of their heads to study the shifting light patterns happening in their very midst. They instantly became more present to one another in spite of their circumstances.

What follows are directions to help you find your own way into the moment. Most people are soon able to dispense with the directions and venture into their own creative ways of experiencing the world around them.

Guided Help for Staying in the Moment

We start with our feelings.

Take some time to center in and reflect on the idea that your strongest emotions are sustained by your own energy. Can you identify a feeling in this moment? Reading has a way of calming the emotions, so put this book down and give yourself a moment to identify a feeling rising from your abandonment situation.

Do you feel anxiety? Calm? Anger? Worry? Sadness? Excitement? Name the feeling and the situation, creating a Truth Nugget.

Truth Nugget: I feel _____ because _____ .

You may have noticed that when your mind is wracked with pain from a Shattering, radio and television don't usually provide enough stimulation to draw you out of your worries. It's too easy to listen to music or watch television and still be into your painful thoughts. At these moments, it helps to use your sense of hearing in a less passive, more focused manner. It's time to turn off the radio and tune in to the background noises so that you can use this exercise to its full benefit.

Focus on the subtle textures of sound in the background until you can detect their origins. As you're doing so, you momentarily leave your painful thoughts. The more engaged in focused listening, the less your panic and grief can take over. When your painful thoughts return, just focus your attention once again on a sensory experience, such as tuning in to the faintest sound you can hear, and hold on to it as long as you can.

Find a relatively quiet place in the house. Once alone, pay attention to what sounds are in the room with you. Can you hear your furnace? The refrigerator? Footsteps in another room? Describe three different background sounds you can detect.

1.
2.
3.

Can you hear any sounds coming from far away? What can you decipher? The song of a bird? A car? The wind?

You are using your sense of hearing as a coping tool to momentarily come out of your thoughts and into a place of peace and calm. The task is that simple.

Make a deliberate effort to study the light patterns in the room in which you are currently sitting. Are there speckles or stripes of light coming through? Are they coming from the sun, a candle, an overhead lamp? Describe the patterns.

Are shadows present? Do they create irregular shapes? Describe.

The emotional crisis of Shattering can make it difficult to turn your attention on what you are seeing. Sometimes it helps to stop gazing and close your eyes and study the light show on the back of your lids. Do you see any stars? Dark forms? Moving figures? Describe.

If it is possible, open a window or step outside. If there is a breeze, feel it blow against your face. Tune in and really feel it. What is its temperature, velocity, effect on your skin? Describe.

Another option is to go for a drive. Roll down your car windows and feel the wind blow across your face. Listen to the engine roar. When you return from your outing, describe your sensations.

Can you feel your hair touching any part of your face? Can you feel its weight on your scalp? Describe how it feels.

Your fingertips have nerve endings that can distinguish subtle differences in what they touch. Rub your fingers across a page of this book. Can you feel the dried pulp of the paper it is printed on? Compare this texture to the paper used on the cover. Describe the difference.

What else can you feel? How do your clothes feel in contact with your skin? Can you feel your socks hugging your feet? Can you feel the textures of the fabrics next to your skin? Cotton? Wool? Silk? Describe the sensations on your skin.

Tune in to your body. Notice whether there is a knot in your stomach. Is it tightening or loosening? Where are you holding your tension? In your facial muscles? For now, don't try to calm yourself—just feel it. Take an inventory of other bodily sensations to discover where else you are tensing up. Forehead? Scalp? Shoulders? Neck?

Can you feel your own energy sustaining this tension? Your goal here is not to relax, but to attend to the sensations, both positive and negative. Describe the overall energy level (or lack thereof) in your body.

Concentrate on the inside of your mouth. Tune in to its wetness, the sense of your tongue against the roof of your mouth, the taste in your mouth. Can you detect the taste of your saliva? Is it neutral? Minty? Bitter? Sweet? Smoky? Coffee flavored?

Feel your chest rise and fall with each breath. Fill your lungs with air and feel your diaphragm expand. Exhale slowly until you have completely emptied your lungs all the way to the bottom. Experience the process, conscious of every sensation. Repeat several times. Describe.

Now let your breath return to normal and concentrate on the muscles that work to draw your every breath. What temperature is the air coming through your nostrils? Describe the sensation of air filling up and exiting your lungs and moving in and out of your nose or mouth.

As you tuned in to these sensations did you feel any peace or calm? Did tuning in help you take leave of your painful thoughts, even if only for a moment?

That's the whole point. You are learning to experience the momentary sensations of life, not in spite of being in an emotional crisis but motivated by the need to withstand it.

Your ability to get into the moment serves as a foundation for the rest of your journey of recovery. As you practice it, you'll learn to stay in the moment for greater lengths of time— from five seconds at a time to five minutes at a time, and eventually for longer periods. Each time the pain distracts you from the moment, just go back and find the moment again.

Staying in the Moment is not just an exercise to use during Shattering but a way to intensify the experience of life at any time. It is a way of being in the world. The more you practice this exercise, the better you become at handling your feelings. For centuries, Zen masters and other spiritual leaders have guided us to the moment as a way of celebrating existence. To learn to live with this kind of mindfulness is to participate in the joy, love, and bounty of life around and within us.

More Food for Thought

 CREATING PRESENCE

When were you most able to get into the moment as a kid?

What lengths do you have to go through to get into the moment now? Does it take listening to background noises?

How do you feel after being in the moment?

Concentrating on skin sensations? Breathing exercises? Describe.

How do you feel after being in the moment?

Are you able to use the moment as an oasis to return to when you're feeling low?

How many seconds, minutes, hours were you able to experience it?

Did you discover self-reliance in the process? Explain.

Which sensory organ did you use to gain entry into the moment?

What, if any, additional senses did you add?

Describe exactly what you listened to or studied with your eyes or felt on your skin or within your body?

How did intense experiencing feel?

How can you use the moment as a tool to enhance your life?

What worries keep you in your head and pull you out of the moment?

What tools help you get back into the moment to manage your feelings?

Q   SELF-RELIANCE

Do you understand the depth and nature of your abandonment wound?

Can you acknowledge its pain? Describe your fears, hurt, and rage.

Do you avoid shaming yourself by accepting your feelings as natural? In other words, can you accept yourself for having such intense and enduring feelings? Or do you tend to fault yourself for feeling out of control? Explain.

Can you affirm your strength for being able to stand alone?

Are you committed to managing your feelings by getting into the moment?

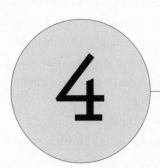

4

Separating

"I didn't ask to be alone."

The Withdrawal stage is when you come to terms with being alone—physically alone, emotionally alone, or both.

Being alone can create desolation and yet provide the privacy you need to work your way through. It can envelop you in a dark cloud of sorrow and at the same time provide an insulated womb of self-comfort. There aren't enough good and bad things to say about being alone. All combined, they add up to the primary challenge of the Withdrawal stage.

During Withdrawal, your body and mind ache for your lost relationship. You don't feel its pull until the shock of Shattering wears off and a sense of wrenching deprivation sets in. Day after day, as more and more of your needs go unfulfilled, you yearn for the security you once took for granted. You're in Withdrawal, addicted to love no longer available to you. There's nobody to ease the pain but you.

Abandonment thrusts you into this isolated state. There is little within your immediate power you can do to make it go away, although many people squander a lot of time and energy in protest, refusing to accept their aloneness. Railing against something you can't change only keeps you stuck in the pain.[1] Your task is to learn how to redirect the energy of Withdrawal to make aloneness work for you.

We're going to devote an entire chapter to the assets and liabilities of being alone—how to cope with it, learn from it, and gain greater connection to self and others from it.

Modern Brand of Aloneness

It's only been the last couple hundred years that we've begun to live in separate dwellings, in relative isolation from one another. For most of us, communal living is not an option. We don't live in a band of people who gather around the campfires at night, each of us playing an integral role in the survival of all. Instead, members of our society tend to board themselves up inside enclosed spaces surrounded by eight-foot-high walls and locked doors.

Millions of people are alone. Less than a hundred years ago most of us still enjoyed the emotional advantages of living in farming communities where large extended families provided support. If we lost our mate, we still had kin living near us.[2] In contrast, today most of our social, interpersonal, and financial needs are vested in the nuclear family—a self-contained unit often stationed miles away from extended family. When we lose our mate, there is no longer a communal society to cushion us, provide on-site social and financial support, and supplant the nurturance we are missing.

Even if we were in constant conflict with our former mate—even if we were the one who ended it— our basic need for security was intertwined with that one person, a need which, like the air we breathe, we took for granted. In today's world, when a relationship ends, the isolation is mitigated only by the care and support of our closest friends and family rather than an enveloping communal society.[3]

> People ask, "How do we cope with this modern world's brand of isolation, that of being *completely* alone? How do we move forward bereft of our primary connection and love?"
>
> I answer: We gain wisdom and strength to reassure ourselves that we can survive on our own one day at a time.
>> We face the situation as mature adults.
>> We broaden our perspective. We grow larger than our problem.

Alone vs. Lonely

When being on your own is your decision, it is a lifestyle to celebrate.

"I wanted out of my marriage for a long time," says Lynne, "but I was afraid to take the plunge. It wasn't until I became involved with a bunch of single women who got together all the time, cooking fabulous communal dinners on weekends, and giving each other constant support, that I finally felt ready to get my own place. My husband begged me not to leave, but I was thrilled to have my little apartment. I celebrated my freedom every night by lighting a candle and taking a luxurious bath—no pressure, just bubbles."

Alone feels good if you chose it, but not so good if it chose you. Aloneness can feel frightening and overwhelming when you've been torn from your ex and are suddenly uncertain about the future. When rejection is involved in the loss, being alone feels like a condemnation—like you're being punished for being unworthy or unlovable. If abandonment is a pattern in your life and you believe you sabotaged your own relationship, the self-recriminations can become a torture chamber.

"Another failed relationship!" says Thomas. "I can't stop beating myself up for being unable to hold on to what all of my friends can take for granted—a love life. I feel so inadequate."

Being physically alone is different from being emotionally alone. You can be in a relationship, but be emotionally disconnected.

"I can't feel any love for my husband anymore—too much water under the bridge," says Andrea. "But I'm not ready to leave. Fear traps me in. I miss the love. Life is flat without it. I'd do just about anything to have those feelings return to my life."

Or you may be by yourself, wishing you had somebody to belong to, somebody who belongs to you, but there is nobody special in your life.

"Everywhere I go, I'm surrounded by couples walking arm in arm," says Jack. "I'm always on the outside looking in."

You try to be upbeat but can't seem to rationalize away the feelings. The bottom line: Since you don't have what you want—a special person in your life—you're not happy. Like millions of people in the world, you feel as if you were going through the motions of life, doomed to loneliness.

Being alone is not the problem. Alone is not loneliness. Alone is a lifestyle many people choose. It is only when feelings of abandonment are present that being alone can create the following situations:

Please check all that apply.

- ❏ I feel loneliness.
- ❏ I feel a drain of life energy.
- ❏ I have separation anxiety, especially in the morning.
- ❏ I have nagging depression.
- ❏ I have a sense of futility in performing the tasks of everyday living.
- ❏ I feel shame—my aloneness means nobody wants me.
- ❏ I feel shame—I am unsuccessful in relationships.
- ❏ I feel shame—I am unable to love someone.
- ❏ I lack daily companionship.
- ❏ I dread vacations—nobody to go with.
- ❏ I lack a helpmate—nobody to help carry in the groceries.
- ❏ I have an empty void to fill on the weekends.
- ❏ I feel isolation on holidays; I feel blue on my birthday because nobody special cares.
- ❏ I am awkward at being a singleton in a couples' world.
- ❏ I feel like the third wheel with my coupled friends.
- ❏ I need to put on a happy act so my friends won't feel sorry for me.
- ❏ I feel less-than at family gatherings.

❏ I have unbalanced friendships—I look to my friends to meet my needs, but they have mates to rely on; I seem to need them more than they need me.

❏ I feel rejected, even though I understand my friends are busy.

❏ I have mini explosions when family and friends seem oblivious to my needs.

Consider the number of items you checked, so that you can appreciate your strength in meeting the challenges.

Q

Describe your own special circumstances that make being alone a challenge to cope with.

Can you see any hidden benefits to being alone? What potential growth does it afford you?

Use this space to give yourself credit for the strength you're using on a daily basis.

Alone Not by Choice

Abandonment creates a state of "involuntary separation."[4] As we've discussed, if you choose to be alone, living separately is a perfectly reasonable lifestyle. But if you were put in that position because you were abandoned, it kicks up your control issues.

We all have control issues—it doesn't mean we're control freaks. Every human being has a need to feel in control, a need begun in childhood and developed throughout life. It's an affront to one's sense of autonomy to be conscripted to a situation foisted on us by someone else's choice. Winding up alone arouses feelings of helplessness and powerlessness. When we've been forced into separation, many of us stage protests into the lonely nights, stabbing our pillows, punching the air, flailing in space—all gestures of victim rage. We rail against a reality we're momentarily helpless to change.

Lynne's situation illustrates how the issue of control affected her feelings about being on her own. About ten months into her foray into single life, her husband stopped calling her every night to check in. At first she was relieved, but when he failed to call on her birthday, she was unexpectedly crushed.

"I told him how angry I was about not calling me. So he responded by sending me a beautiful card and bouquet of flowers. But his daily calls had stopped coming."

About a year later she learned he'd begun to see someone else.

"I confronted him, very upset. He calmly listened and said he was sorry I felt that way. He didn't even bother to argue with me. I knew he had moved on and I was devastated that he was gone from my world."

Lynne's reaction had to do with the fact that she was no longer in control of the options of her life.

"Being alone had been my decision, but now I couldn't go back to him even if I wanted to," she explains. "My husband's new relationship removed the one option I had to fall back on. My little apartment suddenly felt like an isolation cell."

For some people, being on their own was their decision, but a lot of abandonment survivors lead single lifestyles without having consciously chosen to do so.

"I always expected to be married," says Paul. "But here I am in my sixties, never married, no children, living by myself. Maybe being alone was a decision I made subconsciously. This is a comforting thought because it means that I've secretly done exactly what I wanted all of these years, even if I was not aware of wanting to."

One of the most difficult scenarios to cope with is when you've been left for another. It feels unjust because your mate's decision to enter a new relationship automatically confines you to emotional isolation. This places you in extremely inequitable positions to one another. He or she is in the arms of a new lover while you are trying to avoid being devoured by the cavernous jaws of loneliness. You are forced to cope with a lifestyle you didn't choose, while your ex garners a greater sense of power and control, riding off into the sunset in the bliss of new love, knowing that you are waiting in the wings for her return. When you are the one left alone, it's hard not to feel victimized, demoralized, vanquished by your abandoner. Again, it's the issue of control: What you want most is missing from your life. You want love and connection. It's missing. You want your future secured. It's gone up in smoke. You want companionship, someone to care about you. You've been left. You want to regain control of your life. You feel powerless.

"Why Do I Have Control Issues?"

In the last chapter we looked at childhood scenarios that left us with emotional baggage. In exploring the issue of control, it helps to look at childhood experiences that caused us to internalize feelings of helplessness. Many describe having witnessed battles between family members.[5] Having no control over these events, you were suffused with stress, which later translated into posttraumatic symptoms.[6] Now that you're coping with being alone against your will, your old feelings of helplessness resurface.

"I feel so demoralized and helpless now that my wife moved out. I feel as powerless as I used to when I was a kid," says Bob. "I used to cower in the corner of the kitchen when my father browbeat my mother on a nightly basis. I would get very upset but there was nothing I could do. One time my older brother tried to stick up for her and my father knocked him out. My whole world was constantly threatened and all I could do was watch."

As a child, you needed to feel you had a voice, to believe that your needs and feelings were taken into account by parents on whom your security depended.[7] Otherwise you were riding on an emotional roller coaster without any handlebars.[8] Here are excerpts from personal stories submitted to abandonment.net.

"Nobody listened to me."

"My father was a dictator. It was hopeless to assert myself."

"My mother was on top of everything I did. I couldn't breathe without her having something to say about it."

"I had no control over what happened. I was a sitting duck for any insult, slam, or bruise any of my brothers felt like giving me. Nobody interceded."

To bolster your sense of being in control, many of you concocted makeshift defenses. You became finicky about minor things, threw tirades if your routine changed, or balked when your parents tried to get you to put on your shoes.

"When I was in grammar school, my school desk had to be just so. I went berserk if some kid's paper slid over onto the edge of my desk. My pencil had to be in the exact right place and my eraser in another, otherwise I was beside myself."

Some of you developed rituals to give yourself a sense of control.

"I had over twenty dolls and placed them all in a certain way, in just the right order, along my bed. When my mother made the bed, she'd change them slightly, and I'd go haywire. I'd put them all back where they belonged so that I could feel I was back in the control booth."

Some of you rebelled against your parents' attempt to control you.

"I was always in a power struggle with my parents. If they wanted me to zig, I zagged."

Some of you developed a passive-aggressive approach to sustaining control, often a struggle won at your own detriment.

"Dad was hard-nosed about everything, and Mom just went along with it. I couldn't win, so I fought back by not doing. I didn't do as much as I could get away with not doing. Now I torture myself with procrastination. I have library books overdue since 1952 and a car constantly begging me to get it inspected. But I don't budge. I've turned my passive aggression against myself."

When you were children, many of your control defenses, aimed at warding off anxiety, may have turned self-destructive. Your strategies, built on willfulness, laid the groundwork for developing some of the serious problems many of you have described—eating disorders and other obsessive-compulsive behaviors. The conditions known as encopresis and enuresis involve children's control over eliminating their bodily wastes. They can hold back, become constipated, and then eliminate at inopportune moments—such as in school, causing themselves pain and embarrassment. As your need for control went to the extremes, you became your own worst enemy—a pattern that interferes in your adult life and, for some of you, creates conditions requiring psychiatric intervention.

We acquired many of our self-defeating patterns in childhood—patterns that we are now working our way out of through abandonment recovery. Being thrust into aloneness inadvertently throws us into a kind of adult temper tantrum. The more awareness we gain about how we've been overdefending ourselves since childhood about feeling helpless—having no control—the less the past can haunt the present. By recognizing the dynamics of control, we can finally regain emotional composure.

What situations caused you to feel helpless as a child?

What, if any, control issues do you remember having?

Were your parents sensitive to your feelings and needs? Were they controlling?

How did you react?

What situation in your current life causes you to feel helpless?

How do you react now as an adult?

Has anyone suggested that you are too controlling?

Is anyone in your life controlling toward you?

How do you handle moments when you feel helpless and overwhelmed?

What strengths allow you to regain your sense of control?

Abandonment Grief

"I don't know whether I'm mad or sad, I just feel bad."

Being alone against your will isn't the only issue making it difficult to adjust to being alone. Grief complicates the process. After all, you are dealing with loss—a loss just as total as someone grieving a death.[9]

Abandonment creates its own special type of grief—one that has not been officially recognized by society the way bereavement has. This is reflected in the ways your friends and family respond to your situation. They hang in with you for the first month or two, but then harangue you with simplistic advice like, "Just let go" or "You've got to move forward." Meanwhile, your whole being has become as painful as an abscessed tooth and grows more inflamed by the day. You're feeling the agony of rejection and panicking over having no future—and all this mounts just as your friends are losing patience with you. "How could you pine away for someone who treated you so badly?" they logically ask.

How? Because that's how it works. The Withdrawal stage isn't logical. It doesn't matter whether the person you're grieving has shown herself to be an abandoner, a cad, or a ne'er-do-well. You're going through the powerful grief of abandonment. It's a psychobiological process. It doesn't operate according to your friends' or even your own schedule; it has a timetable of its own.

Abandonment is an example of "ambiguous loss"[10] in that it usually involves grieving someone who is still alive. You don't have a body to mourn over. This means that closure remains ambiguous and unresolved. Your wound remains open for a longer period, prolonging your recovery time.[11]

Grief is not limited to those of you going through an actual loss of a person. Many of the people attending my workshops and writing to my website are struggling to deal with a relationship in which they feel chronic abandonment. They are missing the love of someone who is still present.

"We were so in love at first," says Sarah, "but after his first affair, I shut down. I'm in constant grief over the love I am missing. I feel abandoned every day."

Another commonly expressed grief is when you're alone not because you've lost a relationship, but because you haven't found one yet. You are grieving over not having anyone in your life and you feel bereft of that special connection to someone—someone you're still hoping to meet. Many suspect that unresolved abandonment is behind their struggle to find an eligible candidate to fulfill their dreams, but aren't sure how to remove their stumbling blocks.

"When I hit forty," says Lorraine, "it suddenly seemed unacceptable to be single. It was fine in my thirties, but being a single forty-year-old seemed pathetic. Loneliness set in the day after my birthday, and I don't know how to stop singing the blues."

Your grief may not be about losing a person but about losing your lifestyle. Your relationship may have been unfulfilling to begin with, but now that it's over, you're grieving the activities and way of life you had while part of a couple.

"When Sarah and I broke up," says Mark, "it was truly for the better, but I went through hell anyway. My life drastically changed. We used to go to the beach after work every day to walk the dog and watch the sunset. Since she moved out I haven't bothered to go there—it's just too far to make the effort by myself. I miss the things we did together. I miss a coupled lifestyle."

Loss of Background Object

Another factor making it difficult to adjust to being alone is that you were accustomed to having a background object. You may not have realized how much your security depended on having someone to take for granted—someone who is there for you—until that person is gone.

> This is why so many people ask: "If we were so miserable together, then why am I so distraught now that she's gone?"
>
> I answer: Whether your relationship was good or bad, losing your partner means losing an invisible security net—your background object.

What Is a Background Object?

When you were little, your background objects were your parents. In infancy, you progressed from needing Mommy in your sight at every minute to a game of peek-a-boo where you tested to see if she would still be there when you reopened your eyes. You squealed with glee to see her magically reappear and smile back at you. You moved from peek-a-boo to more advanced childhood games designed to test the strength of the security ropes to your parents. Once you learned to trust their constancy, you felt secure enough to play at a friend's house for hours and eventually go on overnights knowing that your parents were in the background ready to receive you the next day.

Many of you were not fortunate to have enjoyed secure attachments to your parents.[12] You've described a variety of conditions that led to disconnections in the bond—your parents' depression, alcoholism, illness, or separation, to recount a few we explored in chapter 3.

Many of you describe feeling plagued with insecurity—an anxiety that intrudes into your attempt to find love. The message here is: Don't blame your parents. First of all, remember that parents were children once and had to cope with disruptions and deprivations for which they might well have blamed their parents. This blame game can go all the way back to infinity.

At the age of fourteen my son, Adam, observed me overreact to a minor inconvenience. He became unusually composed and thoughtful. "Mom," he said, studying me closely. "I just realized that adults are just grown-up children."

Parents tend to pass their abandonment wounds along to their children unwittingly,[13] each generation believing they're making life better for their children than they had it.[14]

Another reason to avoid blame is that your symptoms of separation distress—such as insecurity, hypersensitivity to rejection, social inhibition, or lack of confidence—may have nothing to do with your upbringing at all. Even those of you who grew up in idyllically secure families may have developed these tendencies because of your neurobiological makeup, which might even include the size of your locus ceruleus,[15] a structure located deep within your brain. Whether the cause was biological or the family, the result is the same—you feel vulnerable and insecure.

The Ability to Be Alone

The ability to be alone[16]—the task you struggle with most during the Withdrawal stage—is a skill developed in childhood. A popular theory suggests that if you felt safe and secure with your parents, you internalized those feelings and are able to draw on them for strength when you are by yourself. Your ability to be alone enables you to be industrious and productive without anyone's presence or prodding.

Many abandonment survivors of childhood, given their chaotic family systems, did not have an opportunity to internalize that all-important sense of safety, making it much harder to go through the solo flight of heartbreak now. Some of the people writing to abandonment.net report that they balked at going to kindergarten or being left with the babysitter. The beginning of the school year was a battle as teachers pried them away from their mothers. Therapists working with children know that separation anxiety is usually at the heart of a child's difficulty in completing schoolwork independently. As a child, you needed a parent, teacher, friend—someone right nearby—to help you sustain your ability to function. Now that you're going through abandonment, your anxiety about being alone comes back full force, creating a momentary adult regression.

Even the most independent among us succumb to separation anxiety during Withdrawal. Your task is to use the crisis of aloneness to strengthen your ability to be alone—a skill you began to develop, however falteringly, in childhood. It's never too late and, in fact, now is an optimum time to learn how to be your own separate person.

Do you remember situations that made you insecure as a child? Describe.

Who were you most secure with—your mother, father, grandparent? Describe how it felt being with that person.

Did you have difficulty separating from your parents to go to school, sleepovers, or camp? Describe.

Has separation anxiety intruded into your adult life?

What are your insecurities about today?

How do you rate your ability to be alone as an adult?

How does your ability to tolerate being on your own affect your romantic relationships?

What insights help you strengthen this ability?

SWAN LESSON FOUR
Accepting Your Separateness

In the story, the little girl learned an important lesson about being separate. She had been practicing the previous three lessons the swan taught her—finding her center, pushing the bad feelings away, and finding strength in the moment. But she came up against profound grief over losing her parents and once again beseeched the mystical black swan for help.

> *"I don't want to be alone!" she cries.*
> 　*"Being alone can be safe and beautiful, Amanda. You are learning how to make it be."*
> 　*"But I love my daddy and I want him to come and take me."*
> 　*"You don't have to stop loving him or think unkindly of him to discover how to be separate from him."*
> 　*"That doesn't make sense."*

"It means discovering your separate self—the part of you that does not need anyone else in order to experience life in the moment."

"How do I do that?"

"By using your imagination. Are you ready for me to help you pretend?"

The little girl nods.

"Pretend your father is standing over there on the beach and that you are walking in another direction. Keep going as far as you can in your imagination until you can't see him anymore, until you are alone. Exaggerate your separateness by pretending to get as far away as you can. You can even pretend you are the only person on the earth."

The little girl's eyes are closed.

"Imagine being alone and feeling safe inside. Get inside the center of your separateness and experience its reality. Imagine feeling good that you have your own two feet to stand on, that you are a separate person."

The little girl lifts her face. Her eyelids rest gently closed.

"Yes, Amanda, lift your face to the reality of your existence as a separate human being. Accept the reality that you are alone as we are all alone. The sensations of life are for you to experience alone, all for yourself. You are whole all by yourself. When we are able to appreciate our separateness, we become available to the love of others."

Notice that as the little girl accepted her separateness, she lifted her face—a universal gesture people use when recognizing their separateness as a person.

It helps to spend some quiet time each day centering in and appreciating your ability to be separate. Try it now.

Take a break from reading to reflect on your separateness. Close your eyes and lift your face, as the little girl did. Describe your thoughts and feelings.

When was the last time you felt at peace with the world inside and outside of yourself?

What insights help you strengthen your ability to experience life just for yourself?

Accepting the Single Lifestyle

A primary task of abandonment recovery is to strengthen your ability to be a separate person. This is a first step in accepting the reality of your aloneness. Whether you are emotionally or physically alone, it is where you are right now. As you've discovered, protesting it doesn't make it go away and only keeps you stuck in Withdrawal. The idea is to accept that you are alone for now and decide what you can do to make the best of it.

This requires a huge leap—all the way from focusing your energy on what you wish you had to what you do have. And what is that? You have yourself and your determination to benefit from your abandonment experience.

"I admit I'm lonely," says Patrick.[17] "But I'm not in any hurry to go out and meet someone. I'm still processing my separation from my wife of twenty years. I find being alone too important, too precious, too enlivening. I want to make it productive for me and learn all there is to learn about myself—learn how to be with myself so that if I do meet someone later on, I can meet her as a whole person."

Being alone allows you to face yourself. You open yourself to revelations en route to discovering your higher self.

"I'd never been alone before," says Sophia.[18] "After my divorce, I thought I'd die. I lost not only the love of my dreams but my financial security. Alone, dejected, abandoned, rejected, betrayed—could things get any worse? Don't ask. I was forced to move to an apartment that wouldn't take pets. I couldn't find anyone to take my dog and two cats and had to put them down. As bad as that was, I slowly began to see what an opportunity being alone was turning into. I got to realize how precious it was to finally have me. I'm doing for me for the first time in my life and it feels good."

Being along is existing in a very real way. The layers of security provided by your ex are stripped away. There is no relationship to medicate the feelings that have awaited your attention all along.

"All the static and interference coming from the relationship are gone," says Patrick. "It took her moving out before I got clear reception. Now it's just me. My own existence—it's what I have. I get to turn inside and see what I'm really about—the pure me. It is a death and a birth."

Alone, we face ourselves and the reality of our life with extraordinary clarity. According to psychotherapist Peter Yelton:

To find yourself alone not by choice is the only gateway you'll ever have to really knowing yourself. Only when the deep pain is acknowledged can the truly transformative occur. The painful aloneness creating this transformation is conceptually similar to Bill Wilson's writings of psychic displacement, which when it occurs, miraculously transforms the hard-core addict into a recovering person.[19]

Affirm your strength as a separate person and take actions to prove to yourself that you can stand on your own two feet. Who are you impressing with this transformation? Yourself.

Check all that apply.

BEING ALONE CHALLENGES ME TO . . .

❏ Discover more about myself.
❏ Take a personal inventory of my likes and dislikes, strengths and weaknesses, goals and aspirations.
❏ Learn to connect to my emotional self.
❏ Reorder my priorities.
❏ Restore my emotional reserves.
❏ Discover my very own personal rhythm of life.
❏ Develop new interests.
❏ Question the complacency of my former life.
❏ Celebrate my newly gained emotional independence.

More and more people elect to be single. Over the centuries, people have chosen solitary lifestyles and have explored the virtues of celibacy, hermitage, and vows of silence. I'm not suggesting that you become a hermit, only that these extreme measures hint at the existence of hidden rewards to being alone. Direct your curiosity to the benefits.

Don't let your control issues stop you from discovering the advantages of singleness. Use your willfulness to gain from your aloneness rather than waste your energy protesting it. The idea is to put your situation in a new frame, a perspective broad enough to help you entertain the Power of Possibility. Reframe your reality so that you can maximize the hidden benefits of being on your own.

Here is a thought experiment: A thought experiment is different from a statement of fact. You don't have to believe it is true. It asks that you suspend your rational judgment to consider a proposition designed to help you gain a new perspective. Consider that your abandonment has placed you exactly where you need to be to work on what you need to work on.

What comes to mind as something that's been sabotaging your success and has long needed re-solving?

Having written your first thoughts, give it a little more time.

Refine your idea and finish this sentence: *I am dealing with the challenge of being alone right now because I've needed to work on…*

Now that you have no one to answer to and can do what you want, name three things on your wish list of desires.

1.
2.
3.

Overcoming the Stigma of Being Alone

One of the challenges facing single people is society's tendency to attach a negative connotation to being alone. Look at the terms we gave single women in the past: old maid, barren, maiden aunt, spinster. Due to societal double standards, there aren't any equivalent stigmatizing terms for men. Fortunately, we've dispensed with these terms, but to some extent the stigma remains for both genders. Single moms and dads, as well as others who are divorced, report that they feel societal disregard for their special circumstances. As most of us have come to know, being alone is a position not to be scorned or pitied but honored.

> "I am alone and glad to be," says Janet. "Nobody but me seems willing to understand. I consider it a positive lifestyle choice, but my friends are always trying to get me to hook up with someone. Living alone makes me comfortable. It's a condition I can control. I'm not depending on somebody who could wind up leaving me in the end. Besides, I enjoy my own company."

Many people are thriving without a significant other. It is time to elevate the status of the single life that has so many participants—both willing and unwilling. Whatever challenges single people may face, being alone needs to be understood for what it truly is—a legitimate, rewarding lifestyle that requires personal strength and integrity.

"I love being on my own," says Stephan. "The drawbacks are mostly practical. I don't get to pool my paycheck with anyone or split the rent, and it's hard to dig up someone to go with me on vacation. But I like being able to pursue my career full steam ahead without having to answer to anyone."

"I like the chance to build up my independence," says Martha. "After being hurt, I vowed never to put myself in that position again, at least for a long time. It's been an adventure—being out there in the world and belonging only to myself, taking care of myself."

Unfortunately, though, rather than being seen as a lifestyle of choice, being alone is sometimes viewed as the "default style."

"I love being alone," says Steve, "but when I look at myself through the eyes of society, I appear to be deficient in some way. Being alone just isn't valued. My family worries about me, and my friends feel it's a pity to be alone. But I feel good about my single existence. I am a walking triumph of human spirit."

We should admire the courage, determination, and grit of those who succeed at living alone. Whether you chose it or it chose you, it is anything but a situation to be pitied.

"I'm the only one of my friends who isn't in a relationship," says Roland. "Undoubtedly they have it much easier. They have the security of a family wrapped around them, while I have to reinvent my life every weekend. I plan my time carefully to make sure I feel fulfilled rather than let myself get depressed and lonesome. My lifestyle is not for the faint of heart. Some weekends I feel I'm performing at gold medal levels, but it's always a gratifying achievement."

Granted, from a practical point of view, being alone often requires greater effort than being in a relationship, because everything has to come from your own initiative. It has to be something you're motivated to do all by yourself, as the next example shows.

"There was a Giacometti show at the Museum of Modern Art," says Jackie. "All of my friends were busy, and I just couldn't get up the oomph to go alone. Finally I dragged myself out the door and wound up having a self-welcoming party at the exhibit. I felt like a million dollars for this small accomplishment, like I'd climbed Mount Everest."

The time is overdue for friends, family, and society to acknowledge the special difficulties you're facing and give the credit you deserve, as well as a vote of confidence.

"I'm alone," says Seth, "but I'd love to find somebody. I don't know what I do wrong to scare people away, and that makes it hard. But I know there's a positive side to it. I am living more intensely and

consciously than any of my friends in relationships. I don't take any feelings for granted, or life itself, for that matter. I know that every day is a test of fire and I come out each time more alive. Here I am, just me and prevailing in grand style."

Living alone may not be the lifestyle you've chosen, but it's one you face on a daily basis, at least for now. The key is to stop protesting your current situation. Turn the energy around by choosing rather than railing against your present reality.

 ## HONORING THE CHALLENGES OF SINGLE LIFE

Place a check mark next to the statements you agree with.

- ❏ Solitude is a time for personal reflection.
- ❏ It's all right to be single; it's a viable lifestyle, as well as an alternative lifestyle.
- ❏ Abandonment stigmatizes being alone—the stigma of being dumped.
- ❏ It takes courage to be on my own.
- ❏ Many choose to be alone for spiritual gain.
- ❏ Being alone increases self-awareness.
- ❏ Society has a strong bias in favor of couplehood: it's primarily a couple's world.
- ❏ Many of the benefits of being alone are subtle and go over the heads of those who are in relationships.
- ❏ People gain depth and character from being alone.
- ❏ Some consider individuals without a relationship to be incomplete. I'm pitied, feared, considered less-than—everything but admired.
- ❏ Singleness is an accomplishment because it is so challenging.
- ❏ People who live alone survive by developing personal strengths. It builds self-reliance.
- ❏ People alone don't want pity. They want respect and acknowledgment.
- ❏ Being alone is a condition waiting to be transformed into a positive experience.

Q

Name something of your own to honor about surviving the single style.

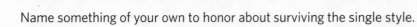

How the Ability to Be Alone Affects Adult Relationships

Your ability to be your own separate person is critical to sustaining a long-term adult relationship.

At the beginning, you can't stand to be apart from your partner. As you enter the courtship period, you do a lot of testing, even when you're not aware of it. You play adult forms of peek-a-boo to determine your partner's staying power. As you both prove your ability to commit, a sense of security sets in.

You break out of the symbiotic phase of the relationship and interact as separate individuals because you're becoming securely attached. Longevity allows you to count on each other for moral support even when you're not physically together. You go about your independent lives feeling you have each other in the background.

The more secure you feel in your ability to be separate, the fewer demands you put on the relationship. The more stable the relationship, the less direct contact you need from your partner to reinvoke the emotional connection. As with children, who need to be securely attached in order to be alone, the surer you are of your partner, the more secure you feel when you're off doing your own thing.

Taking Your Security for Granted

It is often found to be problematic for people to take each other for granted. Yet this is one of the luxuries of a long-term relationship. Contrary to what some people believe, feeling secure with your background object facilitates not dependence, but independence. You make independent strides precisely because you're able to use your partner as a background object. Your ability to be alone grows from the security of knowing that he or she is safely tucked away in your hip pocket.

Just as you are sustained by the air you breathe without being conscious of each breath, you are sustained by the security you receive from having a background object. Your mate provides an invisible security blanket.

Taking your mate for granted is not without a few dangers, however. One, you become careless and risk the relationship through damaging behaviors—such as having affairs, becoming overbearing, shutting down emotionally or sexually, or withholding affection or validation, to name a few ways of sabotaging a long-term relationship. When the relationship is over, you discover too late how important that person was in your life. Many people search the ends of the earth to regain that sense of security.

Two, by taking your mate for granted, you are completely unprepared for the shock and devastation in the event of abandonment. You counted on your partner to be there till death do us part. If he or she leaves you (often for someone else), you are riddled with disbelief and bewilderment. Your whole belief system is shaken to the core, your self-confidence demolished.

Remember Lynne's feelings after her husband started seeing someone else? Her sense of security was threatened because she could no longer count on him being there—in the background.

"I hadn't wanted any part of him for over ten years. But when he began a new relationship, I felt a big hole in my life."

It is common for people in long-term relationships to boast about their independence, unaware of how much extra security they are gaining just from having a background object. Even when they're dissatisfied with their mates, they garner many benefits by having someone to belong to, someone who represents "home" to them.

"Ned and I didn't have much of a relationship, but his being there kept the boogeyman away. Now that he's gone, I wake up daily to that queasy feeling of knowing I'm alone in the world. I feel so unprotected."

Since the support is invisible, many fail to acknowledge the degree to which their independence is enhanced by that safety net. Often it is those who have background objects who remain oblivious to the challenges facing those who don't.

"My friend Alice can't understand why I just don't want to go into the city to see Broadway shows by myself," says Roberta. "She's always saying, 'Why not! I'm completely independent of my hus-band. I go in alone all the time to go shopping. It's no big deal.' Meanwhile, she has no idea who she's talking to here. I'm the one who went off to Europe by myself last summer. At night in Paris, I'd think about how I had nobody to come home to at the end of my trip—nobody who really cared if I ever returned. It got pretty lonely in those hotels night after night."

During the Withdrawal stage, most of you experience what it's like to exist without your back-ground object. You're coping with feeling emotionally deprived—a feeling your coupled friends are hard put to understand. Be assured that this isolation, desolation, and despair are temporary. Living without a background object is a challenge. Your task is to learn how to subsist emotionally without relying on this invisible support. You can do so because you are an adult who can replenish this security through your own resources. You can acquire emotional self-reliance.

Take a moment to review the resolutions we made in chapter 1.

- ❏ I am an able-bodied adult.
- ❏ I can stand on my own two feet.
- ❏ I can survive on my own.
- ❏ I can turn my life in a positive direction.

Cautions

Before we close this chapter, some words of caution.

Rewounding

When adjusting to being alone, people are particularly vulnerable to being rewounded.

Rewounding is a term I use to describe an emotional relapse that can happen when you have contact with your former partner. Since closure usually remains unresolved during the Withdrawal stage, bumping into your ex can stir up a tumult of feelings and elevate your hopes once again. When the meeting ends with your relationship still torn, you feel reabandoned. This rewounding often feels more devastating than the initial tear.[20]

> People ask me: "Why does it seem to hurt worse each time?"
>
> I answer: Imagine how painful it would be if you had a physical wound and someone bumped into the tender sore just as it started to mend. *Ouch.*

A truly painful variation of rewounding is when you've already been through a serious separation or divorce, and now you've tried for a new relationship and once again failed. Now you're going through reabandonment with a *new* former partner.

People tell me frequently, "This time I did it right and still wound up alone."

You thought you'd found a truly sensitive person this time, someone who listened to your feelings, affectionate, a good parent to his or her children, a good communicator—a good person altogether. And you handled your end of the relationship correctly, too—you were nurturing, listened to her needs and feelings, carefully avoided dumping your own emotional needs on her. You were independent, maintained your own interests, practiced the healthiest relationship skills you could imagine. Yet in spite of the idyllic relationship, your partner pulled away, saying, "I just don't have feelings for you anymore." Or "I'm going to try it one more time with my ex." Or "I just need space to figure out who I am. Sorry, but I need to go." Or how about the fatal, "Let's just be friends."

Now you feel you've been robbed of all control. You'd already done everything within your power and still wound up enduring your own worst abandonment nightmare—the loss of love. You feel condemned to eternal loneliness.

The obvious response to this supremely painful situation is that there are never guarantees in life. Things like this can happen even when you function optimally.[21] You have no control over another person. You can only control your behavior. The key is to accept the transient nature of all things in life and move on.[22]

The other answer is that even though you may have done it right this time, there is still a powerful lesson to learn from the experience, one more change you need to make to stabilize your life and fulfill your dreams. You need to dig deeper, bear down, and give birth to the ultimate personal truth. Then you need to follow through with new behaviors—ones you may never have taken before—behaviors we'll be learning about as we continue our journey.

Health Risks

Being alone can put you at risk for both physical and emotional illnesses. According to research, people living alone with limited social support are more prone to heart attacks and illnesses related to lowered immune response such as cancer.[23] Rates are high for depression—often characterized by elevated levels of stress hormones that may be triggered by fears and anxiety attendant to being alone.

While adjusting to being alone, you can mitigate the impact by reaching out to friends who can provide life-sustaining support. Human touch exchanged between friends and provided through contact sports, physical exams, professional masseuses, or affectionate family members stimulate dopamine and serotonin, for example, which help mitigate separation distress. Abandonment support groups* can also help you out by allowing you to connect with others going through what you are going through.

As you work your way through the remaining chapters, you'll gain the awareness and tools you need to succeed in your next relationship as well as strengthen your emotional independence. Your future happiness does not have to depend on any one person—other than you.

Remember the thought experiment: Your life is exactly where it needs to be to work on what you need to work on.

More Food for Thought

Did anyone come along at a significant time in your growing up and save your life or make a difference? Was it a teacher? Aunt? Friend's parent? Peer? Stranger? Parent?

Did you let their positive message in? Were you able to internalize it? What positive message is it sending you today? How is it helping you?

---

*   For directions for setting up support groups, see Appendix A.

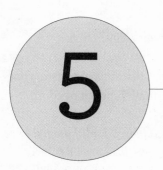

Beholding the Importance of Your Existence

"The heartbreak is endless."

We are by no means done discussing the Withdrawal stage, although I know millions would like to be done with the feelings.

"Finding myself alone after all those years together is tough enough," says Bonnie, *"but I can't take the aching and sorrow anymore. Will I ever get through this?"*

I want you to walk away after reading this chapter understanding what the feelings of Withdrawal are all about, where they come from, and what to do about them. Your primal emotions have great value once you know how to use them as healing tools. They empower you to make internal connections and take back control of your life.

This chapter focuses on a universal conflict that has remained unresolved throughout human history—a battle between two realms—emotional and intellectual. It's all too familiar, you've heard it a thousand times: "Intellectually I know this person is no good for me, but emotionally I can't let go."

The conflict between what we know and how we feel has been raging within the human psyche since time immemorial.

"For me the conflict doesn't just rage," says Keaton, *"it foams at the mouth, turns inside out and upside down, pulls me in two, and spews contradictions at me. I go back and forth between begging Gabby to come back and telling her she's the worst thing that ever happened to me and to stay away."*

The disparity between the emotional and intellectual isn't a problem in itself. The two realms can co-exist peacefully:

"I still have feelings for Marco, but this time I'm looking to find someone who's available—not married."

It's what you do with your feelings that poses the problem:

"I know that being with Jennifer brings me down, but I'm hooked. I can't stay away from her."

It is a common problem—finding yourself compelled to act out emotions that run contrary to your best interests. When you succumb to the dictates of runaway emotions, your life spins out of control.

"I started seeing this guy last year," says Jayne, "but didn't find out he was married until months later. He told me he was separated, but now I no longer believe that. I've seen them together. He's lied so many times." Jayne's face is drenched in anguish. She speaks empathically, the pain palatable to her group mates. "My head knows that I need to break it off with this guy, because it's destroying me, but my heart keeps driving me back to him. Look at me," she implores, "I'm nowhere near the person I used to be. But I have such intense feelings for him and I can't end it. My whole life revolves around when I'll get to see him again. Our lovemaking is the most passionate and intense I've ever felt. I feel like an addict."

Jayne's involvement in this relationship has become abandoholic—that is, she is drawn to the high-stakes drama of unrequited love, addicted to the neurochemistry of an emotionally dangerous liaison. This chapter is going to help you understand the compelling emotions driving your romantic addictions. You will gain insight and determination to help you overcome your cycles of abandonment. Your goal is to operate from your reason, judgment, and wisdom, and to strengthen your adult self.

Another way the discrepancy between what you feel and what you know becomes a problem is that it keeps you pining away for someone who hurt you; you're stuck in the craving of Withdrawal.

"We weren't right for each other, anyone could see that," says Marshall, "but it's been over a year and I think about her all the time and long for her to come back."

The ongoing conflict between emotion and reason drains your energy, confuses your mind, and undermines your ability to move forward.

"On one hand," says Phillip, "I believe from the bottom of my heart that Amy and I will be together again. On the other, I know she's gone for good and that even if she did come back, I could never trust her again."

Throughout our lives we've been faced with the dichotomy between what we want and what is good for us. A lot of the time, we are able to act according to our better judgment, but during Withdrawal, heartbreak's tug-of-war pulls us especially hard in the direction of clinging to our lost love. Consider this conflict in light of your own abandonment scenario and write both sides of this emotional seesaw.

Truth Nugget: Intellectually, I know _____ ,
but emotionally, I feel _____ .

How does having a heart-mind dichotomy affect the overall quality of your life?

How does giving vent to the emotional side affect your behavior?

What does it do to your self-esteem?

What strengths and insights can you use to resolve this conflict?

How Does This Dichotomy Set In?

The brain is my second favorite organ. —Woody Allen

One of the differences between human beings and the rest of the animal kingdom is that we are endowed with a highly specialized cerebral cortex—one that, during times of distress, tries to make sense of overpowering emotions. When it comes to heartbreak, this sense is usually nonsense. The most prevalent false conclusion it draws is the notion that your ex belongs on a pedestal for abandoning you.

> *"I never loved or appreciated Barbara more until after she left."*

Confused by your overwhelming sense of loss, your mind creates makeshift theories to explain why you feel so bereft and concludes that your former partner must have been special.[1] Why else would you feel incessant longing and yearning? Believing in your ex's preeminence is at your own expense, because it causes you to give all of your power to your abandoner. We don't conjure up these overblown sentiments about our ex's worth intentionally or consciously. Our illustrious human brain does it for us.

Thoughts and Counterthoughts

In discussing the dichotomy between thought and emotion, I'm not trying to weigh in on either side of the debate between cognitive behavioral and psychodynamic models of psychology.[2] It is clear that beliefs and assumptions can instigate feelings and that feelings likewise can color beliefs and assumptions. There are neuron bundles leading from the cerebral cortex to the amygdala and back again.[3] Its circuitry is a feedback loop, so it is useless to make a "which came first, the chicken or the egg" determination in every case.

The two worlds—one driven by emotion and the other by rational judgment—are inexorably intertwined, each realm competing for attention, each one seemingly valid: "He is special. He is not right for me."

> *"Gabby is the worst person I ever met and a rare gem of infinite quality," claims Keaton. "I can build a case for either side, becoming both prosecutor and defense of my own love life."*

These co-existing thought worlds become internalized over time and lead to lingering ambivalence toward a heartbreaker. We retain certain special feelings for the person who left us, no matter how hard we resist it and no matter how angry we remain. The fact that an episode of unrequited love can haunt our future is one of the most common posttraumatic stress symptoms of abandonment.*

CAUSES FOR POSTTRAMATIC STRESS DISORDER OF ABANDONMENT

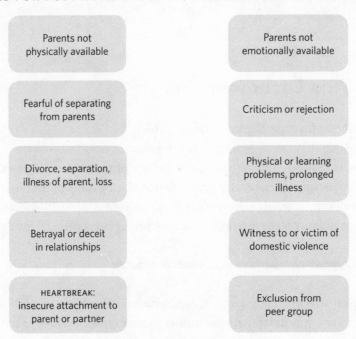

Parents not physically available	Parents not emotionally available
Fearful of separating from parents	Criticism or rejection
Divorce, separation, illness of parent, loss	Physical or learning problems, prolonged illness
Betrayal or deceit in relationships	Witness to or victim of domestic violence
HEARTBREAK: insecure attachment to parent or partner	Exclusion from peer group

---

*   Posttraumatic stress disorder of abandonment is explored in depth in my *The Journey from Abandonment to Healing* (pp. 42–44).

"I still think about my old boyfriend sometimes," says Jeannette. "He was the first to break my heart—all the way back in high school. He was a really lovable guy. When I'm lonely, I feel like calling him."

Fortunately, over time, these idealized notions about your ex integrate with new experiences you've accrued to lessen the heartache (heartache being another symptom of abandonment's posttrauma stress), allowing this idealization to move into the background of awareness. Tucked away somewhere, though, most of us still carry a torch for an old flame.

Does someone still hold a special place in your memory? Who?

What special feelings does this old heartthrob evoke?

Who broke up with whom? Who got hurt the most?

Do you feel it's possible that this old heartbreak contributed in any way to your current insecurity? How?

What insights can you use to put to rest any false conclusions you may have drawn?

The primary task during Withdrawal is to use the resources of your cognitive mind to question the assumptions you've made about your abandoner—especially the ones that hold him or her irreplaceable and omnipotent.

The Scourge of Rejection

Many of you reading this book are struggling with the scorching pain of rejection.

"I felt like I'd been thrown away like yesterday's trash," says Marie. "All the love I had to give to him was worthless. He didn't want me anymore, so I figured I was worthless."

Being rejected by someone you love engenders deep, painful feelings of regret, inadequacy, and self-hatred, causing us to turn the anger we feel toward our partner against ourself. This leads to the unbearable depression that accompanies a loss of love. In chapter 6, we will discuss how this self-anger injures your self-esteem and interferes in relationships, and you'll learn what to do about it.

Being Blamed for the Breakup

I receive e-mails from people all over the world telling me how their abandoners blamed them for the breakup, causing them to feel bewildered, devastated, and demoralized. In most cases, this blame was the ex's way to justify breaking up. Your ex came up with all sorts of plausible-sounding excuses, enumerating ways in which *you* were at fault. It was because *you* were unacceptable. The abandoner is trying to pass responsibility for his actions on to *you*. Being left hurts enough, but being blamed for it adds insult to injury. In spite of this abusive treatment, abandonment survivors continue to put their abandoners on pedestals, accepting the blame as evidence of their own unworthiness.

The idealization of the departed is universal to all forms of human grief.[4] We memorialize the dead, for instance. But paradoxically, when loss involves rejection and blame, we have an even greater tendency to elevate our lovers above ourselves, try as we might to fight it.

"I refuse to believe that someone who acted like such a cad could be so all-mighty special."

Despite our protests, the abandoner usually gets to walk away wearing a lot of our esteem.

Power of Example: Mine

Like millions of other abandonment survivors, six months into my abandonment and knee-deep in Withdrawal, I believed that my mate was extraordinarily unique and supremely special. In spite of all of my years observing my clients idealize their abandoners, I felt that losing my beloved partner of twenty years meant losing the centerpiece of my own worth.

This belief intensified my torment. The well-trained therapist in me knew what I had to do to improve my emotional lot. I had to fight the idealization.

At first my burning-with-love feelings for my partner outweighed all of my attempts to debunk the myth of his preeminence. Withdrawal was pulling me into its quicksand, and I struggled to withstand the pull. I knew my options were: either grab the rope with a tenacious grip or sink into an emotional quagmire of self-debasement.

I found writing to be my lifeline. Pen in hand, I felt empowered to undo the apotheosis of my beloved. My task was nothing short of falling out of love with someone I'd been madly in love with for twenty years. Writing kept me focused. How else could I expect to mitigate the excruciating pain of being left by him? I attempted to prove the pen mightier than the sword in my heart.[5]

I worked long into many sleepless nights trying to convince myself that he wasn't so special after all, that there were always signs of weakness. I enumerated all of the ways in which he now showed himself to be flawed. If he could abandon me without justification or warning, I reasoned, then he was not worthy of me.

To take him down from his pedestal and elevate myself, I told myself that I would never have done this to him (whether it was true or not), that I cared too much about him as a human being to put my own selfish pleasures ahead of his happiness. Sure, I'd been attracted to other men from time to time and could have gone off chasing after someone new—but I didn't. Why, I queried myself, was I climbing onto a high horse? I was a better person, that's why. I would never have left him alone in the woods, like he'd done to me, I insisted. I didn't respect or trust him anymore and never should have, I wrote determinedly: Good Riddance.

My pain eased up somewhat while I was directly engaged in the act of writing. But as soon as I put down my pen, the grief rushed back in and I found myself once again treading water in oceans of hero worship and desolation. Over time, though, with persistence and skill, my writing campaign gradually helped me temper the notion of his being the one and only. I evaluated his merits more realistically.

"He doesn't mean to hurt you, Mom," said my level-headed daughter, Erika, whose sagacity always catches me up short, "even though it does hurt. It's just where he's at in his life for now."

Over time, I began to see him—the love of my life—as just an ordinary person with strengths and weaknesses, who in leaving me for a new love, was only doing what came naturally to him at the time, given whatever needs, lapses in judgment, and human weaknesses he might have. Gaining a more temperate view helped lessen the hurt and longing of Withdrawal enough to dismount from my high horse of self-proclaimed virtue. What I was left with was an ability to survive as a separate person. Thus I acquired a more balanced perspective about what the real issues were in my life and how to channel my emotions productively.

To help you begin this process for yourself, try naming five positive qualities about your abandoner.

1.
2.
3.
4.
5.

Name five positive qualities about yourself.

1.
2.
3.
4.
5.

Lifting the veil of idealization, use this space to describe your ex in more realistic terms—ordinary rather than special, with human faults, lackings, inadequacies, and shortcomings, just like the rest of us.

Make a statement elevating yourself rather than your abandoner.

 Swirling through Withdrawal

The tools of abandonment recovery are designed to reverse this universal tendency toward idealizing the person who broke your heart. Without recovery, people can remain stuck in Withdrawal, indefinitely at loss of their power and self-esteem.

"I refuse to believe he's left me for someone else, that it could possibly be over," says Alicia. "I know I'll love him always and that we were meant to be together. He's the purpose of my life, the only man I'll ever love. My life is meaningless without him."

SCIENTIFIC TIDBIT

Endorphins are known to be released during a runner's high. *Endorphin,* a contraction for *endogenous* and *morphine,* is a class of morphine-like drugs manufactured within the body and thought to be responsible for runner's high and addiction to exercise.

Alicia feels miserable not because her abandoner was special but because extreme discomfort is part of our biological response to breaking an attachment. Abandonment arouses the most primal of instincts—namely, our powerful mammalian instinct to bond. When the drive toward attachment is thwarted, we go through withdrawal symptoms—whether the object of that attachment was a wonderful person or a scoundrel.

Why Do We Have So Much Trouble Letting Go When Someone Leaves Us?

The mammalian brain perceives abandonment as a threat to your existence. The mammal in us is the mouse, elephant, and chimpanzee—the part that thrives on sleeping in proximity to others, touch, cuddling, pairing off, procreating, the warmth of skin-to-skin contact, the safety of connection.

It's the mammal in us that holds attachment.[6]

When your primary attachment is severed, this internal mammal declares a state of psychobiological emergency. Led by your ever-vigilant captain—your amygdala—it throws your nervous system into red alert.

When you are in love withdrawal, your symptoms are as intense as they would be from heroin withdrawal. You are withdrawing from the companionship, security, and sense of belonging you have grown accustomed to. At the neurobiological level, relationships are addictions.[7] When you're bonded to someone, your body produces its own powerful opioid drugs, including endorphins, to which you become addicted—nature's way of promoting procreation. When you are going through separation, your body's production of these powerful, addictive drugs decreases, sending you into opioid withdrawal, which some researchers claim is equivalent to eight milligrams of morphine withdrawal.[8]

> *"I was so strung out and exhausted from thinking about Lonny, listening for his car to roll into the driveway, and imagining his face in every face in the crowd," says Marie, "that if you saw me, you'd think I was having the DTs."*

When you're in the craving, nagging, and yearning of opioid withdrawal, your mammalian brain goes on a search-and-recovery mission. The surges of stress hormones keep your mind hypervigilant, searching for any sign of her approach. This waiting, searching state is universal to all kinds of grief. John Bowlby, pioneer in separation and attachment, called it "searching for the lost object."[9] Your emotional brain automatically scans your inner and outer worlds, seeking a love object it perceives as tantamount to your survival.

> *"I just couldn't stop thinking about every last thing Lonny said to me," says Marie, "going through date books and photographs looking for a clue as to why he stopped loving me. I'd drive by his work all the time, hoping to at least catch a glimpse of his car, just so I'd know where he was."*

Consciously you know your mate is out of reach, but try telling your mammalian brain to accept this fact! Your amygdala relentlessly keeps seeking the object of your obsession.

> *"I'd be ruminating one minute," says Keaton, "hating her the next, and craving a love fix the next."*

These are all symptoms of the Withdrawal stage. But why, people ask, do we want our lovers so badly after they've behaved so poorly?

The explanation lies in the special functioning of that ever-vigilant amygdala. Lovers who reject us become powerful figures to the emotional brain. Abandoners become powerful simply because they inflicted so much pain by leaving us. Pain invokes fear. Fear initiates an amygdala-driven response. Fear

THE MAMMALIAN BRAIN

Your mammalian brain perceives your abandoner as a lifeline as well as a potential procreative partner. Whether you're gay, lesbian, straight, planning to have children, or beyond your reproductive years, your mammalian brain deals in approximations and fails to notice the difference. It just notices that your partner has abandoned the bond, and so it declares a state of emergency, signaling your nervous system to release stress hormones as if faced with a life-and-death battle.

You remain obsessed with this now supercharged figure—your abandoner. Your nervous system is primed for action indefinitely. You interpret this ongoing reactivity as proof of his romantic omnipotence.

leaves its indelible imprint in your amygdala, conditioning you to react to your abandoner, as if he or she were a grizzly bear.

Research on the amygdala shows that fear incubates over time.[10] This explains why you can have an ever-more-powerful response each time you encounter your heartbreaker. Sometimes this response can last for decades.

"It had been twenty-five years since I'd laid eyes on my greatest heartbreaker, Beth. It caught me by surprise. I walked into a luncheonette, and she was walking out with some guy. You'd think we just broke up. I reacted as if I'd just seen a ghost."

This ongoing emotional arousal confuses you into thinking that if your feelings can last this long and feel so strong, your ex must have been omnipotent and indispensable. This perception, of course, is false. In truth, you can carry a torch for an old flame who had nothing at all special to offer you—except a lot of heartache.

When you've had an especially painful breakup, just thinking about your ex or spotting her in the crowd can cause your heart to skip a beat, your stomach to flip flop, and old desires to reawaken. If you see him with a new lover, you can go into apoplexy. But these are all just signs of your mammalian brain trying either to entice you back into the procreative bond or to warn you not to make the same mistake again—to avoid grizzly bears and people who cause intense fear or pain.

"I thought I was going to die when my lover left," says William. "My heart was bursting with love for him every minute of the day. A year later, I still missed him terribly. I believed I could never care about anyone else, that he was perfect for me—my exact love match. It wasn't until I got into a new relationship that I realized that my ex was just an average person, ordinary, in fact, inadequate as a partner for me."

Take a moment to reflect on how you think your mammalian brain reacts to your abandoner.

Check all that apply.

MY ABANDONER IS…

❏ Special
❏ Irreplaceable

- ❏ Indispensable
- ❏ The one and only
- ❏ A cad
- ❏ A jerk
- ❏ Well intentioned
- ❏ Confused
- ❏ Making the biggest mistake of her life
- ❏ Having a midlife crisis
- ❏ Being a bastard
- ❏ A cheat
- ❏ Justified in leaving me
- ❏ Unjustified
- ❏ A liar

Vicky combined these terms this way:

"My abandoner is obviously having a midlife crisis, but I can't help feeling he's irreplaceable, even though the more reasonable part of my mind tells me he's a cad."

Use the space below to express the dichotomy of thought and emotion you hold for your abandoner.

Deidealizing the Wounder

Once you understand where the yearning and aching of Withdrawal come from, you don't have to give credence to the idea that your abandoner is special. You can accept the discomfort for what it is—not as proof of how irreplaceable your ex was but as part and parcel of what it feels like to separate from a human attachment.

If you've been abandoned, betrayed, criticized, or blamed for the breakup, all the more reason to take your ex off the pedestal. Reinterpret your Withdrawal symptoms to salvage your self-worth. It takes knowledge and self-discipline to dispose of your makeshift theories about your abandoner's preeminence. The anguish of unrequited love necessitates this work. What work? The work of deconstructing the myth of your abandoner's specialness.

As you continue through this chapter, you will gain information to empower you to accomplish this task. You will learn how to throw your weight to the side of the equation where your better judgment resides and take back control of your life.

> *"After careful consideration, it occurred to me that Phil was a serial abandoner. He belonged on the ten-most-wanted list. I had to get on with my life and learn from this mistake."*

Use the space below to dememorialize your abandoner. How did your abandoner contribute to the breakup?

What were the warning signs about your abandoner? Were they there in the beginning?

What red flags emerged during the relationship?

Describe your abandoner's behavior during your breakup.

Does your ex fit the profile of an abandoner?*

---

*   The Profile of an Abandoner is posted on abandonment.net. Click on the tab for ABANDONMENT HELP, and then find the button for PROFILE OF ABANDONER on the pinwheel. Please click on CONTACT US to tell us about your abandoner. By pooling everyone's insights, we continue to refine the profile.

The Mind-Body Connection

The more information you have, the better able you are to get a grip on your life. Yes, you feel strung out; but, no, it is not because your ex is irreplaceable and omnipotent. These feelings are just part of going through Withdrawal. Making the mind-body connection helps you reclaim territory lost to the emotional side of the feeling-thought dichotomy and debunk the myth of your abandoner's specialness.

Check the Withdrawal symptoms you've encountered.

❏ I'm obsessed with my ex because norepinephrine (NE), one of my stress hormones, continues to flood my body and brain, causing my attention to stay riveted on the threat at hand—my abandoner.

This is your emotional brain's way of keeping you on task and constantly attentive, enhancing your battle performance.

❏ I have the desire to seduce my abandoner back into my bed.

Remember those Four Fs of Survival? It's that fourth F again. Your body is nudging you in this direction because it is programmed to reestablish your procreative bond. Don't forget, you're in opioid withdrawal. Your body is nudging you to replace some of the missing endorphins it's craving,[11] as well as other hormones and chemicals such as oxytocin,[12] that facilitate sexual reproduction and attachment.

❏ I have a tendency to overtalk about my breakup. I don't mean to go into the details of the story, but I can't seem to cut to the chase.

This is because, as we discussed in chapter 3, each time you revisit the crisis, another stress hormone, adrenaline (also known as epinephrine) is released, causing you to go overboard into a blow-by-blow recounting of the traumatic event. (This is what Truth Nuggets are designed to help you recover from.)

❏ Old familiar feelings of despair, neediness, and panic emerge.

Your crisis triggers emotional memories stored in your amygdala, memories that are reminiscent of your earlier heartbreaks and disconnections. Being equipped with past and present emotional knowledge is your emotional brain's way of enabling your mind to benefit from former experience to aid your self-defense campaign.

❏ I imagine I see him whizzing by in a car or in the faces of the crowd.

When a visual image first hits the eye, the information gives but an approximate impression. To get more detailed information, the sensory input must travel through five synapses as it passes from the back of your brain before it gets to your cerebral frontal cortex. This takes additional seconds before you can appraise the situation more accurately.[13]

❏ I am preoccupied with the relationship—I look at old photos, contact people who knew me and my ex together, and incessantly go over the details of the separation.

The surging stress hormones and depleted opioids cause you to automatically search for the lost object.[14]

❏ I have an impulse to stalk my abandoner. I drive by her house or call his phone incessantly.

Two reasons: (1) because your mammalian brain is bent on its search-and-recovery mission, gearing you to closely hunt the threat at hand, and (2) the decrease in opioids instigates you to look for a fix.

❏ Two to three weeks into my crisis I came down with a cold.

Because energy normally deployed to your immune function is now being diverted to aid your exercise muscles to fight or flee your enemy. (Why waste energy fighting a cold when you're being chased by a lion?) This immune suppression takes a few weeks to manifest into a cold or flu, longer for more serious illness.

❏ I am given to bouts of anger.

Because your emotional brain primes you for the fight response of the Four Fs of Survival.

❏ I feel uncomfortable in my own skin, agitated, queasy, edgy.

The energy usually deployed to aid in digestion and other bodily functions diverts to your exercise muscles to promote action and enhance your ability for fight or flight.

❏ My usual arthritic aches and pains disappear during the worst of it.

This is because of the suppression of your immune system, which has now refrained from sending its usual supply of fluid nutrients. This decreases the swelling around your old injuries, reducing some of your old chronic pains.

❑ Conversely, when I'm not in severe crisis, my aches and pains return.

Because your immune system kicks back into its usual peace-time regimen, once again, deploying fluids to the injured areas to create nutritive, albeit painful, swellings.

❑ I remain exhausted, drained, strung out for months.

You are fighting an intense, ongoing internal battle.

> *"I thought I had some dread disease,"* says Roberta, *"but it was just the long, drawn-out torment I was going through, obsessing over my lost love, missing him."*

Preparing to Overcome: Beyond Withdrawal

Making a mind-body connection is more than just an intellectual exercise. Gathering scientific information empowers you to strengthen your cognitive mind, but it doesn't help all by itself. You have to integrate this information with what is going on inside. It's important to absorb the fact that idealizing your abandoner is an idea not based on your wisdom but driven by your biological instincts. Believing she is the one and only comes from an ill-informed place, written by the blunt instrument of your mammalian brain. Remind yourself that obsessing about him is not because he is irreplaceable but because your mammalian brain has you searching for its lost object.

Accept your emotions for what they are—feelings, not facts. Use your adult cognitive mind to rise above your biological instincts and take yourself in hand.

Use this space to make a balanced statement about your ex. Be sure to lead with your adult wisdom, keeping your mammalian brain in check.

SWAN LESSON FIVE

Beholding the Importance of Your Existence

How to overcome the tendency to idealize someone who has left you is illustrated in the story of the little girl. She had been working on accepting her separateness, even while she cherished and longed for her parents. One day, she accused the swan of not understanding her pain. He pulled back in the water and opened his wings.

"I too have longed for someone's return," says the swan. "I too have known a wounder. Like you, I thought I could not live without her. I yearned for her to comfort me from the very wound she inflicted. But she could never be the one to comfort me. The wounder never can."

"Who was your wounder?" asks the little girl.

"Swans mate for life, Amanda. You will notice I am alone. But I have survived the wounding and so must you."

"Tell me more about her," begs the little girl.

"She, like all abandoners, became powerful just by wounding me so deeply. She brought me to a feeling of insignificance and pain. And all I could do was marvel at her power to accomplish so mighty a task. Pain creates fear, and we give power to those we fear. Reduced to helplessness, I saw my wounder as the more powerful, the more valuable, the more beautiful for having vanquished me. I could only worship my wounder," admits the swan, turning gracefully toward the little girl. "But the pain this caused helped me find my own will to survive and survive separately."

"People keep throwing me away," she cries.

"Only you can throw yourself away, Amanda."

"I'm not special like you."

"It's not about being special. It's about being important to yourself. And only you can become important to yourself."

"But the other swans follow you out into the harbor and make room for you when you come back."

"Yes, they make room for me, Amanda, but it is the caring that I have for myself—the power I have over myself in the moment they make room for."

"But I am nobody!"

"You can learn to become somebody to yourself, Amanda. That is where it begins."

"How?" asks the little girl.

"The way to begin is to use your imagination. I'll show you what to do."

The little girl closes her eyes.

"Find your sacred space within and say your name inside. Fill the whole space with your name. Pronounce it boldly and imagine that your name signifies the importance of your own existence. Know that there is only one you, nobody like you, a separate person, you."

The little girl lifts her chest as she practices the swan's advice.

"Yes, lift your chest, Amanda, to make your sacred space inside larger. Imagine that your name is bursting within your chest, bursting to pronounce the miracle of your own separate existence."

"But it hurts inside," says the little girl.

"Your feelings are important because they let you know you're alive. Fill your chest up with your name so that you know who is feeling so alive. It is you. Your existence is now. Your existence is important because it is what you have and who you are."

You may have noticed that the black swan addressed the little girl by her name—Amanda. In her trauma, she had forgotten her name and then used it to recognize herself. Honoring the importance of your own existence is a life-long journey of self-discovery. Take a moment to close your eyes and lift your chest slightly in a gesture of recognition. You exist now, and there is only one you. Imagine filling the cavity of your chest with your name until it extends beyond its usual boundaries to boldly pronounce the importance of your existence.

As you get in touch with the importance of your existence, bear in mind that the ultimate value of who you are is based not on your attributes—your talents, beauty, financial success, or I.Q. points—but on the miraculous fact that you exist.[15] Take a moment to reflect on the fact that you are alive and that your existence is important.[16]

In spite of pain you may feel, can you behold the importance of your existence?

Can you find elements to celebrate in this moment? Describe.

Describe how you feel while attempting this lesson at this moment.

Like the other Swan Lessons, this one is not accomplished on a one-time basis, but requires daily contemplation and practice. Imagine expanding your capacity to behold the importance of your existence on a daily basis.

How will it benefit your life?

What tools are you using to help you celebrate your existence?

Beholding Yourself

In beholding the importance of your existence it's important to recognize that the feelings of yearning and longing are a persistent call for help—not for your ex to return to take care of you, but for you to take care of yourself.

During Withdrawal, your mammalian brain desperately seeks its attachment. The frustration of seeking and not finding is what Withdrawal energy is all about. When your powerful drive toward attachment is thwarted, it doesn't just give up. It continues its relentless pull—unless you invest your energy in someone else,[17] and that someone is the one person you do have—you. Your drive is nudging you to invest in making a new connection, and that connection is to self.

Check all you agree with to empower yourself to make an internal connection.

- ❏ Before I can really know love, love has to come from myself, toward myself.
- ❏ Going through heartbreak is an opportunity to learn how to perform this critical task: loving myself.
- ❏ My feelings are the gateway to recognizing how important it is to be loved—loved not by my ex or by a new partner, but by myself.
- ❏ The emotional hunger I feel is my yearning for love from myself.
- ❏ The task of self-love is long overdue in my life, something that needed my attention well before the breakup.
- ❏ My life is exactly where I need it to be to work on what I need to work on.*

Accepting the universal need for connection does not mean that you must first find a mate to be happy. It means that you must provide an object of focus for your attachment energy, and that object, first and foremost, is you. Learning to love yourself is critical to recovery.

---

*   This is abandonment recovery's most important thought experiment. Exploring this proposition can turn your life around.

Self-Love: How Do You Get It?

People are always suggesting that we should love ourselves, but this remains one of those easier-said-than-done aphorisms. How to accomplish it? That's the age-old question.

The exercise I am about to explain was borrowed from a book titled *Big You Little You; Separation Therapy*,[18] written by two psychoanalysts, Grace Kirsten, C.S.W., and Richard Robertiello, M.D. What follows is an abbreviation of their life-changing technique. It provides a way to go beyond talking about self-love, to a hands-on method for giving love to yourself. Through incremental steps, you actually administer to your oldest and most important needs and feelings. You perform self-loving actions, rather than give lip service to platitudes.

I've spent over thirty years searching for techniques that work quickly and effectively to heal the primal wound of abandonment and repair sense of self. Big You / Little You Dialogue is the best shortcut I've come across. It works with the energy of the Withdrawal stage and uses your powerful drive toward attachment—a drive that is thwarted during abandonment—to help you make a life-sustaining internal connection.

This approach provides a dynamic alternative to reciting affirmations. Whether you talk to yourself in the mirror every day and say, "I love myself," and "I am great," or find a group of people to chant positive messages at you for hours on end, the use of affirmations proves helpful to only some of my clients. In the long view, many find the results to be ephemeral. The message of self-love just doesn't sink into the abandonment wound deeply enough to effect real change.

It's as if our best-intended messages were being constantly intercepted by internal gatekeepers whose job is to maintain the status quo of our low self-esteem. These inner critics aren't willing to give up their low opinion of you just because you send yourself a bouquet of compliments.

This exercise promotes not placebo relief but real change. That's why I've adapted this technique for use as Ak*e*ru Exercise Two.

AK*E*RU EXERCISE TWO
BIG YOU / LITTLE YOU DIALOGUE

Based on psychoanalytic theory and decades of clinical evidence, Kirsten and Robertiello designed the Big You / Little You exercise to bypass your unconscious gatekeepers and turn self-love into a hands-on activity rather than an abstraction. The technique makes use of separation therapy. It involves separating the part of yourself that contains all of your feelings from the cognitive part where your adult self resides. Separating the two allows you to create a therapeutic dialogue between them.

In keeping with the Ak*e*ru principle, this exercise works with the energy of Withdrawal to create an internal connection. It works as a self-help tool and can be used by professionals. Once you learn how to perform the dialogue, you'll discover remarkable results.

Creating the Big You / Little You Dialogue

Step One

Your first task is to create a vivid picture of what you were like at about four or five years old. The image of your child self will help you personify your emotional self—your inner child, which Kirsten and Robertiello refer to as "Little You." According to the authors, it helps if you imagine your child self standing about five feet away from you on your weaker side, to remind you that Little is more vulnerable and dependent than your adult self, "Big You." If you're right-handed, Little would be on your left.

Little You is going to use the dialogue to express her long-neglected emotional needs and will look to your adult self for help. Through the dialogue, your child self emerges as a separate figure, revealing her fears, hopes, and dreams.

Big You will demonstrate patience and sensitivity, acting as an ideal parent relating to a child's feelings and needs. Many of Little's feelings have been buried within for a long time. The dialogue helps bring them out in the open.

I've developed some Qs to warm you up to the needs and feelings of your child self.

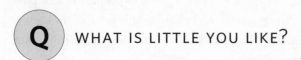 **Q** WHAT IS LITTLE YOU LIKE?

What were you like as a child around four or five years old? What did you look like?

When were your disposition and personality like as a young child?

When you were sad, what were you sad about?

When you were happy, what were you happy about?

When you were mad, what were you mad about?

What were you most fond of doing at that age?

What were you good at?

What were you not so good at?

Whose lap did you feel most safe and secure climbing into?

What were your parents most proud of about you?

What were your parents' disappointments about you?

Did you feel less-than or more-than one of your siblings or peers? Why?

Has Little You ever worried that there's something really wrong with him? Explain.

Which of Little's feelings, needs, and doubts carry through to today?

How does Little react to rejection today?

The child self has been making its feelings known all along, expressing its needs from within. To begin the dialogue, first attribute your feelings, insecurities, self-doubts, and needs to Little. When you feel insecure, it is the child within you who is insecure, the child who feels desperate for acceptance and approval, the child whose anxiety sabotages your relationships, the child who suffers your withdrawal symptoms. Through the dialogue, Big You will administer to Little's emotional discomfort and needs.

Step Two

Form a picture in your head of the adult person you are forever striving to become. Even the highest functioning among us are often hard pressed to picture ourselves as strong, capable adults. To bypass your internal board of critics—those nit-picking perfectionists—try picturing yourself doing the one thing you know you are good at, or one time you asserted yourself appropriately, or one act in which you showed genuine compassion and kindness. Think of times when you were at your best and form a composite picture of them. Big You embodies the higher self you are becoming.

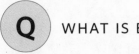 **WHAT IS BIG YOU LIKE?**

What is your greatest moment so far as an adult?

Describe an activity you feel particularly confident performing.

Name another.

Describe some positive attributes of Big You.

Describe Big's nurturing attributes. Is Big able to be understanding? Compassionate? Nonjudgmental? Validating? Supportive? Reassuring? Unconditionally loving? Explain.

Think of your highest aspirations for personal growth. Describe who Big is becoming.

Big's job is to nurture the child's needs, which include being admired and listened to, acknowledged and validated. Big acts like a good parent toward a cherished child. Big provides Little with a sense of belonging and love. Big validates Little's feelings; provides reassurances; and, most important, offers to make changes, where appropriate, to accommodate Little's wishes and needs.

Step Three

You, the individual, sit atop a triangle, mediating the dialogue between your child self, who contains all of your feelings, needs, and wants, and your cognitive self, who can exercise good judgment and nurture the needs of your child self. Little You is on the left, and Big You is on the right.

As the individual mediating the dialogue, you will be conducting a kind of one-person role-play, giving voice to both your child self and your adult self. In creating the written dialogue for the child, you take on the language and attitude of a

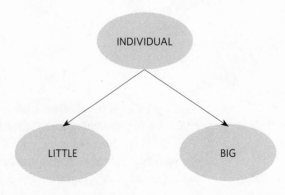

child. When writing the adult's part, you imagine the body language of the strong, sensible adult you are becoming and use language appropriate to reassure and validate a child. Big becomes a caring parent who administers lovingly to and guides your helpless inner child.

Daily Dialogues

To help you get started, I've developed a few sample dialogues between Little You and Big You for you to free-write.* *Free-write* means to run your pen across the page without care about spelling, form, handwriting, or logic. The samples** are intended to give you an idea of how the process works. As soon as you get the hang of it, it's best to dispense with my script and free-write your own dialogues in your notebook or journal. This way, you are not just reading prescribed questions, but getting inside the personalities of Big You and Little You.

Sample Dialogue One

ISSUE: LITTLE'S NEGLECTED NEEDS

BIG: Ask Little how she feels about your life right now, what feelings she needs help with. You might need to coax her out of her shell—she's not used to anyone caring. Big, use your own words.
LITTLE'S RESPONSE:

BIG: Show your concern by asking Little to elaborate more. Get her to be honest, to really open up.
LITTLE'S RESPONSE:

---

*   You'll get a lot of benefit from reading Kirsten and Robertiello (1977). My books *The Journey from Abandonment to Healing* and *Taming Your Outer Child* also provide additional instruction.

** You can share these dialogues in your support groups. Write them during the group or at home and bring in highlighted sections to share. For example, members can share responses to "What did I learn about myself (Little, Big) from this dialogue?" "What surprised me most from doing the exercise?"

BIG: Ask Little how you can make things better for her.
LITTLE'S RESPONSE:

BIG: Ask Little what other needs she has.
LITTLE'S RESPONSE:

BIG: Ask if she is angry with you for neglecting these feelings for so long.
LITTLE'S RESPONSE:

BIG: Promise you'll make this up to her. Let that sink in for a minute and ask if she trusts you to keep your word.
LITTLE'S RESPONSE:

BIG: Ask Little what you can do to prove you mean it.
LITTLE'S RESPONSE:

BIG: Make a commitment about the specific changes you plan to make. Big, use your own words.
LITTLE'S RESPONSE:

BIG: Ask Little if she has confidence in you to actually carry them out.
LITTLE'S RESPONSE:

BIG: Reassure Little that you will always love her and never leave her alone again. Ask her if she believes you.
LITTLE'S RESPONSE:

Continue this dialogue in your notebook, writing out Big's part in a free-form way using your own words until Little feels reasonably reassured.

Sample Dialogue Two

ISSUE: LITTLE'S BASIC NEEDS

BIG: Ask Little what he wants from your life.
LITTLE'S RESPONSE:

BIG: Ask Little how he thinks things are going—is he happy, fulfilled, disappointed, worried, emotionally hungry?
LITTLE'S RESPONSE:

BIG: Tell Little to be honest, to really open up with his needs.
LITTLE'S RESPONSE:

BIG: Show how concerned you are by asking him to elaborate even more.
LITTLE'S RESPONSE:

BIG: Give reassurance that you will take care of Little's needs from now on. Ask whether he trusts you to keep such a promise.
LITTLE'S RESPONSE:

BIG: Ask Little why he feels that way. Ask him how you can make it better in the future.
LITTLE'S RESPONSE:

Continue in a free-form way until satisfied.

Sample Dialogue Three

ISSUE: IS LITTLE YOU LOVABLE?

Little's fears, neediness, and internal seething may make it hard for you to succeed in your love relationships.

BIG: Can you still love and commit to Little in spite of the nuisance she creates in your love life?
BIG'S RESPONSE:

BIG: Tell Little you'll always love her unconditionally—warts, barnacles, basket-case fears, and all.
LITTLE'S RESPONSE:

BIG: Ask Little if she believes in your sincerity.
LITTLE'S RESPONSE:

BIG: Ask Little to tell you more about what she feels. If she resists, coax and reassure her, ask sensitive questions until she can be convinced of your sincerity.
LITTLE'S RESPONSE:

BIG: Do you feel closer to Little now that she has told you her feelings? Tell her this in your own words.
BIG'S COMMENT:

Continue this free-form dialogue until you feel strongly connected to one another and reasonably assured that Big and Little's new bond will continue.

Sample Dialogue Four

ISSUE: YOUR CURRENT LOVE LIFE OR LACK THEREOF

BIG: Ask Little how he feels about your current (or lack of) background object.
LITTLE'S RESPONSE:

BIG: Ask Little what kind of emotional support he'd like from another person to make him happier and more content.
LITTLE'S RESPONSE:

LITTLE then asks Big (if applicable): How come you don't get this for me?
BIG'S EXPLANATION:

BIG: Ask Little if he is angry with you about this.
LITTLE'S RESPONSE:

BIG: Ask what you can do differently to make this up to him.
LITTLE'S RESPONSE:

BIG: Ask Little if he trusts you to do the right things to get these needs met.
LITTLE'S RESPONSE:

BIG: Reassure Little that you will never leave him alone with these feelings again, that you will always be there for him. Big, use your own words.
LITTLE'S RESPONSE:

BIG: Ask Little if he believes you. Invite him to really be honest and not to spare your feelings.
LITTLE'S RESPONSE:

Continue until mutual satisfaction is reached.

Sample Dialogue Five

ISSUE: LITTLE'S UNSPOKEN, BROKEN DREAMS

BIG: Ask Little what secret dreams and desires she has.
LITTLE'S RESPONSE:

BIG: Ask Little how it feels to wait so long for you to express interest.
LITTLE'S RESPONSE:

BIG: Ask Little what old hankerings and new interests and activities she would like to see you get involved in now.
LITTLE'S RESPONSE:

LITTLE: Ask Big, How come it took you so long to ask?
BIG'S RESPONSE:

BIG: Ask Little if she trusts you to follow through this time.
LITTLE'S RESPONSE:

BIG: Reassure Little that from now on you will listen more closely to her needs, wishes, desires, and dreams. Big, use your own words.
LITTLE'S RESPONSE:

BIG: Ask Little if she believes you.
LITTLE'S RESPONSE:

BIG: Ask Little what part of your unlived life she wants you to begin living first.
LITTLE'S RESPONSE:

Sample Dialogue Six

ISSUE: EMOTIONAL HUNGER

Attribute your emotional hunger to Little.

BIG: Ask Little to describe his most urgent emotional needs.
LITTLE'S RESPONSE:

BIG: Ask Little to elaborate.
LITTLE'S RESPONSE:

BIG: If Little is holding back, say what you need to get him to open up and express his long-neglected needs. Big, use your own words.
LITTLE'S RESPONSE:

BIG: Reassure Little that from now on you will listen to these feelings and not ignore him. Ask if he trusts that you will keep this promise.
LITTLE'S RESPONSE:

BIG: Ask what you can do to show Little you mean it, that you care.
LITTLE'S RESPONSE:

BIG: Ask Little what you can do differently to make this up to him.
LITTLE'S RESPONSE:

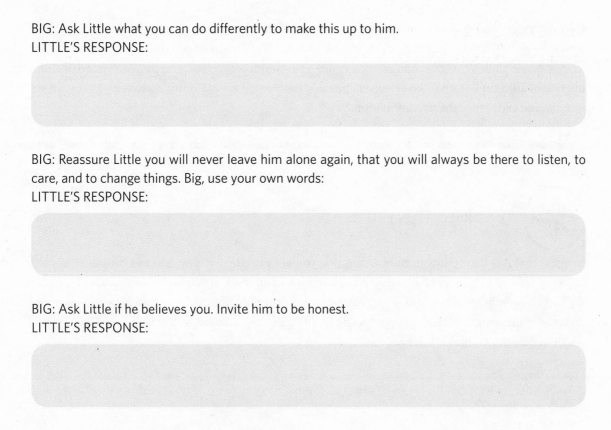

BIG: Reassure Little you will never leave him alone again, that you will always be there to listen, to care, and to change things. Big, use your own words:
LITTLE'S RESPONSE:

BIG: Ask Little if he believes you. Invite him to be honest.
LITTLE'S RESPONSE:

You can use this technique anytime. Whenever you become aware of an uncomfortable feeling, just attribute it to your child self and begin the dialogue.

At first Little may go blank and fail to divulge her deepest feelings without a lot of coaxing. Big has to be very sensitive, persistent, and committed. Big asks caring questions, always demonstrating sincere interest in understanding and helping.

The outcome: Big becomes stronger, Little less intrusive.

Once you get going, you might use up half of your notebook, as your first dialogues can get lengthy. Surprisingly, once Little's feelings start to come out, it's often hard to shut him up. No matter how emotional Little might get, Big's job is to reassure Little that everything will be all right. Getting your child self to express his feelings is the most effective way to lift his mood (and yours along with it), even during the worst of times. The idea is that Big becomes stronger as she administers to Little's most despairing feelings. You strengthen your adult self and give love to yourself all at the same time.

If the dialogue gets too intense, it is up to you—the individual at the top of the triangle—to end it. At a later time, when Big feels capable of handling Little's profound despair and neediness, you can resume the dialogue with greater strength and commitment to say and do what it takes to comfort and reassure Little.

Psychoanalysts are trained to bring unconscious conflicts to the surface. Three months of steady dialoguing brings your primal feelings right to where they need to be, allowing you to attend to them—a process easily worth years of therapy, in fact, a process that enhances psychotherapy.

When your primal emotional needs and fears remain submerged inside the individual, Little is able to interfere unconsciously. When Little is separated from the individual through this dialogue, you are no longer driven by unconscious (Little-submerged) fears and hungers, but by an ever-stronger, more-capable adult. As Big becomes strong enough to administer to Little's needs, you resolve lifelong internal conflicts and learn to love yourself, possibly for the first time. Do this exercise every day for six months and experience the transformation.

 Back to the Future

Imagine that it is six months from now and that you are extremely happy. You feel confident in your ability to operate from your adult wisdom rather than remain stuck in your emotional quagmire. Imagine that six months from now you've gained control over your life. Your child self is a glowing emotional presence within you. Little feels supported and loved by Big. Big, in turn, feels strong, capable, and confident in facing all of life's challenges.

How does having a strong adult in control benefit your life? (Imagine that it is six months from now.)

What emotional obstacles did you have to overcome to achieve this future success?

Working backward from the future, how did you overcome them?

What daily changes on a behavioral level enabled you to make this change?

Action Vow: I will take the following action within twenty-four hours as a baby step in the direction of this change: _____.

Action Bullet

Action Bullets are a lot like Action Vows. Action Bullets give you, the individual mediating the dialogue, the opportunity to integrate emotion (Little) and reason (Big) and translate them into action. Action Bullets are Truth Nuggets with an action attached to the end.

Action Bullets are also different from magic bullets in that Action Bullets recognize that any magic existing in the world exists inside you. You may wish there were a magic bullet or someone outside of yourself who could perform some miracle treatment to absolve you of your problems. You may even hope that just reading through this workbook and answering some of the questions will lift you from your self-defeating patterns and change your life. This kind of wishful thinking is highly prevalent.

People are always holding out for a magic bullet, expecting that one more book, one more tape, one more lecture will finally free them. But the magic is not in any book, exercise, lecture, or guru. The magic bullet is not even inside this workbook, but inside your ability to take action. It is entirely up to you to change your life. Just reading words on a page, no matter how much wisdom they contain, cannot transform your life. You must integrate their wisdom with action. Commit to change.

Action Bullet: I feel _____ because _____,
and I am going to _____.

Maria completed the Action Bullet this way:
"I feel scared *because* I'm afraid of being alone *and I am going to* look up the number of the Women's Center."

More Food for Thought

What are you feeling today?

[ ]

Truth Nugget: I feel _____ because _____.

Can you remember an earlier time you felt this way?

Go back even further. What is your very earliest memory of having this feeling?

What situation created it?

Who was this feeling with? Your mother? Father? Someone else?

Describe the situation and feelings.

How were those feelings different from your current ones?

How were they similar?

How was the problem resolved?

Are there any residual feelings left over? Name the feelings.

Does this unfinished business relate to where you are currently stuck? What's the connection?

How can using the Big You / Little You dialogue help you resolve this issue?

Action Bullet: I feel _____ because _____,
and I am going to *write the dialogue to work through this feeling.*

6 Accepting the Unchangeable

About six months into my heartbreak, I had a rude awakening. I was sitting on my bed pulling up my stockings. A mirrored door was ajar and its reflection caught me off guard. In a flash, I recognized the woman hunched over her feet, glowering at the mirror. It was me, caught in a moment of self-revulsion.

I undertook an immediate reality check. I'd always considered myself to be a reasonably attractive woman, and my friends and lovers had thought so too, I told myself. And besides, I'd just lost at least fifteen pounds of abandonment weight, and I knew I looked better than ever. It was unmistakable what this sudden negative image of myself meant: I had managed to internalize my partner's rejection. My abandonment wound had become infected.

For decades I had watched this same process in my clients after they survived a breakup. They'd take their rejection to heart, as evidence of unworthiness. But how had I, a therapist with over twenty years of experience specializing in this issue, managed to fall prey to the same dynamics?

Internalizing is the *I* in the middle of the S.W.I.R.L. Process—the eye of a hurricane wreaking destruction on the self. Internalizing is the most critical stage of abandonment, when your body and soul incorporate the deep personal wound of losing someone's love. Without recovery, this wound can leave permanent scarring. It burrows beneath the surface where it continues to generate insecurity and undermine your self-esteem for decades to come.

Internalizing is what distinguishes abandonment grief from all others. You grieve not a loss of someone's life, but a loss of his love and, in the process, doubt your own worth. Peter Yelton, a friend and personal guru, says that abandonment is a profound enough trauma to implant an invisible drain deep within the self that works insidiously to siphon off self-esteem from within. The paradox for abandonment survivors is that no matter what they do to build their self-esteem, the invisible wound of abandonment is always working to drain it away.[1]

Although its appearance in my mirror caught me off guard, as a therapist, I understood what my sudden bout of self-loathing was all about. Abandonment is a cumulative wound, containing all of the disconnections, disappointments, and heartbreaks of a lifetime. My current heartbreak had reopened that wound and bombarded me with emotional memories of a painful past. The ugly duckling phase I'd gone through as a child had come back to haunt me full force. Between the ages of eight and eleven, I'd been obese. Not only was I gigantic, but my teeth managed to grow in crooked. To make matters worse, I suffered through 365 bad hair days per year. I was always getting home perms to improve the situation, but these experiments created bald spots on one side of my head and frizzy puffs on the other. The only thing that changed was which side they were on.

Now as an adult, I avoid perms and I zealously diet and exercise to keep myself trim. Though more slender than usual and appropriately coiffed at the time of my abandonment, that glimpse into the mirror revealed what I was feeling about myself on the inside. In a split second of awareness, I witnessed my damaged self-image rise up from the ruins. It was heartbreak's ghost staring me down. A negative self-image is an apparition of abandonment grief.

Having already scoured the psychology shelves over the years for all available information on abandonment's ability to diminish one's self-esteem, I was now living proof that its wisdom was insufficient. I searched in adjacent fields for answers. Finally, in an improbably obscure journal called *Social Subordinance*,[2] I found what I was looking for.

I learned that when alpha males—the head honchos of baboon societies—become stricken with grief following the breakup or death of a mate, it causes their glucocorticoid stress hormones to skyrocket. With elevated glucocorticoids, they no longer demonstrate dominant behavior. In other words, alpha males let their lower-ranking troop mates get one over on them. I identified with the plight of these grief-stricken alphas who'd become so debilitated by increased glucocorticoids, they stooped to asking permission from lower-ranking males for a share of the food supply.

When alphas become wimpy with grief, the others begin jockeying for new positions within the rank and file. The ensuing mayhem causes all of the baboons' glucocorticoids to rise, but with intriguing differences. The males who fight to gain higher rank show a smaller increase in glucocorticoids than those who fight to defend their existing ranks.

This told me what I had to do. I had to act like the upstart baboons who fought, not to protect their present position but for higher gain. I'd have to fight my own internal restrictions and barriers to avenge my abandonment wound. I'd prove the old maxim correct: the best revenge is success. I'd raise my esteem and lower my glucocorticoids by fighting my way out of the lockstep patterns that held me in place. I'd forge onward to higher ground.

Fighting was the last thing I felt like doing. "Fake it till you make it"—a trusty slogan borrowed from twelve-step programs—proved true. I forced myself through the motions of building a new sense of self, acceding to my highest goals, and I developed a whole new technique in doing so, which I outline in this chapter and the next.

Can you think of a higher gain worth fighting for?

What would higher achievement look like in your life? A promotion? Change of careers? Obtaining a new degree? Describe where you can go from here to reach higher ground.

What barriers must you first overcome?

Can you think of a time when you forced yourself to exceed your highest capabilities? Describe.

How did it feel?

What strengths do you have for pursuing higher goals?

Action Bullet: I feel _____ because _____, and I am going to _____.

Swirling through Internalizing

We talked about the importance of deidealizing your abandoner in the last chapter. Remaining stuck in the myth of your abandoner's specialness causes your symptoms of Withdrawal to overlap with the self-debilitating process of Internalizing—a painful mix. Yet many people still fight tooth and nail to keep their beloved on a pedestal.

"How dare you suggest that my Danielle wasn't the most precious, exquisitely beautiful woman in the world?" declares Thomas.

There are several reasons why people resist debunking the myth, even though it is at their expense.

First, convincing yourself that your partner is omnipotent and irreplaceable is a way of justifying the intensity of your despair. It allows you to say, "It's not because I'm weak or lowly that I'm still drowning in grief. It is because my beloved was so unbelievably special." You don't feel as out of control for succumbing to the emotional excesses of heartbreak if you believe that you've lost the whole kingdom.

Second, putting your beloved on a pedestal is a way of sustaining the emotional connection, although now the relationship takes place only in your mind. As painful as the yearning and self-doubts are, remaining obsessed allows you to feel attached to your abandoner, delaying the moment at which you must face the abyss of total disconnection—of having nobody special to think about. Your unconscious reasoning is, "It's better to pine away than to have no one to think about at all." Being obsessed beats being totally alone.

> People tell me: "But I'm still in love with my abandoner."
>
> I explain: It is normal to have these feelings, but they are feelings, not facts.

This chapter is going to show you how to use your persistent heartache to motivate positive change. This begins with examining the negative assumptions you've made about yourself.

There's Something Wrong with Me

On some level, most of us worry that there must be something fundamentally wrong with us. This deep-seated fear emerges in childhood and lingers throughout life. As children, we worried about whether we were up to par. We compared ourselves to peers and identified areas where we came up short.

Check all that seem familiar.

AS A CHILD, I MAY HAVE FELT DISAPPOINTED IN MYSELF FOR...

- ❏ Allowing another child to bully me.
- ❏ Making a fool of myself when trying to impress someone.
- ❏ Overreacting to things that didn't seem to ruffle the other kids.
- ❏ Feeling intimidated by other kids' show of confidence.
- ❏ Doing something impulsive and then regretting it because I got in trouble.
- ❏ Becoming inhibited around those who seem free and spontaneous.
- ❏ Craving attention, but getting it at my own expense.
- ❏ Being more emotionally sensitive than others.
- ❏ Being unable to get someone to stop teasing me.

❑ Feeling invisible.
❑ Feeling frozen with fear when a situation called for me to take action.

The impact of these mini-crises—nearly universal to childhood experience—lessens as you develop social competence, but the worry that there's something wrong with you lives on, plaguing the unconscious. Going through an adult breakup inflates those old doubts, causing them to float up to the surface. During Internalizing, they smack you in the face. The situation creating them now may be different, but the feelings remain the same.

Check all that apply.

I WORRY THAT...

❑ The loss of control over my emotions now proves me weak and defective, just as I've always suspected.
❑ There must be something fundamentally wrong with the impression I leave in the hearts and minds of others; otherwise why would someone discard me?
❑ I'm missing an important attribute.
❑ I'm endowed with an unlovable trait over which I have no control.
❑ I'm destined for perpetual victimhood—an accident waiting to happen—and now with this heartbreak, it finally did.
❑ I'm inherently undeserving of love. I'm not attachment-worthy.

It is easy to internalize these self-injurious ideas. Without recovery, they burrow beneath the surface and commingle with earlier self-doubts. Then they get ready to pounce when you attempt a new relationship. The ensuing identity crisis is powerful enough to sabotage your love life for decades to come.

During Internalizing, as your self-esteem plummets, it is also a time to rebuild. Ak*eru* refers to "ending" and "beginning," as well as "the empty space created when someone leaves." Your task is to use this Internalizing energy to fill the empty space with positive images. We're going to learn how to refurbish our sense of self with invincible principles that cannot be felled by someone's rejection, changes in our status, weight, age, or any other life process that befalls human beings. This rebuilding begins with understanding what self-esteem is all about.

Scrambling for Self-Esteem Points

People need direction in reversing abandonment's deep personal injury. Otherwise they resort to scrambling for their lost self-esteem points by comparing their looks, pocketbooks, and academic degrees to what others have. We're not interested in this counting/measuring game in which you tally up your trophies, miles jogged, years of sobriety, pounds lost, stocks gained. No matter how high your points, they still won't fill you up. For all of your acquisitions and attributes, unless you feel wanted and desired by significant others in your life, you're likely to continue to question your self-worth.

"When Jake left me for another woman," says Patricia, "I felt disqualified, as if I had no worth at all. I did everything I could to feel like a woman again. I went out and bought lingerie, flirted with men, but I continued to feel gross and undesirable for a long time."

Learning to feel good about yourself is not about making a tally of your attributes, as the little girl in the story learned.*

"Feeling good about yourself" says the black swan, "has nothing to do with whether you're talented, or beautiful, or strong, or smart, or any of these things. These have nothing to do with the value of your own existence. They are only attributes—the spokes of the wheel—not its center."

When you see yourself through the shattered lens of rejection, it is as if the very center of the wheel—the essence of the self—had been disqualified.[3] In the center of us exists raw human substance with which to build a new sense of self. Rebuilding from the center on outward is a primary focus throughout this workbook.

Self-Esteem and Self-Image

There is a lot of confusion about self-esteem and self-image. The discussion about what these terms mean and how we are supposed to apply them remains ethereal. I'm going to make it practical. *Self-esteem* is something you give to yourself. That's why it's called *self*-esteem. *Self-image* is based on how you imagine others perceive you. It's based on your perception of their perception, all of which is subject to distortion.

Abandonment survivors are famous for needing external validation. Self-help wisdom counters this, suggesting that you aren't supposed to look outside of yourself to feel good about yourself. After surviving the loss of love, however, abandonment survivors face deeply personal and complex problems as they try to reconstruct their lives. Under such circumstances, the need for external validation is understandable. My message is that when it comes to abandonment, self-help's one-size-fits-all prescriptions don't always apply. The edict against looking to other people for reassurance may discourage people from the very thing that helps them most during this difficult time.

If you've been left, you've been externally *in*validated. You feel demoralized because the most important person in your life presumably no longer loves, wants, or needs you. So you look to the *external* world to take away the awful feelings of unworthiness. The line from the old song, "You're nobody till

---

* See my *Black Swan* (p. 43).

somebody loves you," feels painfully true after surviving abandonment. You feel desperate to be reassured that you are still lovable, romantically desirable, and socially valued.

It may seem as if I were committing self-help treason for honoring the route of external validation, but nature won't send a thunderbolt out of the sky to strike me dead for sedition. Nature recognizes the universal need for fellow human beings to give each other positive feedback. Supportive social intercourse is the ever-present nurture from which we derive our sense of security, value to others, and the life-sustaining feeling that we belong.[4]

Seeking recognition from others does not mean that you expect them to bestow self-esteem on you. They cannot. People can give you the responses you have positioned yourself to receive from them. They can stroke you in a way that feels good. But after receiving validation from them, you must bestow esteem on yourself.

We're going to send the self-esteem police away with their lofty ideals and staunch prohibitions about not looking to others to help you feel good about yourself. This chapter will show you what you can do to feel better about yourself, and it may involve seeking feedback from others. You will learn to channel your need for external validation in a positive direction.[5] In chapter 8, you'll learn the third Akeru exercise for working with the Internalizing energy to build your self-esteem. Here, you'll learn to go *with* its energy rather than against it and use external validation as a tool.

Name a time you patted yourself on the back for an accomplishment that was acknowledged by your friends, family, or community.

How did getting their feedback feel?

What do your friends seem to value most about you?

What do you value most about yourself?

Think of a cherished friend. What do you value most about him or her?

Is there anything about yourself you value that your friends don't appear to recognize?

Do your friends' appraisals of you match your own? How?

What additional assets would you like them to recognize?

Are you satisfied with the impression you think you make on others?

How would you like this impression to improve?

Action Bullet: I feel _____ because _____,
and I am going to _____.

Self Is a Social Construct

Self-esteem is very much a social construct. It's about how we perceive ourselves in relation to how we perceive others.

"I'm getting my body back in shape," says Jane. "I know I wouldn't bother to go through this torture if I lived alone on a desert island and nobody could see me. But I'm going back out there into the dating world and I want to look good. So I signed up at the gym."

A few months later…

"People keep telling me how great I've been looking lately! I feel so much better about myself."

Indeed, if we all lived alone on separate islands and there were no other people around to compare ourselves to, we would most likely love ourselves unconditionally. Why? Because we would have only ourselves to love. Self-love would translate into "survival instinct." We would love ourselves for all of the things we accomplish to survive another day. It's when we compare ourselves to how well others are doing that we decide whether to feel good about our accomplishments, or not so good.

Social Niche

We all have a social niche we identify with—a reference group within whose ranks we evaluate our own worth, even though we're usually not conscious of it. This niche becomes our own personal hall of mirrors[6] reflecting back a composite image of how we believe we're coming across to others. Everyone's niche consists of a unique constellation of people. Mine probably overlaps with yours to some extent, since it fits into a larger society. Social niches are circles within circles. For example, Jennifer Lopez, Meg Ryan, Whoopi Goldberg, and Diane Sawyer are women celebrities who've caught my attention; but I don't know them, and thus I am not forced to compare myself to their level of talent, beauty, or fame. But they are part of my larger world, and they serve as standard bearers of a sort, so you could consider them on the periphery of my social niche and perhaps your own.

Do you feel accepted by people? Explain.

Name someone you consider to be your peer.

Does this person consider you to be his or her peer as well?

Name three people you consider to be within your personal social niche—and three you do not.

On what did you base these selections? Which attributes (or lack thereof) influenced your choices?

Name someone you know who seems comfortable within his skin and within his social standing.

Does this person exemplify your ego ideal? Is there anything that prevents you from feeling comfortable within yourself?

Name three celebrity figures who serve as standard bearers.

What personal strengths allow you to feel good about yourself in relation to others?

What aspects of personal growth are you working to improve to feel better about yourself?

The Hall of Mirrors

You can think of your social world as an ever-available Hall of Mirrors, yielding a composite picture of how you come across to the collective eyeball of others. The people in your life reflect back an image of you as they see you. Depending on the variety of others' likes and dislikes, these reflections can range from flattering to not so flattering. Your image, as it comes across to them, has as much to do with others' quirks, values, pet peeves, and preferences, as it does with your own assets and liabilities. We try to control the way others perceive us through adjusting our styles of hair and clothes, by adopting the right attitude, or by accruing more accomplishments, but we can't guarantee we'll get the response we want. Since we can't control the way others respond, what we can try to control is our own side of the equation—the actions we choose to get a favorable response. The key is to use the Hall of Mirrors to our own benefit.

"My son's been diagnosed with attention deficit disorder (ADD)," says James, "but I think he got the disorder from me. Unless I'm really concentrating, my own mind flies all over the place. This explains why I've never been a good listener. I recently decided to work on my attention span. I began listening intently and responding to whatever people say to me. I force myself not to interrupt every five minutes with stuff about myself. I'm noticing all kinds of new people warming to me and my old friends opening up more and more."

By seeing his reflection in the responses of his friends, James got positive recognition just by changing a single behavior—listening.

The following two examples represent vanity issues. Given the emphasis our society places on women's physical appearance, both testimonies come from women.[7]

"I'd worn my hair in the same flip since high school," says Sarah. "After my breakup, I needed a change, so I cut it short. Of course, I hated it at first. So I did damage control by accentuating my strongest asset—my eyes. I started wearing subtle shades of eye shadow and I restyled my hair a bit and it worked like magic. I look better now than twenty years ago. I had been stuck in old ways and felt good about rebuilding a new me, letting the outside-me show people what was going on inside. I get lots of compliments, which reinforces the fact that I am changing for the better."

"I get feedback from my jeans," says Janet, "never mind the Hall of Mirrors, but from my smallest jeans—the ones I haven't been able to get up past my knees since the birth of my son. These old power jeans gave me a big compliment by sliding right up my hips. I felt really hot wearing them. Lately I've been strutting around exuding new confidence."

How do you feel about the fact that so much of a woman's sense of self-worth is based on her physical appearance?

How does society's emphasis on women's and men's looks affect your life?

How does it affect the way you feel about yourself?

How can changing this better your life?

What can you do to change it?

Gain Self-Esteem by Working on Your Inner Self

"I was the one to blame for my breakup," says Larry, "and the remorse is killing me. Missing Joyce so badly has completely cured me of being the demanding and critical guy I used to be. I don't want to be self-centered anymore. I'm working on myself and becoming a more giving person. I feel good about who I am becoming."

The personal work you do is reflected in the Hall of Mirrors. As you extend yourself to others in a new way, they respond to your evolving higher self. The ultimate reward is the deepening bonds you are establishing with the significant others in your life. Reach out to make new connections.*

Action Bullet: I feel _____ because _____, and I am going to work on _____.

---

*　See page 238 for Community Projects, a way to reach out to isolated members of your community, build your self-esteem, and help others at the same time!

How Does Self-Esteem Get Damaged in the First Place?

Learning how your self-esteem gets damaged makes it easier to rebuild it. One of the goals of this workbook is to take complex psychological theory and break it down into bite-size pieces so that you can understand the workings of your mind without having to get your Ph.D. in neuropsychobiology.

What Is Self?

There are many technical definitions of *self*,[8] but for the purpose of our work, we'll define it as your inner core, the sense you have of yourself as a separate person—the sense of where your needs and feelings leave off and other people's begin.

Sense of self begins from a center of awareness—the point from which you peer out to register the world around you. This peering out involves neurobiochemical activity taking place in the present tense of your mind, what neuroscientists call "working memory." Awareness is always occurring in the present. Even if you are thinking about what happened twenty years ago or wondering what will happen twenty years hence, you are thinking about these things in the present. This present tense of awareness is the center from which we engage life. Onto that center of self, we eventually learn to attribute certain qualities, such as being likable, popular, good, bad. This is how we derive a sense of that self.

We are not necessarily in touch with our *sense of self*[9] until something lifts it from the background of experience and makes us pay attention. Likewise, we are not aware of our feet as we're walking along until we stub one of our toes. The throbbing reminds you of that toe's existence. Or someone may lavish your toes with loving caresses, and the pleasurable attention elevates your feet to the top of your awareness.

This is how it works with self. You might not become aware of that internal center until it is stubbed or stroked into self-consciousness.

Are you aware of having a sense of self?

Could it use sprucing up?

What negative thoughts do you have about yourself?

How would you like to feel about yourself?

Self-Consciousness

If someone dismisses your deeds, ignores your existence, or rejects your love, your focus turns inward to ponder your worthiness. Or if someone lavishes you with compliments, you might turn inward to congratulate yourself. The variety of our life experiences triggers many sojourns into the self, where sometimes we feel good about ourselves and other times, not so good. Being self-conscious means you're preoccupied with "how you're doing" or "how you're coming across to others." This self-evaluation can become obsessive and causes some to feel inhibited in the company of others, and others to put on a show. Either way, self-consciousness interferes with your ability to authentically be yourself.

Essence of Person

We gain a lot of our self-image through observing others. In childhood you begin to notice that some of your classmates seem more popular than others. As you interact with them, you tend to gravitate toward some more than others. Over time, you form an impression of each person based on various nuances and subliminal responses of their personalities—their facial expressions, interests, physical appearance, voice quality, and achievements—combined with your comfort or enjoyment level in relating to them. From all of this and more you gain a sense of them, about the essence of their personalities.

If each person you encounter creates a certain unique impression in you, it is inevitable that at some point, you wonder what impression you create in others. You realize that you too come across to people in a certain way. But how do they perceive you? You want the impression you make to be positive. You look for signs in the Hall of Mirrors, hoping to discover that your own essence of person is being accepted.

"My older brother, Brad, had this charisma," says David. "Everybody loved him. He lit up the room, but nobody seemed to notice me. He had flair, and I apparently didn't. I decided I didn't have as good a personality as his. I was acutely conscious of how everyone—my family, kids at school, people on the street—reacted to me. When they weren't giving me lots of strokes, I felt bad about myself."

When you feel rebuffed, you worry that you are not coming across to people as well as you'd like, and you're not sure why. You don't know what you might have done to warrant this dismissal, so you invent reasons, the way David did when he believed he didn't have enough flair. You become conscious of yourself in a worrisome way. You feed your self-consciousness with a lot of self-depreciating assumptions.

"In high school I was always trying improve my personality to get people to like me more," David continues. *"I figured it was because I wasn't gregarious enough, didn't make a big enough splash. I put on bravado to cover up my insecurity. To this day I'm conscious of the way people respond to me, always trying to figure out if I'm being accepted."*

Your self-image accumulates its bumps and strokes along the way, without your realizing it. At some point, many of you accumulate enough negative experiences to create deep worry. If you could give voice to this internal gauge, you might hear yourself saying, "I must be inherently lacking essential worth. I am internally afflicted with something that makes me unacceptable."

As you grow, you continue to examine yourself with a critical eye, using external validation as a Hall of Mirrors to help you make adjustments along the way. You incorporate the misgivings you have about yourself into the inner core of yourself—that peering out part of you. In this way, the negative messages you receive go directly to the core of the self.

"This kid lived three doors down from me," explains Ruthann. *"There was something about her I liked. It seemed she was everybody else's favorite too. When she had somebody else over to play and I couldn't come in, I felt like a nobody, like I didn't have enough worth."*

We don't usually form our self-image in a conscious or deliberate way. Most of us tend to plod along without knowing we are taking score.

Think back to when you were in elementary school.

Name the person you gravitated to most.

Second most.

Who sought you out as a friend?

Can you remember feeling slighted or ignored by a friend, parent, teacher? Describe.

What impact did this have on the way you felt about yourself?

Did you fit in socially? Explain.

Can you remember any worries you had about yourself? Express your doubts.

Can you think of a friend or classmate who represented your ego ideal? How?

How did you rate yourself compared to him or her?

What strengths do you have for resolving these outdated assumptions?

How Nonmutual Relationships Can Damage Self-Image

Unrequited love wreaks havoc on self-esteem.

"I like Kimmy but she never wants to play with me."

"I'm attracted to Cindy, but she sees me only as a friend."

"I love Ed so much, but he doesn't desire me and isn't interested in working on our marriage anymore."

These are examples of nonmutual liaisons that lead to deep-seated feelings of what one psychological theorist, Michael Balint, calls the "limited capacity to perform the work of conquest." He defined conquest as "the work necessary to transform an indifferent object into a participating partner."[10] In other words, when someone you're attracted to doesn't return the compliment, it causes you to feel sexually powerless and romantically invisible—as if you had a limited capacity to establish mutual attraction.

Beyond romantic disappointments, there are many other letdowns that cause you to feel powerless and insignificant.

"I pledged Delta Omicron Pi sorority in my freshman year but they didn't take me," says Jennifer. "I felt my image must have lacked something or that my personality was weak or unacceptable or that I must have given off some bad vibes. Why else would they reject me? I battled these worries throughout my college career—and now that I'm going through a divorce, the old doubts are consuming me all over again."

False Attribution

Blaming someone's rejection on your supposed weaknesses is an example of false attribution. False attribution is a granddaddy of a topic.[11] It is responsible for most of the fiction we create about ourselves. It's how we idealize others at our own expense. It burrows itself deep into our relationships.

False attribution is a type of mistaken identity. It's when you misidentify the cause of an event. The event affecting us during Internalizing is abandonment. In the last chapter, we discussed the tendency to attribute the yearning and longing of Withdrawal to the alleged specialness of your partner. During the Internalizing stage, you attribute your rejection to not being good enough. This oh-so-common tendency to make false assumptions about yourself is responsible for the lingering damages to self-esteem incurred during the Internalizing stage.

"I was the only child of Asian descent in my school. I noticed the other children were confident and laughed and spoke a lot. I noticed qualities about them that made them likable and fun and special. I liked to be around them, but they didn't seem to notice whether I was there or not. I thought it was because I wasn't as special as they were, not as important or interesting. It wasn't until I grew up that I realized that my only real shortfall was that I'd been raised to wait my turn before speaking—probably a cultural trait. The other children and I were all just dealing with difference, and I'd taken it personally. Now I have my work cut out for me—ridding myself of those bad feelings—a whole lifetime of work."

False Attribution of a Second Order

It is not only onto the self that we attribute blame for the slings and arrows of everyday life. We frequently blame our feelings on other people, places, and things. Following are some examples.

EXTERNALIZING UNCOMFORTABLE FEELINGS ONTO YOUR JOB

"I'd gone through a breakup about five years ago and I was in the dumps," explains Cassandra. *"The clothing store I'd opened was a financial success, but I hated going there day after day. I was fed up with the customers, the paperwork, having to be on top of it seven days a week. I decided the place was making me depressed, so I finally sold it and got a job managing a store for someone else. After that, my depression dipped even lower. I blamed it on my new job—on not being accustomed to working for someone else and for half of the money. Then I ran out of things to blame. I realize what a salvation owning my own business had been. I'd falsely attributed my chronic heartache onto the store, and I realized it too late."*

PROJECTING INSECURITY ONTO YOUR MATE

"I accused Jack of being withholding," says Elaine. *"He'd try to please me, but I always raised the bar on him. When he couldn't keep up with my needs, I'd accuse him of making me needy and turning me into an emotional beggar. One day he said, 'I can't make you happy. All you do is abuse me. I'm out of here.' It took me a long time to realize that the problem was not Jack but my own insatiable needs."*

PROJECTING FEAR OF ENGULFMENT ONTO YOUR MATE

"I pursued Sylvia for a year and finally I convinced her to move in. Three days later, I shut down sexually. I remained indifferent to her for the six months we stuck it out living together. I attributed my lack of interest to the weight she'd gained, the way she yawned without covering her mouth, the glow-in-the-dark face cream she applied at night. Thanks to the fact that I neglected her, she eventually took up with another guy. I was devastated. At this point, I can see that my emotional shutdown was about me—not about her looks or personality. I would cherish every one of her traits, if only she'd just come back—even the glow-in-the-dark night cream. It took her leaving for me to realize that I had a real problem with commitment."

ATTRIBUTING UNCOMFORTABLE FEELINGS ONTO YOUR BODY PARTS

Somaticizing is the clinical term for a common form of false attribution in which you attribute your uncomfortable feelings onto somatic sensations—twinges of pain and weakness that seem to emanate from within your body.

"I've been alone for years and it's really getting too much already—having to do everything by myself without anyone to share it with. I wake up every morning feeling tired, drained, and achy.

I've been to so many doctors trying to get to the bottom of it. They've diagnosed me with everything from fibromyalgia to chronic fatigue syndrome to Epstein-Barr. I've finally come to recognize that a lot of it was coming from my anxiety—that lingering lovesickness I've felt ever since Jacob left me to survive all alone. Why? Because I don't notice the aches and pains as much when I'm visiting my daughter and surrounded by my grandchildren. There I'm brimming with get-up-and-go."

Why Do We Falsely Attribute?

One of the reasons we appropriate blame to the wrong cause is that most of us don't know what to do with our uncomfortable feelings. We either internalize them (blame them on ourselves) or externalize them (project them onto someone or something else).

Feelings are neither good nor bad. Having uncomfortable feelings does not reflect on your worthiness as a person. It is how you handle your feelings that should determine whether to give yourself esteem or not. Feelings are given; they just are. Having the feelings in the first place? Over that, you have no control. What to do about them? Over that, you are master.

It is the very fact that you have no control over whether to feel or not to feel that makes many people want to disown feelings. It's those control issues once again. During abandonment, both men and women feel ashamed of not being able to control the intensity of their feelings.[12] You believe you're supposed to avoid getting stuck in its grief, that you should be able to control it the way you control your words or actions. This is an unrealistic expectation to impose on yourself, and it causes you to damage your self-esteem.

Believing that you should be able to control negative emotion is one of the reasons people suffering with clinical depression feel stigmatized. They believe (as do many of their friends) that they should be able to snap out of it. When they can't, they falsely attribute feelings of weakness and powerlessness onto the self, adding a layer of shame to their depression. For most of the sufferers of this very real illness, quite the opposite is true. Depressed people are demonstrating Herculean strength in coping with the emotional burden of their symptoms.

Going through abandonment mimics the anxiety and despair of major depression. The link between grief and depression is reflected in a quote by Andrew Solomon from his groundbreaking book on depression: "Depression is a response to past loss, and anxiety is a response to future loss."[13]

The acute depression following abandonment is the result of losing your primary relationship. Your grief is compounded by the fact that you inflict the rage you feel about being rejected against yourself. It is important for psychotherapists to distinguish the profound despondency and negative self-obsession of abandonment from the protracted state we call clinical depression. During the acute phase of abandonment grief, the difference is negligible, and the risk of injuring yourself is as high as it is for clinical depression.*

---

* Mental health professionals can get more information by going to the Professional Page at abandonment.net.

IS THERE NO WAY TO LESSEN THE PAIN?

When you make good choices and take actions to change your personal life for the better, your uncomfortable feelings may dissipate and even transform into positive feelings. But most people fail to take this route. Rather than change the self-defeating patterns that give rise to their uncomfortable feelings, many try to make the feelings go away. Since this is an impossible task, they blame themselves or displace their unwanted feelings onto a perceived target—someone or something else. Attributing your unacceptable feelings onto the wrong cause drives them underground, further complicating your recovery.

SWAN LESSON SIX
Accepting and Confronting Your Reality

The issue of reality over false attribution is illustrated in the story about the little girl. She found herself with a particularly difficult reality to face. Unless she did, she would continue to blame her father's profound rejection on her already shattered sense of self. She beseeched the black swan for help.

"My daddy doesn't want me!" she cries. "I want him to come and get me."

"Wanting and wishing will not bring him back," says the swan. "You can accept this reality or fight it, Amanda. But fighting it only prolongs your pain and grief. Trying to change the unchangeable keeps you in a powerless place. Go inside and find the sacred space where you can accept the reality, one moment at a time."

The little girl closes her eyes and takes a deep breath.

"That's right, Amanda. Take a breath and face your reality. Accept your life as it is in the moment—all in one gulp. Belong to the reality of now."

"I am alone." She sighs. "But I don't want to be."

"It may not be the reality you want, but it is the reality you have—at least for the moment. If aloneness is the reality facing you, you must face it back."

"It hurts," whimpers the little girl.

"Yes," says the swan. "Pain is when the future and the past overlap and squeeze out the present. You must carve out a path between them. You must find the moment. Get into its groove, Amanda. Use all of your will to cross over into your present life and accept its realities. Once you do, you will be filled with the power of existence, free to act, to move forward. Fill yourself with the reality of your life, even the reality of your momentary aloneness, and experience the sensations of life all around you in this moment."

Name an aspect of your current reality that is difficult to accept.

Do you fight accepting it? If so, does fighting it change the circumstances or spare the pain? Does it hinder your progress? Express your thoughts on this.

Take a deep breath—a gulp of reality—and face what you need to face. In so doing, you are not condoning the reality, not excusing it, not making any other judgment about it, but simply acknowledging the simple fact of it.

Q

Using a short phrase, name the reality facing you.

What feelings come up as you face it back?

What strengths are you using to deal with life on life's terms?[14]

Truth Nugget: I feel _____ because _____.

Reality Leads to Realistic Solutions

Gaining a clear perspective on yourself and your situation allows you to use your energy to move forward. We discussed the need to feel in control in chapter 4. After surviving a loss, choosing to take positive actions is one way to increase your personal power and take back control.

> *"After my wife packed up and left," says Frank, "I felt pretty low. I knew I could use some female attention, but I was unemployed and fifty pounds overweight. Who was going to want me? So I did three things: I busted my hump to get a decent job, forced myself onto the treadmill every morning until I lost some weight, and signed up with a dating service. I didn't meet anyone special for a long time, but taking these actions gave me a sense that I was controlling my own destiny. My life was once again in my own grip."*

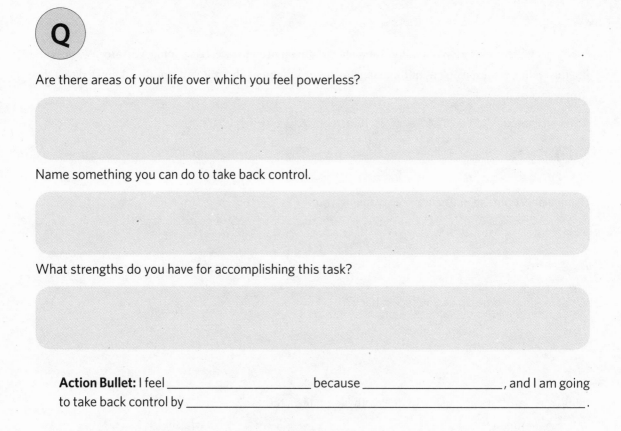

Q

Are there areas of your life over which you feel powerless?

Name something you can do to take back control.

What strengths do you have for accomplishing this task?

Action Bullet: I feel ＿＿＿＿＿＿＿＿＿＿ because ＿＿＿＿＿＿＿＿＿＿, and I am going to take back control by ＿＿＿＿＿＿＿＿＿＿＿＿＿＿＿＿＿＿＿＿＿.

The Effort Needs to Be Continuous

Self-esteem isn't about achieving a goal once and letting it end there. You need to keep moving toward your highest potential. This effort sustains your ability to value and respect yourself.

Janet quit smoking over twenty years ago:

"It did a lot for my self-esteem back then because it helped me recognize my inner strength. With-standing those horrible cravings and all of the peer pressure with everybody smoking around me made me feel good—then. But I need to accomplish something now to feel okay about my life again."

One cynical friend of mine insists that achievement is to be avoided at all costs because it means losing a goal. He gloats over having 3,719 unfinished projects stacked up in piles all over his house and yard—all to ward off that sense of loss. If achievement marks the end of a goal, then you need to constantly create new goals. Life can feel flat and self-esteem can droop unless you find a new mountain to climb.[15]

It isn't achievement that rewards us; it's the process of getting there that keeps good feelings flowing toward self. When you're actively working on things, you earn the right to give yourself credit, not for the end product of your efforts but for the efforts themselves. Get in touch with your strength. Commit to action. Regain control.

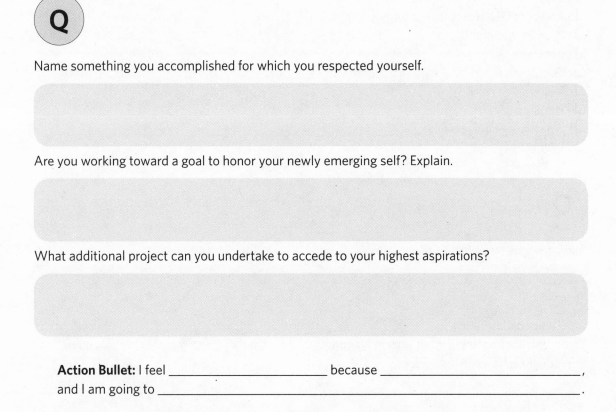

Q

Name something you accomplished for which you respected yourself.

Are you working toward a goal to honor your newly emerging self? Explain.

What additional project can you undertake to accede to your highest aspirations?

Action Bullet: I feel _____ because _____, and I am going to _____.

As you change within and without, you'll see improvement reflected in the responses you receive as you parade through the Hall of Mirrors. Remember, you are not expecting other people to give you self-esteem. You are validating yourself by using the Hall of Mirrors as a tool for reinforcing your own accomplishments. Being in tune with the responses of others offers a reminder that the positive feedback isn't about your sexy jeans, new job, or flat stomach. It's about the positive energy other people see you exuding. And it's contagious—a highly valued social commodity.

Check all of the qualities you recognize in yourself.

- ❏ Inner strength
- ❏ Willpower
- ❏ Integrity
- ❏ Ability to delay gratification
- ❏ Heartfulness
- ❏ Effort
- ❏ Wisdom
- ❏ Honesty
- ❏ Ability to face reality no matter how difficult
- ❏ Positive intentions
- ❏ Gratitude
- ❏ Compassion
- ❏ Determined spirit
- ❏ Humility
- ❏ Emotional endurance
- ❏ Warmth

Add a few positive qualities of your own.

This is only the beginning…self-esteem is addressed further in chapter 7, where we see how it relates to increasing your capacity for love.

More Food for Thought

Do you feel on par with most people you associate with or do you perceive a hierarchy in which a lot of other people seem to be on the top and you on the bottom? Explain.

How do you feel about your relative position in the pecking order?

What holds you back from having higher status?

Are you satisfied with where you are or are you striving to climb higher?

Are these goals in your best interest? If so, describe the insights and tools you can use to achieve them.

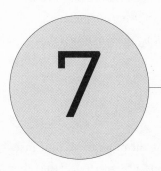

Increasing Your Capacity for Love

I ponder "What is hell?" I maintain that
it is the suffering of being unable to love. —Dostoevsky

Love Challenged

Whether single or involved in a relationship—people are looking for answers to a common conundrum—how to love.

So many people in the world are love challenged.[1] Some are struggling to find someone to love; others, to love the person they're with. Being unable to love—to feel and give love—is a major problem plaguing relationships all over the world.

This chapter explores this issue for two reasons: First, many of you are at the receiving end of your partner's difficulty with love. That's what brings most of you to this book. To assuage your feelings of hurt and rejection, it helps to recognize that the love failure was your partner's, rather than evidence of your own personal failings. With this insight you can not only salvage your self-esteem but use it to create a new dialogue with your ex, and finally address some of the real issues underlying the breakup, empowering you to reach better resolution or closure.

Second, maybe you are the one who has difficulty being able to love and have yet to recognize it. Perhaps you choose unavailable partners to mask this problem. This chapter is going to explore yet another layer of the abandonment cycle—those abandoholic patterns that cause you or someone you care about to break your love connections out of confusion and false beliefs.

A Lot of Love Problems Occur in the Middle Stages

As you've no doubt noticed, romantic love tends to flow more easily at the beginning of a relationship. After you've been together for a while, the novelty wears off. The constant availability of your partner can dampen romantic intensity. After coming down from the initial infatuation, you both stand face to face with all of your imperfections glaring in the daylight. You enter the middle phase. Indeed, some people are very good at beginnings but very poor at middles.

"I seem to go about three dates before I start getting itchy," says Rebecca. "I don't feel the attraction anymore, so I start pulling back. I know this is a pattern of mine, so I try to stretch it out for another couple of dates. Eventually my relationships all end the same—with me telling them to take it slow. 'Let's get some space,' I tell them, trying to be as anesthetic as possible."

Top-Heavy Relationships

During the middle period, one side of the partnership can pull back, causing the other to become insecure and hang on more tightly. These roles are exchangeable; each partner gets a chance to feel the other one pulling away. Reciprocally feeling the pull of the attachment allows both sides to develop staying power. Frequently though, one side of the equation pulls back more than the other, tipping the power to the side of the more detached partner. As the relationship unbalances, one side feels engulfed, the other abandoned.

When our partners dangle love in front of us but don't follow through, we tend to give over our control. All of the energy keeping the relationship together comes from us—we feel the love and attachment for both parties. At this point, the craving and desperation we feel begin to seem more like an addiction than a relationship.

Distancers tend to remain oblivious to their partner's plight. By withholding what you want most—love and commitment—they gain emotional power over you. They keep you on a string, exploiting your love to fill a gap in their lives. What gap? The one created by their own difficulty with love. They fill the gap with power and control instead of love.

Being love challenged is a common but difficult problem to diagnose. People generally conceal this truth from themselves and their therapists under the guise of not having found the right person. People's penchant for false attribution allows them to blame their difficulty with love on a multitude of inadequacies their partners supposedly have. When you're at the receiving end of this—being blamed for someone else's love deficiencies—your self-esteem can take a beating.

"I felt criticized all the time," says Sarah. "I tried to be perfect, more desirable, change the things he didn't like. But I could never seem to get it right. I wished I'd realized then that his constant complaints were just excuses for his own problem with commitment. It would have saved me from doubting my worth for so many years."

Love Obstacles

Here are some situations that may have caused you or someone you know to disconnect from a relationship when it entered the middle stage.

Stuck in Neutral

In an extremely common scenario, people complain that their relationship is stuck in neutral. You or your partner wants to move forward, the other one doesn't. Let's say, this time it's you who wants to end a relationship. Imagine it: You don't want to hurt your partner because there is real caring between you, you just want a chance to find somebody better. You've become ambivalent, critical, fault finding, and nitpicky, and you lose sexual interest. You've built a case against your partner to justify your emotional shutdown.

Your friends know how ambivalent you feel, and so does your therapist. You've already regaled them with your laundry list of your partner's faults and inadequacies.

"Why do you stay in situations that aren't right for you?" your friends ask. Bolstered by this support, you finally get the courage to break up with this person. Of course, your friends recite the expected congratulations for doing so: "You were right not to stay in a relationship that wasn't giving you what you needed." Or, "It was about time you moved on." Even your therapist supports your decision, suggesting that ending your relationship constituted real growth on your part, a real breakthrough. Indeed, you may feel empowered by it, a sense of triumph. After all, leaving your partner put you in the vanquishing position. You feel badly about causing pain, but at least you're not the victim this time.

Why then, a few months later—when your ex has found somebody new—do you feel so devastated? In many cases, you feel regretful and lonely because although you feel that breaking up was right for you, it just takes time to get through the separation process. But it's important to ask yourself some questions to see if there is more you can learn from the experience.

Check all that seem plausible.

COULD IT BE THAT...

- ❏ Love showed up and I wasn't ready for it?
- ❏ I decided to break up just as it was becoming a real relationship?
- ❏ I couldn't handle the emotional intimacy that was developing?
- ❏ I've falsely attributed my own internal struggle to my partner's supposed inadequacies?
- ❏ My cycles of abandonment or some other unresolved abandonment issue got in the way?
- ❏ I have trouble giving, feeling, and receiving love but have yet to realize it?
- ❏ I have trouble with "middles" of relationships?

If any of these could possibly be true for you or for your ex, confronting the issues now may keep love from eluding you the next time.

Mutually Injured Parties

In another common relationship malady, you feel abandoned by your partner during the relationship, so you feel justified in pulling back. Each one abandons the other in a different way. But before you opt out, stop to consider the following.

Check all that seem plausible.

- ❏ I have difficulty taking responsibility for my own feelings of insecurity, fear, and dependency.
- ❏ Though I admit to being a bottomless pit of emotional needs, I want my partner to fill the hole.
- ❏ My own neediness has caused me to give too much power to my partner; I've volunteered to play victim.
- ❏ My uncomfortable feelings are triggered by my partner to be sure, but I'm confused into thinking he created them.
- ❏ I'm blaming uncomfortable feelings accumulated from previous abandonment wounds on my partner.
- ❏ What feels like my partner's emotional neglect is really my own vulnerability—emotional hunger left over from childhood.
- ❏ Little Me has become so needy that no one outside of myself can possibly fulfill me.
- ❏ I've placed my partner in a no-win position.
- ❏ My anger spurts out of control when my partner can't instantly remove my feelings of desperation and neediness.
- ❏ When my partner falls short of accomplishing these impossible tasks, I falsely attribute my insatiable needs to something missing in her.

Why Do We Blame Our Love Issues on the Person Who Wants to Be with Us?

For most abandonment survivors, just being close to someone can throw us into an overblown emotional response. Love makes us vulnerable. When someone gets close, she bumps into our love wounds and hits against the tenderness and pain left over from past abandonments.

The insecurity you feel is painful and can cause you to feel angry, turned off, blameful, or insatiable. Who's right there to blame? The person who reached out to you and inadvertently set off your love pain.

For people who have been through heartbreaks and losses in the past, it is common to develop panicky feelings of insecurity when attempting a new relationship—one of the symptoms of posttraumatic stress disorder of abandonment.[2]

POSTTRAUMATIC STRESS DISORDER OF ABANDONMENT

Intense fear of abandonment	Tendency to repeat abandonment themes in your life
Intrusive anxiety from past losses	Memory blocks of childhood
Extreme sensitivity to rejection	Tendency to shut down emotionally
Difficulty letting go, excessive need for security	Tendency toward self-defeating or self-destructive behavior

Trying to understand the cause of your lovesick feelings is fraught with confusion. You think you want out, but you're not sure if it's you or your partner who's causing the problem. After all, there is such a thing as justifiable abandonment—when you want out because your partner is an alcoholic, emotionally or physically abusive, cheating on you, or won't commit, etc. To separate false attribution from reality, it helps to ask yourself some questions.

Check all that apply.

- ❏ Might the problems in the relationship be caused by having unrealistic expectations of my partner?
- ❏ In pulling back, am I the one being emotionally difficult this time?
- ❏ Is my own insecurity creating the instability in the relationship?
- ❏ Am I projecting my own vulnerability onto my partner?
- ❏ Is my partner guilty of emotional abuse?
- ❏ Is it possible that my partner isn't guilty of emotional abuse but is just getting too close to my old abandonment wounds?
- ❏ Am I able to assume responsibility for my own posttraumatic stress symptoms—those lovesick feelings?
- ❏ Am I the one being the abandoner this time?

The cloud of confusion rising up from the turbulence of a new relationship can truly obscure real issues. Being rigorously honest with yourself helps pull back the veil of self-deceit. Indeed, the first step in dismantling your love barriers is recognizing your side of the equation.

Identify the patterns that keep short-circuiting your attempts to find love. The more awareness you gain, the more you can inoculate yourself from breaking future connections when a new relationship reaches the middle phase. Below are more examples of what can go wrong.

When Security Turns You Off

Have you ever been in a relationship in which you felt entirely sure of the other person's love? If so, you had an opportunity to discover whether security turns you off. It is easy to feel the pull of attachment when your partner remains detached because the emotional challenge sustains your interest. The ultimate test is when someone becomes fully available. When you feel secure, you can take your partner for granted, at which point, the dynamics can go from fireworks to no spark at all. With the emotional challenge gone, you can become bored, shut down emotionally, or lose sexual interest. Feeling secure may empower you to feel in control of your life for a change, but the restlessness may tempt you to look elsewhere for romantic excitement.

It's not always easy to draw the fault line.

"I thought I had Prince Charming, but I began to see him as a needy person. Every time I'd go out with my friends or feel too tired to go over to his place, he'd complain that I didn't want to spend time with him. I was all set to accuse him of being too dependent on me. Then something someone said in my abandonment support group got me thinking: Am I creating this neediness in him? If the tables were turned, wouldn't I feel in need of more attention?"

Having a partner who wants to be with you can kick up your fear of engulfment, and distort your perception of him. It helps to check in with yourself to assess the real issues before you run away.

Have you ever felt so secure that you took your mate for granted?

Did this dampen the emotional or sexual dynamics of the relationship? Describe.

Have you ever felt engulfed or pressured by someone's attachment to you, and wanted to end it? Describe.

Action Bullet: I feel _____ when _____, and in future relationships I plan to remind myself _____ _____.

When You Have the Edge

When one person has more of an edge than the other, the relationship can become unbalanced. Maybe this time it's you who is not sure you want the relationship. Maybe you're the one who's got the edge. Maybe you're more experienced, more confident than your partner. Maybe you're the one with the better career. Maybe you consider yourself more eligible and desirable than him. So your fear of loss is less pronounced, making the emotional stakes that much higher for him. Your take-it-or-leave-it attitude toward the relationship puts him in the emotionally disadvantaged position. When one side is more invested than the other in holding on to the relationship, the dynamics of push and pull set in.

Q

Have you ever had the edge in a relationship? When?

What did it feel like?

What were the emotional advantages to you?

What were the disadvantages?

When You Think You've Loved Before

One of the things that makes it difficult to recognize whether your lack of feelings indicates that you might be love challenged is when you believe you've felt intense love for previous partners, just not this one.

> *"I keep trying for a reasonable relationship with an eligible woman," says Michael, "but I can't seem to get over Jeannie, the one who trampled my heart about two years ago. She constantly blew me off, lied, cheated, and played with my emotions. I've tried to start new relationships, but at some point I lose interest and hit the wall and then go right back to obsessing about Jeannie. She's the only one I've ever seemed to love."*

Michael's case illustrates people's confusion about being love challenged. They haven't figured out yet that they can only experience that intense craving for unavailable partners.

When the Love Is Gone

Sometimes in a long-term relationship, it feels as if the love is gone. Your spouse imagines she is no longer in love with you. The hitch is that the love she felt at the beginning was intense and compelling because she was pursuing love, not attaining it. By now, she's secure with you and feels bereft of all that emotional excitement.

Remember, insecurity is an aphrodisiac. When you're not sure of your partner's commitment, your fear of abandonment kicks in and causes you to feel that lovesick craving. This feeling is very different from the more stable feelings that develop when you feel secure.

When You're Involved in Triangles

Take a moment to think of all the triangles[3] you've been in since birth—between your mother, father, and you; between mother, sister, and you; between your best friend, her other friend, and you; etc. Triangles create a good deal of competition.[4] The players compete for exclusive rights to a prized parent, friend, or lover. When you feel like the odd man out, it means you've become triangulated.[5]

Many of you have written to me about your painful triangles.

"My boyfriend has an old girlfriend who keeps coming into the picture. When she's buzzing around, he treats me like chopped liver. All of my friends consider someone else to be their best friend, instead of me. It seems I'm always at the short end. Some days, I feel abandoned by everybody."

Getting into triangles can become a pattern for the love challenged. You need to be competing for someone's love to feel any pull. If there's no third party to compete with, there's not enough challenge to keep your romantic juices flowing.

"I fell madly in love with Heather—one of the wives at the club. Her husband was a distant kind of guy. I could tell that she wasn't completely happy in her marriage. I pursued her relentlessly and finally won her over by being more attentive and supportive than he was. All during our affair, I tried to get her to leave him and come with me, but she remained elusive. Then there was a tragic turn of events. He was suddenly killed in a skiing accident. Now I had Heather all to myself. No more triangle. Somehow that changed the dynamics—with her looking to me for support more and more—and I've lost my attraction to her. That's when I knew I needed help."

Howard's example is unusual. Most people have a difficult time recognizing their addiction to the competition involved in love triangles.

What triangles have you been in? Was there a triangle involving mother, father, and you? Sister, mother, and you? Father, uncle, and you? Spouse, mother-in-law, and you? Name two people involved in one of your earlier triangles:

_____ and _____

Did you get triangulated (the short end of the stick)? How did it feel?

Are you involved in triangles today?

Do they arouse feelings of insecurity, jealousy, inadequacy?

Or do you enjoy the sense of competition they stir up?

Does this cause you to get hooked? Explain.

How do you handle your triangles?

What insights do you have to better manage your triangles?

"Why Can't I Fall in Love Like Every Other Man? What Kind of Fool Am I?"

Since the distinction between *pursuing* love and *having* love is lost on most people, it's easy to see how confusing this love game can get. You don't suspect that you have trouble loving because you remember having felt intense love for previous partners. What you fail to realize is that the love pangs were really conquest, competitive pursuit, and insecurity all mixed together. You loved before, but only when your partners were withholding something you wanted, and this withholding generated a release of love chemicals to keep you in heated pursuit.[6] You forgot that in the end, they wound up leaving you. By failing to understand the dynamics involved, you conclude that you have no problem loving, but that you haven't found someone who turns you on.

"I never felt bored with my former lover," explains William. "Not that we had such great communication. Jason was always avoiding issues by running off with his friends or getting involved in

time-consuming projects. Our sex life wasn't that great either—I was usually more interested than he was. But I always looked forward to coming home just knowing he'd be there. When he left me for someone else, I was devastated for over a year. Until I met Sam. We really hit it off at first, but now I'm unsure. He's responsive and giving, but this time the problem is me. I don't feel turned on anymore. A part of me wants to go back out there and seek someone who excites me the way Jason did."

William's problem is a common one. He felt intense feelings toward Sam during the early stages of pursuit and then lost those feelings when he became sure of him. William isn't able to recognize his feelings toward Sam as love because they don't match his reference point about what love is supposed to feel like. Does William feel respect? Yes. Does he care about Sam? Yes. Does he trust and admire him? Yes. But he doesn't feel the emotional hunger he's used to from all those years of trying to win over an emotionally unavailable partner, so he doesn't think he feels love. He's looking for the wrong feeling, one he's misidentified as love.

Defining a Narrow Path for Love

One of the leading causes for this national epidemic—the inability to love—is that, like William, we tend to define a narrow path for love. Many people in our society have misconceptions about love.

Check all you are familiar with.

I BELIEVE LOVE IS…

- ❑ Something I'm supposed to fall into.
- ❑ A feeling of magical proportions.
- ❑ Something that can happen at first sight or at least by the second date.
- ❑ An altered state of consciousness.
- ❑ A blissful kind of trance that overtakes me when I meet the right person.
- ❑ A warm feeling that delivers me from the doldrums of everyday life.

The above feelings pertain to the initial infatuation and are not prevalent during the middle phase. I'm not knocking these ebullient feelings, because they are highly pleasurable and represent a perfectly legitimate natural high.[7] But infatuation is highly combustible and can easily go up in smoke. In many cases, infatuation can turn your life into a roller coaster with soaring emotional highs and stomach-churning lows.[8]

Infatuation is temporary. When one or both sides of the couple come down from euphoria and the relationship enters the middle phase, trouble begins to erupt in paradise—especially if one of you crashes before the other one does. At this point, those of you who are love challenged get to find out whether you're able to tolerate secure love, or whether your love capacity goes belly up.[9]

Becoming a Love Junkie

Lots of people are infatuation junkies. They move from relationship to relationship, always looking for a new partner to trigger that emotional high. They seek romantic love because they know how effectively it medicates them from loneliness, depression, and their chronic concerns. New romance lifts the spirits. Belonging to someone is a welcome relief from the chronic malaise associated with heartache, loneliness, and feeling not so good about yourself.

Remind yourself to hang in there. Long-term relationships offer more substantial benefits and even have a chemical incentive in that they stimulate a steady production of endogenous opiates that reward you with a feeling of warmth and well-being, bringing stability to your life.[10]

Love and Depression

Some of you have described being depressed, even though you have a working long-term relationship providing you with all of the security and support you need. Depression and distress can cut you off from your ability to feel and cause your emotional life to go flat. When you're depressed, it becomes difficult to create love for your partner—to feel, give, express, or experience love. Your creative energy—love's greatest resource—momentarily stops flowing.[11] Some depressed people blame their lack of love feelings on their relationship or on their mate. Couple counseling, individual therapy, and psychiatric intervention are ways to take responsibility for overcoming the problem.

Is It Love or Self-Abuse?

When you feel unworthy of love, you tend to seek partners who treat you the way you feel about yourself—poorly.

> *"I married this guy who cheated on me within the first year, but I kept giving him another chance. Then he began hitting me, apologizing profusely afterward. You guessed it. I kept giving him another chance. I'd been my father's scapegoat, and this guy just fit right into my picture of myself as a powerless victim. I felt too much contempt for myself to get rid of him, almost like I deserved to be treated this way."*

Unrealistic Expectations

One of the greatest barriers to love involves having unrealistic ideas about what a relationship is supposed to be. We want all of our emotional needs to be met in one basket.[12] When this one person doesn't live up to our romantic ideals, we either overtax the capacity of the relationship and bring it to its breaking point or run away to pursue someone else in hopes of satiating our needs.

It is reasonable to expect your primary relationship to meet some needs, but you are responsible for the balance.

"I'm with this new guy and I have real affection for him. We get along great. He doesn't happen to be an intellectual. Ten years ago, that was the most important thing—the guy had to dazzle me with his intellect to turn me on. If he couldn't cut the mustard in debating theoretical physics or something, I'd get turned off. With my new guy, I cherish his warmth and tenderness. He is a good person. I never get bored; but if I did, I have plenty of ways to get intellectual stimulation—from my other friends, and all kinds of stuff going on in the city."

When you're caught up in romantic frenzy, you could easily live in a shack on a desert island with no food or water and still be happy, as long as you had your romantic partner. But when you become securely mated and your love chemistry returns to "normal," you go back to desiring the material comforts you were accustomed to, such as friends, family, career, and amenities, etc.

Having more realistic expectations to begin with can help you better appreciate the person you are with. It means you are responsible for a larger portion of your own fulfillment. The message is to continue to pursue your independent life while pursuing a new relationship.

Shifting Values, Adjusting Expectations

Sometimes our expectations shift as we get older. Many in your late forties and above have written to me about how much the criteria for who you consider to be a good mate have changed.

"When I was younger," says Bernadette, "a prospect had to be a bit wiser and more successful than me and about three years older, to be ideal. My first husband had an engineering degree and was the major breadwinner. But now in my fifties, I don't care about those things. Why? Because I have my own success. That's why. Now, the guy could be a lot younger and a lot less accomplished than me. None of that stuff matters as long as he's a decent human being. It's not that I've lowered my standards; it's that I have my own success and I've evolved."

"My former girlfriends had to have polish, sophistication, regal beauty—all of that," says Steve. "Now I see that as packaging, plastic, lamination—decorations on the person, not the person themselves. I'm living my life now based on different values. I'm so glad I'm past the false-value stage of life. What turns me on now is the essence of the person inside—her sweetness, her trustworthiness. It doesn't matter what college she went to, what kind of family she grew up in, or whether she uses pluperfect verbs correctly. It took years of experience and self-love before I came to realize that it's the human qualities that count—and I don't need someone to match every one of my own attributes."

Let your primary relationship be what it is rather than burdening it with expectations it isn't designed to meet. Don't let your concept of love stay mired in your old beliefs. The task is to resist conforming to your friends' or society's values. Sometimes it takes getting older to feel that you have enough personal authority to rewrite the rules. Seek fulfillment through multiple resources—not just through your partner. That is what the outside world is there for.

Stuck in a Romantic Ideal

A great deal of your love response involves conditioning.[13] Your parents and other early experiences conditioned you to respond to certain stimuli. Maybe you tried to win over a mother who was emotionally unreliable. Later you associated the insecurity and emotional hunger you felt with romantic love. In high school you didn't feel any chemistry unless your date evoked these old yearning feelings.

During adolescence and early adulthood, these romantic notions get played out and reinforced by crushes and heartaches. Some of you have a hard time letting go of your high-school values, even when they prove to be at odds with your adult needs.

> *"My ideal type is Gwyneth Paltrow," says George. "Thin, blond, and elegant. I've dated a few women like this, but so far no one stayed. My most recent girlfriend is Mandy. Even though she's a brunette with a stockier build, we hit it off. She is really a match for me—successful, great personality, beautiful inside and out. All my friends love her. My family thinks she's great. It was really intense between us at first—but I can't get used to her body type. I'm still hoping to find the tall, blond woman of my dreams, and I resent Mandy for not being that person. I've tried to talk sense to myself—we get along great and I know she's perfect for me, I really know that. But try telling that to my sex drive. My body started reacting to her like she's just a friend. I've lost interest and don't know how to get it back."*

Married People with Love Wounds

It isn't just single people who are love challenged. Many suffer this incapacity within a committed relationship. Marriage can place walls around your love wounds—walls restricting you from gaining access to the outside world of possibilities.

> *"I don't love John anymore. I guess he's been so distant and noncommunicative for so long, my own feelings finally just went cold. The woman in me is desperately lonely. With no love, I feel no hope. I feel trapped."*

Sometimes recovering from love loss involves scaling your prison walls and leaving the marriage behind. But if you want to treat yourself as a responsible physician would, you'll want to rule out all other possible causes for your symptoms. Physicians rule out other diseases by performing diagnostic tests. You do this by subjecting your feelings to careful self-examination. One of the first things to consider is whether you may have attributed your uncomfortable feelings to the wrong cause.

Check all that seem possible.

- ❏ Am I blind to the potential for love with my current companion because I'm chasing after a romantic ideal?
- ❏ Do I have difficulty loving when I feel completely secure?
- ❏ Have I lost access (due to depression, perhaps) to the creative process of love?
- ❏ Am I displacing my dissatisfactions with life onto my partner?

What is your own explanation for your love issues?

What insights can you use to resolve them?

Universal Source of Love

Going through heartbreak means that you're going through a loss of love. But it's only your ex's love you're missing. Love itself is all around and within you. Abandonment recovery provides both opportunity and incentive to tap into the universal source of love—the kind you can generate within yourself. Self-love holds the power of connection to others.

SWAN LESSON SEVEN
Increasing Your Capacity for Love

In the story, the little girl was bereft of love and returned to the swan for help. He showed her that she already possessed this precious commodity within.

"You have the capacity for love, just as I do, Amanda. Its warmth is waiting for you."
   "But I don't have any."

"Yes, you do," says the swan, "and it's there waiting for you to discover it."

"How?"

"Begin with the idea of love, Amanda. Press the idea into your chest. Feel the warmth of your hands and hold the idea of love in your heart at the same time."

"But I want love and nobody wants me," cries the little girl.

"I too have felt others pull away," explains the swan. "At first the other swans did not welcome me—until I found my capacity to create love." The swan stretches his long graceful neck and turns in the water. "I generated love inside myself until it grew so bright and bold that it shone upon them. But I did not need them to receive it. My capacity for love was free for them to take or leave. Love has become my beacon, guiding my way through the giant ocean ever since."

The little girl presses her palms upon her heart. "I have nothing to love!" she cries. "I am alone."

"So am I, Amanda, but I love."

"Love? What is there to love?" she demands.

"I love life. I love existence. I love me. I love the idea of love."

"But that goes in a circle," says the little girl.

"It's the circle of love," agrees the swan, "a perfect circle."

The little girl closes her eyes once again and burrows within herself. She presses warmth from her hands down into her heart.

"That's right, Amanda. Whenever you need love, press your palms against your chest and create its warmth inside yourself. Imagine that this is love. Hold on to the idea and let it radiate outward to others. It takes lots of practice and time, but each time you become master of its power, you connect to others. You deepen your own experience."

We all have a capacity to increase love—a capacity that allows our human worth to expand on a daily basis. We live our lives using only a fraction of our capacity to express and experience love. During abandonment we feel bereft of that precious commodity altogether. Take a moment to consider that love can grow and expand within—whether you are alone or in a relationship. It is the kind of love you can feel for a fellow human being, spiritual being, child, pet, lover, life itself. It is the kind of love you give to yourself.

Love is a creative process. Starting from ground zero, you can learn to create that love right now in your current life, whether you're alone or part of a couple. Express it by being caring, considerate, and emotionally present with others and with yourself. Create it by discovering that you have the capacity to generate love from within.

Try the little girl's gesture yourself. Press your palms against your heart and feel the warmth. It's a gesture we perform during heartfelt times, even when we're not conscious of it.

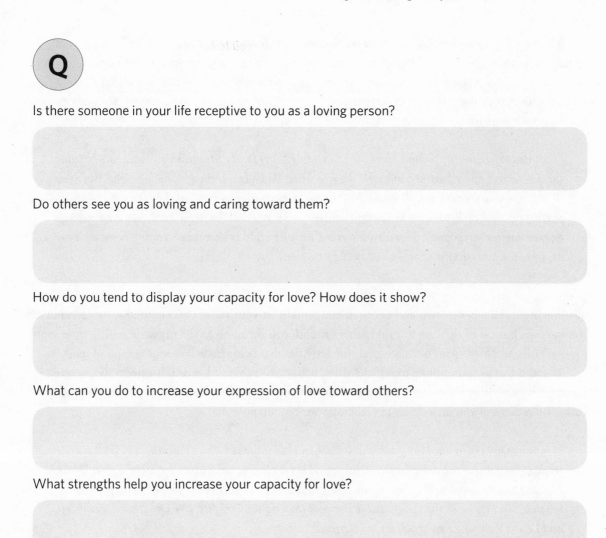

Q

Is there someone in your life receptive to you as a loving person?

Do others see you as loving and caring toward them?

How do you tend to display your capacity for love? How does it show?

What can you do to increase your expression of love toward others?

What strengths help you increase your capacity for love?

Self-Control versus Immediate Gratification

We constantly hear: to love somebody else, you have to first love yourself. The second *Akeru* exercise, discussed in chapter 5, allowed you to put this aphorism into practice. As you continue performing the Big You / Little You Dialogue on a daily basis, self-love becomes not an abstraction, but an action you practice toward yourself—Big You to Little You.

The greatest boon to sticking to an exercise regimen is self-discipline. Not coincidentally, self-discipline is also a critical component in the ability to love.

Put another way, one of the biggest stumbling blocks to loving yourself or anyone else is the difficulty in delaying gratification. You want things to come to you by way of a magic bullet, rather than by exercising the self-discipline it takes to forgo immediate pleasures and work toward longer-range goals.

The need for immediate gratification is common among abandonment survivors of childhood. To assuage uncomfortable feelings stemming from your accumulation of losses and disconnections, you grab for quick fixes, even when you know that doing so sabotages your ambitions. Getting stuck in this pattern causes your dreams to drift farther and farther away. You grow anxious and guilty about not reaching your potential.

"I wanted to lose twenty pounds for my son's wedding," says Linda. "It meant giving up my bedtime snacks—a bad habit I formed after my divorce when I'd be languishing alone at night. But even with the wedding coming up, I couldn't resist the potato chips in front of the television. I'd keep putting off the diet till tomorrow. Tomorrow never came. With all the stress, I did, however, manage to gain another ten pounds. This meant torture, because I had to share the wedding event with my ex, who had his skinny new wife constantly by his side."

During internalization, when your self-esteem is at an all-time low and your glucocorticoids at an all-time high, you feel depleted and defeated and tend to let your more challenging life projects fall to the wayside. Instead of fighting to gain higher ground, you succumb to the urgencies rising from your love wounds. You forgo your ultimate goals for activities that bring instantaneous feel-good relief.

The antidote to succumbing to self-defeating behaviors is to build your self-esteem by engaging in constructive activities. Once you raise your sense of worth a notch or two, your ability to delay gratification increases and you inch closer to reaching your human potential.

"I never drank much until my girlfriend left. Then I got into the habit of meeting my friends after work at the pub. I ordered drink after drink until I wasn't feeling any pain. One night, I got a D.W.I. I knew I had to stop drinking, but I was lonely and needed to be around people. I still go down to the pub, but I try to be the designated driver—at least on some nights. I've just started a new job, and I don't want any new problems to interfere."

Why Is Achieving Goals Such a Struggle?

It is easy to get stuck in the Internalizing stage and get mired in feelings of low self-worth, especially if you've been through rejections and heartbreaks in the past. By internalizing feelings of self-doubt, you come to believe you're not entitled to what you really want. Emotional hunger from past wounds urges you to seek insubstantial rewards; the equivalent of candy, which pleasures your mouth but leaves you malnourished and stimulates greater hunger later on. Laden with self-doubt and depleted of confidence, you don't feel strong enough about yourself to sustain the ongoing effort it takes to achieve higher-reaching goals. This explains why abandonment survivors are notorious underachievers.

"I wanted to become a doctor," says Holly. "I had the academic qualifications and my adoptive parents had the bankroll, but with all of the abandonment I'd been through, I didn't feel grounded enough to keep up the constant studying. Med school turned out to be all work and no play, so I gave it all up to go out and party with my friends—the ones who didn't have such high aspirations.

Now we're all pretty much in the same boat, struggling to get out of dead-end careers and other bad habits."

Self-Love versus Self-Indulgence

Self-love does not mean self-indulgence. Many people confuse the two. Self-indulgence means you're buying an extravagance you can't afford, having one cookie too many, or wallowing in your misery. Self-love means nurturing your needs by doing something that's good for your growth and development.

Name the last time you grabbed for a quick fix—an indulgence that didn't help you in the long run. Was it chocolate? A third glass of wine? Sleeping through your alarm clock? What?

How did this self-indulgence make you feel?

Name a long-range goal you've put by the wayside.

Name the temptations that thwart you from achieving this goal.

Name a time when you were able to delay immediate gratification to accomplish one of your goals.

How did having self-discipline make you feel?

Name a time you engaged in a pleasurable activity, but one that did not interfere in your long-range goals—taking a bubble bath or visiting a museum.

How did this make you feel?

Action Bullet: Although I feel tempted to _____,
I will _____.

Procrastination—Abandonment Survivors' Number One Downfall

Procrastination is another form of indulgence. You keep postponing positive action.

"I figured out the only things I say no to are the ones I should be doing," says Keaton. "The stuff that's no good for me? I say yes. Cigarettes? Yes. Booze? Keep it flowing. Sex with a stranger? Sure. Junk food? Second bag of Fritos, please. But how about finishing my degree? No. Getting my car inspected on time? No. Raking my leaves? Not until tomorrow. Finishing my paperwork? No. I'm a master at procrastination."

Abandonment survivors tend to procrastinate because they've internalized negative messages of rejection. Their sense of entitlement has been breached. So they forgo the opportunity to feel good about themselves and their achievements.

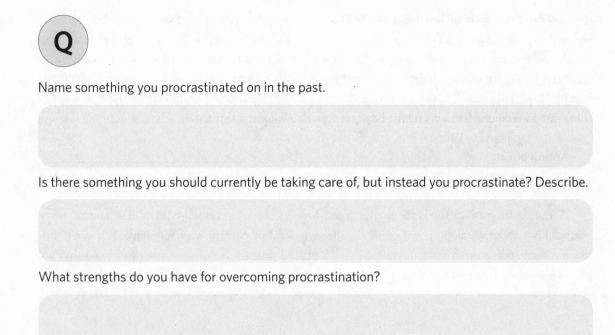

Q

Name something you procrastinated on in the past.

Is there something you should currently be taking care of, but instead you procrastinate? Describe.

What strengths do you have for overcoming procrastination?

Action Bullet: I feel _____ because _____,
and I am going to _____.

Self-Control and Self-Esteem

Nothing is harder on your self-esteem than feeling as if you were your own worst enemy. Nothing erodes self-respect more than feeling you can't help yourself from doing what you know isn't good for you.

> *"My credit cards hit the max," says Juliana. "I thought I was on top of the problem, but I still wanted to go out to dinner every night and buy clothes and things whenever the spirit moved me. When I splurged really bad, I felt horrible and woke up in cold sweats in the middle of the night, afraid I'd wind up losing my house. I felt like I had no control over my life."*

Giving in to your impulses at the expense of achieving your goals brings on overwhelming feelings of fear, shame, embarrassment, and guilt. Depreciating yourself in this manner intensifies your desire to medicate the anxiety with more immediate gratifications, higher doses of alcohol, food, or shopping. This need for quick fixes creates a downward spiral leading to self-contempt.

> *"I feel too down to meet with my personal trainer today. I know I should go because I paid in advance and besides, he's waiting for me. But I just don't feel like getting out of bed." Later that day... "I finally got up, but I am so far behind in my day. I feel wasted and low."*

You can't magically make your down feelings disappear, but you can control your behavior. Force yourself to go to the gym; get into the moment; perform the Big You / Little You Akeru exercise, perform the Dream House exercise (described in chapter 8), or pick up the phone to talk out your feelings with a trusted friend* or therapist. Any of these initiatives can lead to a more positive emotional climate within. How? They are all ways of delaying the need for self-destructive gratifications. By doing something good for yourself, you create the basis on which to commend yourself.

> **Action Bullet:** I feel _____ because _____,
> and I am going to _____.

If immediate gratification is the enemy of self-love, its best friend is self-control. The control we've been talking about all along is *self*-control—the only kind of control we really have. You can't control another, you can only control yourself. Self-control's domain is not over your feelings—they are givens—but over how you handle them.

How to Love

Self-discipline is an important component in the ability to love. Love isn't supposed to be "emotional candy" but something more substantial that hinges on self-control. Love involves your ability to make commitments and follow through.[14] The following IQ list is designed to help those of you who by now suspect that you are love challenged and are willing to delay gratification and use new insight and tools to get there.

The actions described below come naturally to those who don't have difficulty loving, but are much more challenging for those of you who have been caught up in patterns of reabandonment.

ADVICE FOR THE LOVE CHALLENGED

Check the items you need to work on, and circle the ones you're already practicing.

❏ The first step is to recognize that I have a problem.
This can be the most difficult step owing to all the layers of self-deceit and false attribution that have been confusing you all along.

---

* Go online to abandonment.net anytime, day or night, to share your situation with us. Click on HELP CENTER and submit your PERSONAL STORIES.

❏ I will redefine love for myself.

Love is not an absolute feeling, nor is it confined to infatuation. When it comes to love, one size doesn't fit all. Love is a set of feelings unique to the two people involved in forming a bond.

❏ I will decide to make *love* an action, a verb.

Don't rely on love to be an all-powerful feeling that motivates you to be loving. Motivate yourself.

❏ I will recognize that love is a creative process.

Be open to discovering your ability to create loving feelings.

❏ I will learn to make the connection between self-discipline and love.

Recognize that achieving love involves following through with loving actions on a consistent basis.

❏ I will carry out caring actions toward my partner.

The expression "Fake it till you make it" doesn't quite fit the bill here,[15] but I am suggesting that even when you feel at a loss for romantic feelings, walk yourself through the motions of caring. There is no dishonesty here, as you will see in the next step.

❏ I will honestly talk about my feelings with my partner—even if it means explaining that I have a
     problem with feeling love for him.

It is best to talk about the difficulty, since it is real. Holding back only hurts your partner more in the long run as he senses your rejection and blames it on himself.

❏ I will be responsible for my difficulty with love.

Tell your partner that this is a problem you have and that you're working on it. Again, don't blame your love issues on your mate's inadequacies.

❏ I will begin sentences with "This is about me, not about you" when I bring up my issues about
     the relationship so that my mate won't feel she's responsible for my struggle with love.
❏ I will show caring, not only when I feel the romantic desire for doing so but also just because I
     know it is the right thing to do.

You are investing in your own creative process of love, reinforcing *love* as a verb.

❏ I will plan to be completely in the moment with my partner.

Show up not just physically, but emotionally. Carefully attend to everything he or she says and does.

❏ I will create special moments with my partner.

Set the stage and atmosphere for optimal communication, intimacy, intensity, and joy. Remain in the moment.

❏ I will initiate conversations designed to get underneath the surface emotions.

Draw your partner out by asking gentle, caring questions to learn more about her emotional issues, such as how she feels about the relationship or about herself.

❏ Then I will share my own feelings—both about the relationship and about myself.

❏ I will initiate reciprocal conversations about our childhood experiences.

❏ I will initiate reciprocal sharing of current issues.

❏ Later, I'll ask follow-up questions to show that my interest carries through, that I continue to care about my partner's problems and interests.

❏ I will discuss our relationship.

Reciprocally sharing vulnerable feelings builds intimacy and trust.

❏ I will create new experiences with my partner, ones that only the two of us share.

Build your own personal legacy that belongs not to the individuals alone, but to the relationship.

❏ I will be open to a new range of feelings.

Remember, your old reference point for love might be based on feelings of infatuation or love conquest. Your love gauge is skewed by the fact that you were used to pursuing unavailable partners.

❏ I will tune in to the positive feelings I do have.

By now you should feel some closeness and caring. You might feel trust, respect, security. Rather than dismiss these feelings as not romantic, include them in your new definition of love. Sometimes it is hard to recognize love even when it's there working for you. Yes, feeling secure, caring, and comfortable may not be very intoxicating, but it is emotionally nourishing. Consider that this may be what it feels like to experience mutual love—love discovered anew.

❏ I will make myself sexually available.

This is an important step. Understand that your sexuality may be specifically conditioned to respond only to those who present an emotional challenge. Be patient with yourself; make allowances for the fact that insecurity is no longer serving as your aphrodisiac,

❏ I will share my sexual struggle openly with my partner.

Talking about it builds intimacy and relieves the pressure to perform. Within a relationship, sex becomes a way to consummate commitment and caring. The old you consummated love conquest. The new you is learning to consummate more substantial feelings, like mutuality and trust.

❏ I will try to open up to the wide range of feelings within the creative process of love.

When you're not holding back, your energy flows between you and your partner. Be open to receiving the sparks she sends back.

❏ I will remain consistently available and stay open to new feelings.
Keep making *love* an action verb.

Does following a list of regimented suggestions like these mean you should force yourself to stay with someone you have no feelings for? No. The list is helpful only if you've recognized that you have a problem with love, and that you're focusing your love energy on a worthy person. If these two conditions fit, then following this path can help you build toward a love that has eluded you in the past. Love is hard to recognize when you're accustomed to pursuing emotionally unavailable partners. Self-discipline overcomes these habits.

Nature Creates Love

Take an example from the billions of people around the globe who abide by the code of arranged marriages—a highly stable structure that provides love and nurture. In these societies, people do not rely on infatuation to initiate a bond.

Nature does not frown on arranged marriages any more than it does on marriages based on romantic attraction, nor does it bestow less love and sexuality. There are many mechanisms in place to ensure that two people who demonstrate loving actions toward one another on a regular basis can form an attachment and share pleasurable feelings. We discussed some of them in chapter 5—the powerful drugs within your body that promote attachment to your partner and to your social group—oxytocin, phenylethylamine (PEA), opioids, dopamine, prolactin, etc.,[16] as well as becoming addicted to each other's pheromones.[17]

Over time, being in a relationship and engaging in creature-to-creature behaviors—such as sleeping together, snuggling, sex, touching, thinking about the person—lead to mutual attachment. As two people's psychobiological systems meld into each other's, they create one interwoven neurohormonal system.[18] During your breakup, these intertwined systems go haywire. The connecting wires are pulled apart and go off sparking.[19] If your partner is in a new relationship, she has the advantage of hooking up her loose wires to a new lover and is spared feeling the shocking pain of disconnection. If you've been left alone, your mammalian brain continues searching for its lost object—truly the other half of your hormonal regulatory system.[20]

Your attachment energy creates extreme discomfort while you're still searching, but it also motivates you to increase your capacity for love. Abandonment strengthens this capacity, because it brings you in touch with your feelings. It forces you to recognize the power of human attachment. Vulnerability is a human condition. Your most painful feelings remind you what it

SCIENTIFIC TIDBIT

Ironically, the fact that your relationship became a "mutual regulatory system" is most apparent when it breaks apart. The pain is your first sign that you'd grown addicted to that person. That addiction is biochemical. You have been breathing in each other's pheromones, which are known to be habit forming. Your pupils dilated in synchrony, your breathing patterns synchronized, as did your speech patterning and your electrocardiographic (ECG) rhythms. Your cognitive mind incorporated your partner into your sense of future as well as in every aspect of your current life.

means to be alive and to need love. They teach the value of unconditional love—and you don't have to wait until you've found that special someone. You can begin practicing it right now with your friends, your family, and yourself.

More Food for Thought

What are your current thoughts about why you shut down emotionally or sexually when someone grew to need you?

What caused you to become so needy and upset, unbalancing your former relationships?

What insights and tools can you use to overcome these cycles of isolation and abandonment?

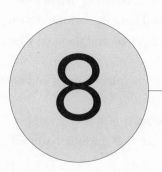

8 Letting Go

Letting go is the first step in bringing closure to your lost relationship. It allows you to relinquish your tenacious emotional grip on your loved one and accept the reality of loss. Only then can you grieve and move on. In letting go, you surrender to the positive forces of change. Reality is in flux, forever changing. Appreciate the transience of life by facing your reality in the moment.

Letting go reinvests your energy in new opportunities. Until you face an ending, you delay the beginning of your new life: Akeru. Letting go is the beginning of acceptance. The serenity prayer[1] is all about acceptance—learning to distinguish what you can change from what you can't. Once you gain acceptance of the unchangeable, you can move forward.

Acceptance doesn't mean grin and bear it—although in the early stages of abandonment, it may feel that way. Acceptance involves facing facts and letting go. Borrowing another piece of twelve-step philosophy, it means "accepting life on life's terms."[2]

Human beings are famous for going off half-cocked to do battle with the unchangeable. We all have a little Don Quixote in us, driven to tilt at windmills. The message is to stop railing against what you can't change. Protest prolongs heartbreak's pain. What is the opposite of protest? Letting go of trying to change it. Letting go redirects your energy from the past to the present.

Letting go allows you to stop fighting your feelings—especially anxiety, grief, and insecurity. Accept these feelings as belonging to a precious inner presence—to Little You. Little You needs your love, acceptance, and devotion. Rather than fight her feelings, address them. Administer to the needs that underlie them—work through them—rather than wage an internal war against them. Remain deeply committed to Little.

According to twelve-step philosophy: "An unrealistic expectation is a premeditated resentment."[3]

Let go of unrealistic expectations of others. This means letting others be who they are without the need to control.

This is a big step. It means giving up the need to have other people fill your hungry hole. Relinquishing people from your needs and demands sets up the dynamics for healthy relationships. It allows you to love people unconditionally for who they are, rather than who you need them to be.

Let go to focus not on your partner but on how you handle your side of the equation. Tell her your feelings, treat her according to your needs, but let go of your need to control her response. Over that, you have no control. Letting go allows you to interact with her as a separate person and stand on your own two feet.

Let go of your unrealistic expectations toward yourself. Accept yourself as you are, warts and all. This strengthens self-love.

Let go of your need to control the future. Do what you can each day to maximize your life opportunities and then let go of what you can't control—the outcome. When you arrive at the future, you will face it one day at a time.

The importance of letting go is illustrated in the next lesson of the black swan.

SWAN LESSON EIGHT
Letting Others Be Who They Are

In the story, the little girl had been practicing love, pressing her palms against her chest and using her imagination to generate warmth from within. As a new presence of love expanded within her, she noticed another child. His name is Jonathan. One day, he called out to her, and his loud voice frightened Amanda. She felt bruised from this encounter and sought guidance from her beloved swan.

"Jonathan was not nice to me!" cries the little girl.

"And you are hurt, I see," says the swan.

"Yes, I am, and I don't know what to do."

"Try using the Golden Rule. It's a powerful way to be with others. Treat them as you like to be treated."

"But I want him to be nice to me."

"The Golden Rule is not about how people treat you, but how you treat them, Amanda."

"But he doesn't deserve it. He was mean."

"It's not about what he deserves," says the swan. "It's about following the simple rule of treating others exactly as you like to be treated."

"But if I do, he will still be mean to me," says the little girl.

"You cannot control how he behaves or responds to you. You can only take care of yourself and let others be who they are."

"I want someone to care about me," cries the little girl.

"Be the one to care. Try the Golden Rule on the boy—treat him as you would like him to treat you."

"What if he is still not nice to me?"

"You have no control over how he feels or acts," says the swan. "Just practice the Golden Rule

and let go. Walk away knowing you lived up to your own idea of how to act toward people. Let people be who they are. It will help you be connected to them."

As the little girl takes in the swan's advice, she opens her hand in a gesture of letting go.

Think about the last time you were disappointed by someone's response to you. Describe.

Do you usually feel good about your side of the equation—how you treat others?

Are there strings attached when you are treating someone well? In other words, do you deliver kindness free of expectations or do you hope to get some recognition in return? Explain what usually motivates your kind deeds.

Do your expectations of others ever lead to feelings of frustration, resentment, hurt? Explain.

Consider a time when you were kind, generous, or loving to someone without having expectations of how they responded to you. Were you able to honor yourself for your positive behavior instead of looking to them for acknowledgment? Describe.

Think about what is unchangeable about your current situation—at least in the moment—and open your hand in a gesture of letting go. Describe the feelings that come up.

Can letting go help you reach better closure? How?

How can you apply letting go to other areas of your life?

Abandonment Grief

The special conditions of abandonment make the task of letting go especially challenging. Like anyone grieving a death, abandonment survivors have lost a loved one—a loss as complete and as life changing. But as we discussed in chapter 5, your closure remains incomplete because your loved one didn't die, but in most cases chose not to be with you. The feature that distinguishes abandonment grief from all others is the damage that feeling unloved does to your self-esteem.

For some of you, abandonment's special type of grief is evoked over and over, as you attempt yet another relationship, which falls by the wayside. The torment can erupt even when you've had a single date and he didn't call back. You had high hopes and now you feel unloved all over again.

In running abandonment recovery workshops, I find that one of the topics abandonment survivors appreciate hearing about most is the difference between abandonment grief and other forms of bereavement. They are relieved to have the unique circumstances of their special type of grief—the terrible blow of rejection and love loss—recognized.

We've already touched on the way rejection complicates your grieving process. Yearning for someone who has discarded you creates a deep personal injury. During Internalizing, you turn rage about being left against yourself. In attacking yourself for being unworthy and unlovable, you incur severe depression (often mistaken for clinical depression)—a depression that can leave residual damage. Insecurity, diminished self-worth, and emotional hunger reign for the duration of the Internalizing stage and can undermine future relationships.

These factors are nearly universal to abandonment, and yet society does not recognize this grief the way it does bereavement over death. It recognizes divorce as disruptive and stressful,[4] and it sympathizes with burdens carried by single parents; but beyond these logistical problems lies the demon at the root of the emotional disruption—the primal pain of abandonment. Losing someone's love—being left behind—makes going through divorce, separation, and isolation extremely difficult.

Not all relationships are cloaked in the time-honored institution of marriage and family. Perhaps you'd been together only a few months. In this case, your grief—recognized as heartbreak—may seem trivial to the larger world. As bereft as you feel, your heartache doesn't entitle you to wear black, attend a funeral, and receive bereavement cards from your co-workers and acquaintances. If you were to cry a lot in public, people who didn't know you well would think you had psychological problems, rather than displaying legitimized grief.

Abandonment creates an "ambiguous loss."[5] Because death was not involved, there is no finality to your loss—no absolute closure. This delays the process of letting go. Ambiguity generates false hope and prolongs the agonizing period of searching and waiting. You wait for your lost love to return well beyond what your friends and family may deem appropriate.

Following is a list of additional elements that make abandonment grief especially difficult.

HOW ABANDONMENT GRIEF DIFFERS FROM OTHER FORMS OF BEREAVEMENT

Check those you identify with.

❏ My loved one is not lost to my friends or family, but only to me.
This further isolates you in your grief.

❏ I am not granted bereavement leave from work.
Unless you seek consideration for extenuating circumstances—and usually only if you were married or have children to make arrangements for—this won't happen.

❏ I feel disinclined to tell co-workers and acquaintances about the circumstances of my emotional crisis.
This can be particularly true when your heartbreak is over a personal relationship. Your grief, which is nonetheless disabling, must be handled on your own time, shrouded in privacy.

❏ Because I'm not grieving a death, I feel embarrassed about my sudden weight loss and red nose, caused by crying on and off during the day.
❏ I don't have the status of widowhood.
Instead you're suddenly alone because someone's rejected you. In many cases, you've been replaced by someone else. Being dumped adds shame and humiliation to the burden of heartbreak.

❏ I feel like a victim—not of a natural life process like death but of my own alleged inadequacies and poor choices.
❏ There is no societal outreach for my kind of grief—no bouquets of flowers from distant relatives and no clergy at my door to offer consolations.

❏ I can't even visit a spiritual medium who conveys loving messages from the departed.
There would be no comforting message that he still watches over you with loving care. He's not on the other side, but going on with his life without you.

❏ I've suddenly been conscripted to single life against my will.
Being thrust into this aloneness kicks up your control issues. Widows have control issues too, but abandonment survivors feel them with a vengeance. Railing against the circumstances of your loss prolongs the protest, anger, and hurt.

❏ I wear out my friends and family with my pain and obsession.
They have difficulty remaining in empathy with you for the duration, because—until now—the prolonged nature of abandonment grief has been neither sufficiently understood nor acknowledged.

❏ Yearning for someone who has treated me poorly doesn't make sense to my friends. I feel judged and pressured to snap out of it.
Letting go is more difficult without a body to mourn over, so you remain in purgatory longer.

❏ I obsess and pine for my ex to stave off the torment of love loss and to stay plugged into the hope of regaining love.
❏ My friends want to fix it and give me simplistic advice, like "move forward."
This only makes you feel worse because it implies that they think they'd get over it more quickly than you. You think they must perceive you as emotionally feeble for staying in the pain so long.

❏ I sometimes blame myself for not being able to contain the pain.
❏ Deep down inside, though, I know I am doing my best, so I harbor anger toward my friends for failing to understand.
❏ I suspect that the emotional wound created by abandonment is more serious, more destructive, than society is willing to admit.

Add elements of your own experience with grief.

You have two jobs with respect to abandonment grief. One is to accept the pain of loss. The other is to reverse the injury to your sense of self. As you will see, the end of this chapter is devoted to these tasks.

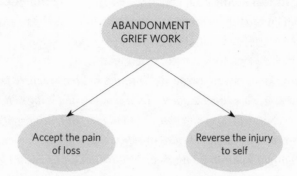

Hanging by a String

This story is about abandonment grief that occurs when the couple is still together, but barely. The elements of rejection and ambiguity make it extremely difficult to let go.

Jill's husband, Barton, had always been a loyal husband and devoted father, but he began having an affair after twenty-two years of marriage.

"When I found out, I was grief-stricken. I confronted him and he confessed. He pleaded with me to give him another chance. He said he'd get over the other woman—that he loved me too much to lose me. This did not ease my grief and turned me into a wreck.

"I agreed to let him stay, but he became more confused and morose by the day, saying he felt increasingly emotionally dead at home. He became dreadful toward me. I realize now this was because he resented me for being in the way, blocking him from being with her.

"It got unbearable for me and for him. He said he felt more and more torn, especially when he saw what the agony was doing to me. He finally decided to move out so he could find out what he really wanted. He insisted he'd continue to work on resolving things between us to resume what had been our happy marriage.

"He moved into a studio apartment and called me every day and I saw him every week at marital therapy. During the sessions, he confessed that he still had feelings for her. He said he tried to end it but just couldn't cut the cord.

"Meanwhile I've gone from being this independent woman to a complete basket case who no longer has control over her life. The pain is excruciating.

"There's a lot at stake here. I work part-time. I'd given up my career to be a wife and mother. To get a full-time job—to get back into my field—the options are really bleak at this stage of life.

"I love my husband. We have three kids who need him at home. What do I do? He says he's trying to work things out and that I am the most important woman in his life. One minute he seems ready to come back and the next, farther away. In the meantime, I am still married. I can't go on dates. I still feel like Barton's wife."

Barton's emotional vacillation keeps Jill in suspended animation, hanging by a string. The ambiguity of her situation makes it difficult to channel her energy productively—working on her marriage on the one hand or grieving its loss on the other. If Jill were sure that Barton was never coming back, she could face facts and put an end to the torture. Grieving the loss would be painful, but it would help her move on.

> *"But he gives me hope. I know he says encouraging things to keep me there for the sake of his own security. He's using me as a spare tire. He doesn't realize it, but he's being selfish and manipulative. I also see that he's more confused, torn, and obsessed than ever. But, he's trying. He's seeing a shrink now and taking all sorts of medication. He also still shows up for couple's therapy every week. How do I know whether he might wake up from this nightmare and come back? I want to let go but the situation won't let me. I have to wait and see what happens, which keeps me in purgatory, dangling above the fires of hell."*

In sharing Jill's feelings with you, I want to make the point that there are no easy answers to this type of dilemma. Jill is dealing with some of the most challenging elements of abandonment's special type of grief. She's battling the following foes.

Check items that hold you back from letting go.

- ❏ Ambiguity
- ❏ Lack of closure
- ❏ Confusion
- ❏ Continued contact with the person who abandoned me
- ❏ Double messages, creating false hope
- ❏ Prolonged feelings of rejection, betrayal, isolation, and fear

What to Do When Faced with Such a Difficult Task

Face it in the moment.

In Jill's case, the future is up for grabs. It is only in the moment that she can regain the power to take back control. In the moment, she can face the bottom line: Barton is not emotionally there for her now. Regardless of what he might do tomorrow, in this moment, she is alone. There is nothing she can do to change his position for now. So she can face this moment's loss, accept her powerlessness over that one fact, and let go. She is letting go not for all time, but for this moment. This letting go releases her from the protest, eases the torment.

Like Jill, most people have difficulty facing an ending where there is a high degree of ambiguity. It is too large a job to accomplish once and for all. Face your loss in the moment, rather than try to face it for all time. Let go for the moment. Doing so strengthens your emotional self-reliance and releases pain.

AKERU EXERCISE THREE
Building a Dream House

To close one connection is to open another from the very center of your conscious being to interconnectedness with the world within and without. The third Akeru exercise is called Dream House. It was designed for the Internalizing stage because it taps into the inward-bound energy of the Internalizing process to inculcate confidence and self-worth. It fills abandonment's cavern of emptiness with gifts from your imagination. Through this exercise, you reinforce your growth, set new goals, and steadily move your life in a positive direction.

Once again, the key to success lies in your ability to employ self-discipline—because you must practice this exercise three times per day for several months to produce the changes you desire.

Fortunately, Dream House is easy to do—even pleasurable. Once you learn the basics, it takes less than a minute each time. It can be practiced while doing other things, like driving the car, taking a walk, or getting your teeth cleaned at the dentist.

Dream House is a Gestalt exercise that I've modified to include some additional elements to direct your meditative and creative energies toward accomplishing life goals and increasing your sense of self. Fueled by the power of your imagination, this exercise facilitates the process by which you redirect the energy of your grief toward increasing your capacity for life and love on a daily basis: Akeru.

The exercise involves conjuring up the Dream House, picturing yourself within it, and feeling grateful for the possibilities of life. That's it. As long as you consistently practice it three times a day, you will begin to see major results within a few months, smaller ones even sooner. Your sense of self-worth improves, because you're accomplishing things in the world and within yourself to help you feel good about yourself.

People surviving abandonment find it hard to dream hopeful dreams. Their diminished sense of entitlement makes it difficult to imagine getting what they want. They feel they don't deserve more, aren't worthy of their dreams. An old adage proves true: "If you can't visualize it, you can't achieve it." All great accomplishments—the Eiffel Tower, for instance—began with a vision in someone's mind, driven by the Power of Possibility.

Dream House automatically lifts the ceiling above what you currently think is possible in your life. It uses your imagination to scale the prison walls that have long barred your success. As you visualize your Dream House, your creative energy moves you out of complacency and beyond your comfort zone, all the way to the confidence you need to reach for your dreams.

How Does Visualizing the House Bypass Your Internal Gatekeepers?

As I said when I explained Back to the Future, when karate masters prepare to break a cinder block with the side of their hand, they must first visualize the space beyond the block, not the block itself, in order to break through. Visualizing the house of your dreams places your psychological energy in the space beyond your own blocks—those restrictions and low ceilings you've imposed on yourself—and places it there three times per day. Your actions become more effective because you're directing your energy to the solution rather than the problem.[6] Your creative energy remains focused on breaking your own blocks.

Your creative energy remains diffuse, disorganized, and undirected, until you harness it. Dream House contains this energy within a structure that you've custom-designed to define, reinforce, and exemplify your goals and dreams. The process transforms you into a goal-directed, energized individual, ascending to your highest potential.

What Is This Energy?

By energy I don't mean anything particularly ethereal. The energy I refer to is the energy behind work—the force required to make something happen. For instance, there is energy involved in the Internalizing process. To internalize someone's rejection is to perform work—to use your energy, however unwittingly, to inculcate new (negative) beliefs about yourself. To reverse this process, Akeru suggests using this inbound energy on your own behalf to inculcate positive messages.

The feelings involved in abandonment are all about energy. Internalizing is attachment energy that, in seeking an object it can no longer find, turns frustration inward against the self. When you internalize someone's rejection, the energy uses your imagination to conjure up matching images of yourself as being unworthy and unlovable. The feelings of self-doubt created by this process feel real precisely because your imagination created such vivid pictures of a negative you. The Dream House redirects this energy, appropriating your imagination to repair the damage you did to your self-esteem.

Dream House organizes your creative energy according to your ultimate dreams to overthrow your fixed ideas about what you consider to be realistically attainable. It helps you move beyond what you think you are capable of. It focuses your energy, not on restrictions imposed by your self-limiting self-appraisal but on your true needs and capabilities. Through your imagination, you bypass the self-defeating notions holding you back.

Check all that apply to you.

These self-defeating notions are holding me back:

- ❑ Skepticism
- ❑ Fear
- ❑ Guilt
- ❑ Feelings of inadequacy
- ❑ Low sense of entitlement

Dream House overcomes obstacles to build your self-esteem.

Why Visualize a House?

If I were to ask you to spell out what you want from life, you'd most likely hold back a great deal of information—both from me and from yourself. Why? You might be afraid your desires are too far afield from what you think you deserve. You've already given up hope of reaching your ultimate goals, so you are reluctant to put yourself through the disappointment all over again. You've downsized your wants, limited your goals, and forsaken your dreams. You've calibrated your sense of entitlement downward, and you're reluctant to hope for more.

But if I ask you to suspend your realistic mind and use your imagination to play a harmless game of pretend, you're not bound by the same unconscious rules. Under these conditions, you're able to suspend your notions about what is realistic. Since we're not talking about you, but about an imaginary house, you are more likely to give vent to your hidden desires. Using your imagination, you project your needs, aspirations, and hopes onto a nonthreatening image—a Dream House. Over time, this house comes to embody your secret needs, capabilities, and desires into its structure, environment, and embellishments. The house is a fantasy, but the personal power you develop is quite real.

I have observed the positive impact of Dream House clinically for over twenty years. It has helped me move many mountains in my own life. Exactly why it works so effectively, though, cannot be completely explained.[7] It has to be experienced.

How to Begin

Begin by closing your eyes. Imagine that you've somehow acquired unlimited financial resources. You have millions or even billions of dollars (depending on your needs and tastes) at your disposal. Maybe you've won the lottery? Think about what you might do tomorrow if you had this kind of money.

Name three things you'd do immediately.

> 1.
> 2.
> 3.

Fast-forward to the future—about a year or two from now. What do you suppose your life would look like, assuming your financial resources have remained unlimited? Imagine that you're spending a good deal of time in an idyllic, beautiful environment. This scene may be some place you've visited or always wanted to. Maybe it's the setting you've been envisioning when performing Back to the Future. What country or part of the world would your Dream House be in? Remember, you are wealthy enough to have your own jetport and pilot (if you'd like) so that you can touch base with family and friends anytime, anywhere in the world.

Describe the location, environs, and country of your Dream House.

Where do your family and friends stay in relation to your new location? Do they stay in a guest suite within your mansion? In separate dwellings you've built nearby? Or do you fly back home to visit them? Describe where your family and friends stay.

What does your Dream House look like? Is it a Victorian? Cobblestone cottage? One-of-a-kind contemporary? Converted barn? Spacious loft? Renovated castle? Yacht? Rustic beach bungalow?

No matter how outlandish or humble, describe the house of your ultimate dreams.

What materials is it made of? Brick, stone, bamboo, tile, concrete, tin, wood?

Describe the materials and textures.

Stop to consider the overall shape and size of your Dream House. Remember, money is no object. If you'd like your home to be cozy—just large enough for your needs—then build it accordingly. If you'd like it to be so large that you can go for a mile walk within it without having to go outside, then build it the size of a gymnasium. For that matter, build a gymnasium, monastery, or skyscraper, if you'd like. Describe the overall structure of your house.

What are the most important functions you perform within your imaginary house? Do you conduct a career from your house? Entertain people? Do you house family members? Do you use it as a personal retreat? A love nest? Do you have a yoga or meditation room? A massage room? A bathing room? Describe the different functions your house is designed for.

What rooms do they take place in? Describe.

Now that the construction is nearly complete, walk directly through the front door to your favorite spot—the place where you feel most relaxed and centered—the heart of the house. This is the place you are most likely to plop yourself down to do your relaxing, thinking, reading, reflecting on life, talking on the phone—even when construction is going on nearby. To help you decide where the heart of your Dream House is located, think about where you spend most of your time within your current dwelling. Where is the heart of where you currently live?

Now, imagine where this central spot might be in your Dream House. Would it be the kitchen, living room, den, library, observatory?
Describe your central spot.

Imagine that you are sitting in the heart of your Dream House in a wonderfully comfortable chair. Is it a bar stool in the kitchen where you can sit and gaze out the window? Or are you nestled into a comfortable chair in the library? Lounging on the deck? Kicking back on a sofa in the living room?
Describe your favorite chair within the heart of the house.

Imagine that as you sit in your luxurious chair, you face a spectacular view—the view of your dreams. Describe the focal point of this view.

Describe other elements of this view.

Think about where the other rooms might be located (assuming there are to be other rooms). Where might your kitchen be, relative to your position in your chair? Is it behind you, to the left, right, or are you *in* the kitchen?
Describe your kitchen.

Imagine where you'd put the bedrooms (relative to your center spot). Are they above you, on either side of you, up one level, down the next? In a separate building? Adjoining building?
Describe where your bedrooms are placed.

What about other rooms, nooks and crannies, guest quarters, or outbuildings of your Dream House? Describe other rooms and buildings.

When you're first attempting this exercise, it is not necessary to specify the exact location of all of the rooms and outbuildings. For now, just get a general idea of where the most functional rooms might be and what they might be like. With repeated use of this exercise, you can add or delete rooms to your heart's content. Renovating to include additional space comes into play as you perform this exercise over many months.

It's important to conjure up an image of your Dream House no less than three times a day for at least three months—that is, if you hope to see appreciable improvements in your personal growth. Frequent contemplation of the visual image focuses your energy on the space beyond your blocks.

MY DREAM HOUSE
Draw or describe your Dream House—in its current stage of design.

Renovate Your House Regularly

The house's design is not static, but constantly changing according to your latest interests, desires, or needs. In fact, to promote this flexibility, begin one of your thrice-daily visualizations by asking, "Since I have unlimited resources, what would I add or change to my Dream House today?" Some people select a different location every time they visualize their house. Some visualize a house they already live in, imagining only minor modifications. As long as you're sure that it's not your low sense of entitlement trying to limit the scope of your house (or of your ultimate dreams), it makes no difference whether your house changes every day, resembles a palace, shack, or rowboat.

Your Dream House Becomes a Crucible for Forging Love

For those of you who desire to find love, your house can become a crucible in which to forge internal changes that help you build toward love. All you have to do is imagine that it's sometime in the future and that you already have found someone special to share your life with. To make this feasible to your imagination, you'll want to imagine a time anywhere from six months to a few years from now, making sure to give yourself enough lead time to make whatever internal changes this will require.

Place this relationship in your Dream House. It's best not to give your Dream Partner a specific physical appearance. Imagine him or her as a vague presence, securely situated somewhere within your dream environs. The exception to the "vague features" rule is when you have a viable relationship and have reason to believe that this person stands a good chance of being in your future.

Remember, you cannot control another person, only yourself. So when you picture your Dream Partner, be sure the success of the union does not hinge on changes the other person makes or any superhuman traits he or she needs to have to be able to be in a relationship with you. The only real control you ever have is over yourself. Any changes must come from you. Your growth might trigger your partner's growth, but you have no control over if, when, or exactly how he or she might change. Visualize the relationship that you are able to create as a result of making your own significant changes, even if you're not sure what these changes might be. You can use Back to the Future to figure out what actions to take.

When you visualize your lover situated within your dream environs, give yourself enough time to allow for your internal growth to take place—sometime in the future. This homes in your energy to the task of unconscious problem solving. As you visualize the Dream House, your actions begin to move in the direction of your desired goal.

Set up a scene in your mind in which you are sitting in your favorite chair, feeling the presence of your special someone. He or she is not in the room with you at the moment, but somewhere within the environs of your Dream House.

Where would your significant other be? In the driveway, coming home? Backyard? Tennis court on your property? In a separate dwelling, thinking positive thoughts about you?

Think about the other people in your present and future. Are there children? What about friends? Neighbors? Pets? Think about who you'd like to have living with or near you.

Where are these people relative to your position in the center of your Dream House? Describe.

 Back to the Future

It's sometime in the future and you're within your Dream House, sitting on your comfortable chair before your beautiful view, feeling happy and fulfilled because you resolved your need for love. You feel good about yourself for being able to make the changes necessary to take this momentous step in your life.

What obstacles have been blocking you from finding love all along?

How did you remove them?

How did your behavior change to accomplish this?

Action Vow: In the next twenty-four hours, I am going to take the following baby step in the direction of increasing the love in my life: _____

Other Uses for This House

Dream House is a change vehicle. It provides a psychic infrastructure in which to embed the Akeru exercises, the twelve Swan Lessons, and the other healing balms of the program, as I'll show you. Conjuring up your ever-changing house on an ongoing basis reinforces all of the tools of abandonment recovery.

For example, sitting in your Dream Chair helps reinforce "centering in"—something we explored in chapter 1. You can also use Dream House to strengthen your ability to get into the moment.

In designing your house, create a structure so spectacular, that just living in it draws you into the moment. Imagine that the house is so complete, it brings you out of your head and into the sights and sounds of life around you. So compelling are its views, so breathtaking its landscape, so satisfying its interior atmosphere—that you are able to spend most of your time experiencing life rather than thinking about it.

Describe the changes you'd need to add to your house to inspire you to stay in the moment.

The house can reinforce the work you are doing with your Big You / Little You Dialogues. Imagine that it has everything to satisfy your child self. What special features would you need to add or delete from your house to help Little feel safe, secure, and happy in this house?
Describe the renovations you'd need to enhance Little's contentment when nestled into the environs of the house.

Imagine that within your Dream House Big You feels strong and capable of resolving lifelong problems. What special features do you need to add to the house to enable Big to feel capable and strong while living there?

The house you've created is you. It contains all that you know, all that you are, all that you need. Structurally, it contains all of your capabilities as well as the internal barriers you are overcoming. The renovations and details you put into it reflect who you are becoming and the direction in which you are taking your life.

Describe your Dream House in one paragraph. Include its overall structure, the environment, the newest renovations, the emotional goals you achieved living within it, the problems you solved, the obstacles you removed, and the initial actions you took to set the changes in motion—all in one gulp.

Is the Dream House a Magic Bullet?

Although the Dream House exercise gives profound results, it does not work by magic. For example, there is no sense in which visualizing the house means that you will actually receive the house. The house is not supposed to materialize physically. This palace of your dreams is strictly for your imagination to live in. You have control over your choices in the real world.

You gain a lot of benefits by letting the Dream House do its work unconsciously, but you must practice it three times a day. By setting your sights on the house of your wildest dreams, you project your greatest needs and goals into its structure, furnishings, and ambience. Over time, this process automatically opens up new windows in your awareness and clarifies your goals.

Indeed, new goals seem to set themselves.

Visualizing a structure that contains your hopes and dreams directs your visionary power to your unlimited capacity for life and love. That is what this exercise seeks to capitalize on—your creative energy focused at the level of solution rather than the level of the problem.

To make your goals materialize into achievements, you must take constructive actions in your daily life, and you will find this tendency increases as you perform the exercise on a daily basis. The confidence you gain, enhanced by your visionary powers, helps you overcome procrastination and follow through. Taking positive actions increases your self-esteem.

Is It Necessary to Analyze Your Dream House?

The less you analyze your house, the less opportunity you give your internal gatekeepers to censor the size and scope of your vision. It is not necessary to make a connection between the design and the specific goals you are working on. True, there may be clues about these goals slipped into the structure, size, shape, climate, or atmosphere of your Dream House, but it is not necessary to identify the correlations. Maybe you want more security and your house reflects this by being built into rock. Maybe you want more lightness of spirit and relaxation in your life, and your house reflects this by being perched on the beach with windows galore. Maybe the size of the house expresses your desire to expand something in yourself you have yet to admit that you want. Maybe you expressed your desire for elegance, beauty,

Peut-être

and luxury in your dream decor. Maybe you're expressing a sentimental wish in the objet d'art you've placed on the table next to your Dream Chair. No matter. You do not need to figure out the whys and wherefores of your Dream House's design, location, or embellishments. Just use your imagination and dream away.

Keep your energy focused on, say, deciding what kind of tapestry to use in your Dream Foyer, rather than wondering what goal this tapestry might or might not reflect. You don't need to know the reason you're moving the central staircase, or relocating your Dream House to a cooler climate, or downsizing from five bedrooms to two, or going from sleek to quaint. Just make the changes you desire and know that your creative energies are working for you internally.

The bottom line is that this house becomes a crucible for forging internal changes, helping you to launch the ever-changing you. Be sure to take advantage of each opportunity the real world offers. Keep visualizing three times a day, and you'll find motivation to follow through.

Some people get attached to their Dream Houses and worry that they will never get an opportunity to acquire the actual house. This exercise helps you acquire, not the house itself, but progress toward the goals, desires, needs, and dreams you've unwittingly built into it.

In using this exercise over the years, both personally and professionally, I've noticed that many people acquire a lot of the elements they'd built into their Dream Houses in their real-life dwellings. But the real changes are found in the quality of life and love they've attained.

The house represents who you are and who you are becoming. Visualizing your Dream House works subconsciously on your behalf. It opens your future to all possibilities. In performing this exercise three times per day for a few months, you channel your unlimited natural power to move your life forward.

Without overanalyzing, can you glean anything from the structure of your Dream House about your dreams; the obstacles you are overcoming; the direction in which you're taking your life; or your goals, constraints, and strengths? Explain.

The house focuses all of your positive energy on all that you are, all that you need, all that you are capable of, all that you're becoming.
What clue does your Dream House give you about where you want your life to go?

What part of this growth is realistic to achieve within a few years of growth, if you were to start within the next twenty-four hours?

How will it feel to make this a reality?

How badly do you want it?

Is your existence important enough to go out and get it?

What impact will it have on your self-esteem?

What is currently blocking you?

What insights and strengths can you use for overcoming?

How can you use Dream House as a tool for ascending to your aspirations?

More Food for Thought: How to Use the Dream House to Incorporate the Four Cornerstones of Self

The house becomes a crucible for incorporating the principles of self-esteem we've been discussing: Separating (chapter 4), Beholding the Importance of Your Existence (chapter 5), Accepting Your Reality (chapter 6), and Increasing Your Capacity for Love (chapter 7).* Combined, these principles are what I call the Four Cornerstones of Self.

To help you incorporate the first cornerstone, Accepting Your Separateness, think about your Dream House. What design changes in the house would it take to create an ambience to make you feel completely at peace and fulfilled, even if you lived there all by yourself? Come up with renovations dramatic enough to make living alone as happy an experience as if you were with a partner.

This requires a lot of thought.

Think about what you need to change in your Dream House to create an ideal environment in which to embrace your separateness. Do you need to move it to another location? Do you need to change the view? The furnishings? Create new functions in the house? Go ahead and make whatever renovations are necessary to create an environment in which you could live as happily all by yourself as you would with a Dream Partner.

Describe the renovations to your Dream House that would make this possible.

For the second cornerstone, Beholding the Importance of Your Existence, what additions or embellishments would help you truly appreciate the importance of your existence? Think about what it means to be alive. Think about the precious opportunity it is, the miracle of existence itself. What renovations do you need to make to your Dream House to help you truly appreciate this miracle?

Describe the changes in location, decor, design, size, or function you need to add to your house to help you behold the importance of your existence.

---

*   These Four Cornerstones are the same as Swan Lessons Four (Separating), Five (Beholding),
     Six (Accepting), and Seven (Increasing Love). See my book *Black Swan*.

For the third cornerstone, Accepting Your Reality, imagine that your surroundings are so complete that you are able to face your current reality squarely, with peace, calm, and strength. The details of your favorite room are so compelling that just by sitting on your Dream Chair, you are able to face any reality that may come to you. The view you've imagined is so spectacular that gazing on it fills you with strength to accept any challenges life throws at you. What additions or deletions would help you accept any reality no matter how challenging?

Describe the changes in structure or embellishments.

For the fourth cornerstone, Increasing Your Capacity for Love, imagine that your Dream House is constructed and decorated in such a way that just by living within it, your capacity for love increases every day. Others can feel the warmth and connection emanating from you all the way from where you sit in your comfortable Dream Chair. Living within this house, your capacity for love increases toward yourself, the people you know, and those you have not yet met. Soon your capacity for love radiates to all of the people in your life. What design changes do you need to make in your Dream House to help you increase your capacity for love just by living in it day by day?

Describe the love-inspiring renovations you need to make for this growth to take place.

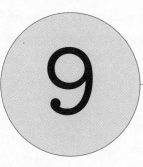

9 Reaching Out

"Reach out? There's nobody there! Doesn't anybody get it?"

I can remember the anger. I didn't realize at the time that all of the agitation I was feeling meant I was in a pivotal stage of recovery. It felt more like I was going backward than nearing the end of the grief process.

"I felt like a human boil forever on the verge of exploding," says Janet. "I'd warn my friends to watch out and sure enough, anyone who dared to spend time with me, I spewed on."

That's the Rage stage—an extremely turbulent time of transition when you can barely contain your feelings or your will to break free of the pain. I was truly perplexed by the amount of frustration and rage I felt.

"I can't seem to tone it down," says Roberta. "It feels as if I were being followed by a gang of hornets who make me and everybody around me miserable."

Abandonment's Rage gets more intense just as you're hitting bottom. It still feels like you're falling into the pit of hot coals, only this time you hit a springboard that propels you upward. In the midst of the descent into Rage, it's hard to envision your ascent to a higher level of functioning. But indeed Rage is a launching pad, charging you to take action to repair your life.

Rage's energy is externalizing rather than internalizing. Its outbound energy empowers you to actively refute the messages of rejection you've accumulated. You revoke the power you gave to your abandoner and garner it for your own use. The work you began in the last chapter (restoring your dreams) gives you maximum lift when you touch down on abandonment's trampoline—that taut, spring-loaded bottom of Rage.

Throughout this workbook you've been preparing to take this step. You're learning to center yourself. You've gained awareness of your self-defeating patterns, learning about the obstacles blocking you

221

from finding love, and repairing damage to your self-esteem. You've engaged in an ongoing dialogue to administer to your primal needs and feelings. You've created a Dream House in which to forge new goals. Now in the Rage stage we'll learn about a self-awareness tool that helps you use Rage energy constructively.

What Is Rage Energy All About?

Unlike sadness and fear, rage is energizing and exhilarating.[1] Its rocketing energy propels you back out into the world. When your drive to bond was initially thwarted, this energy turned inward against yourself. Now, during the Rage stage, your embattled self finally stands up and says, "Enough! It's not my fault. I don't deserve this much pain!" This active resistance sends the energy back outward. Rage, then, is attachment energy that has rebounded against the self. It is attachment energy pushing outward, still seeking an object it can't find, but no longer willing to take no for an answer, no longer willing to take it out on you.

You Rage because you feel deprived of the one commodity you need most: love. Rage thrusts forward to find it.

Are you currently in touch with your anger?

Does your anger or frustration have anything to do with feeling deprived of love? Explain.

Use a Truth Nugget to identify the situation causing your rage.

Truth Nugget: I feel _____ because _____.

Do you feel good about the way you cope with your anger?

How would you like to handle it?

Rage occurs in two waves of arousal.[2] When something first ticks you off—a date cancels, for example—you experience Wave One. Adrenaline and norepinephrine (NE) are released, and you feel an initial surge of aggressive energy. Wave One lasts for a few minutes—enough time for you to mobilize your energy for swift action (your mammalian brain assumes you're in a life-and-death crisis). Wave Two occurs as your glucocorticoid stress hormones build up in your bloodstream, and its effect lasts for hours and even days. So, even after you've gotten past the initial urge to strike out, your body sustains a background tone of rage, keeping you in a constant state of action readiness. This background tone creates a foundation on which subsequent responses build more quickly.

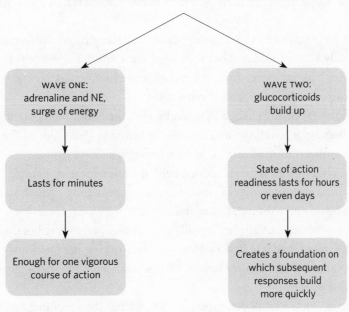

ANGER'S TWO WAVES OF AROUSAL

WAVE ONE: adrenaline and NE, surge of energy	WAVE TWO: glucocorticoids build up
Lasts for minutes	State of action readiness lasts for hours or even days
Enough for one vigorous course of action	Creates a foundation on which subsequent responses build more quickly

The key to change is learning to use Rage energy constructively rather than destructively. You've no doubt heard people suggesting you should be proactive rather than reactive. But how do you channel anger in a positive way? That's the real question.

You need a tool.

I'm going to introduce you to a new voice of your personality: Outer Child. Outer Child is a self-awareness tool that helps you get a handle on how your Rage has gone underground to subvert your relationships. You learn to put your needs and dreams in the hands of your adult self—Big You.

In the hierarchy of self, Outer Child stands between the inner child and the adult— between Big You and Little You. Unlike Big or Little, Outer is a nemesis.

INNER CHILD
OUTER CHILD
ADULT

Whereas the inner child is all about feelings, Outer Child doesn't want to feel Little's feelings and chooses to act them out instead. When you enter the Rage stage, you come face-to-face with this saboteur.

Big's role is to take charge of Little's needs. Outer interferes. Outer doesn't have enough self-control to delay gratification and do the right thing. Outer wants what Outer wants *now* and isn't particular about how it goes about getting it.

Outer doesn't come from Big or Little but is borne of inappropriately channeled anger.

Outer Child is the part of the personality that is driven to act out Little's anger and fear about being abandoned. The seething, burning feelings of rage activate Outer Child, forcing it out of the closet. Once Outer Child is exposed, you're able to pinpoint its traits and defects. The Outer Child tool empowers you to undertake the first in-depth personal inventory[3] of your lifetime. You identify traits and character defects most people prefer to deny—traits that until now created an invisible dysfunctional infrastructure.

Outer isn't about taking constructive actions, but about taking impulsive, headstrong, pigheaded actions. Developmentally, Outer Child is about nine years old. Outer's main role is to interfere between Big and Little. Until you separate Outer from the rest of your emotional core, Outer weakens the Big-Little bond, forcing your feelings underground once again.

Outer fights change—especially change initiated by you, the adult. Outer stands in opposition to what's good for you, bent on frustrating Little's needs. By bringing Outer out of the bunkers and into the daylight, you get to subvert its mission, rather than letting it subvert yours.

Without recovery, Outer Child remains hidden behind Little's most vulnerable feelings. The good news is that Outer's constant trouble-making motivates Big to get strong enough to take care of Little. That's how Big gains power—by wresting it away from Outer.

Outer is an actor. It poses as your ally but is really your gatekeeper. Herein lies the challenge of dealing with Outer Child. Outer Child has had a covert agenda, working unconsciously to maintain your patterns. Becoming aware of Outer Child's defenses helps you adjust the mechanisms that have been causing you to spin your wheels.

The key to disarming Outer Child's defenses is to acknowledge the anger fueling them. Anger can be a constructive force, but not when it is in Outer's hands. Outer bungles anger, not only by overreacting, but by underreacting as well.

Abandonment survivors tend to have trouble with anger. Some feel too needy and insecure to get in touch with healthy anger. The reason: Their fear of abandonment is so pervasive that they can't tolerate any break in their connections. They're afraid that expressing anger will cause others to pull away. Outer takes advantage of this fear and lack of assertiveness and gets you to take your anger out on yourself.

It often manifests in convoluted ways.

"Why was I showing up late for appointments?" asks Debbie. "I can't stand it when my customers are mad at me. But I was giving them every excuse in the book to yell at me, fire me, hate me. Then I realized that I was somehow funneling my heartbreak into business. I was getting my customers to beat me up so that I could get some of the anger expressed, even if it was twisted."

Not all people going through heartbreak have trouble expressing anger. Many are able to vent it directly at the source.

"Every day, the anger got hotter and hotter until it felt like I'd explode," says Gary. "So I called my ex-girlfriend up and told her about how lousy she treated me and how contemptible her cheating and lying was. It was for my benefit, not hers, because it helped me move on."

In Gary's case, his adult self chose to express his anger through appropriate action. By contrast, here's an example of Outer Child being in control and performing an overreaction:

"It didn't go well for me. I called Jimmy to give him a piece of my mind and wound up going haywire and got myself more worked up. He hung up on me, so I drove to his job and harassed him in front of his staff, who now see me as a mad woman. It felt like the right thing to do at the time, but I feel worse than before and now he doesn't speak to me at all."

The first step in gaining control of your behavior is to separate your feelings from your actions. With Outer Child in your sights, your adult wisdom has an opportunity to guide your behavior, rather than this unconscious amygdala-driven nemesis.

Identifying Outer's many behaviors helps you locate your emotional triggers. Keeping tabs on what Outer Child is doing empowers you to become the self-possessed adult you always wanted to be.*

"I have a habit of letting people step all over me," says Beth, "because I'm too timid to speak up for myself. When I have a grievance with someone, I don't say anything. I just disappear on them. I know this is wrong, because it leaves people confused, hurt, and angry with me. It isn't good for them, and it's even worse for me, because it means I keep repeating my abandonment from childhood over and over, making myself even more isolated.

"But I'm more aware of my feelings from doing the Big You / Little You Dialogue every day. I'm in tune with how frightened Little feels with people. I work on this dialogue every day—soothing

---

* See my *Taming Your Outer Child*. Also, click on OUTER CHILD HELP at abandonment.net.

Little, reassuring her that she's a good person and that I would never take advantage of her and that I will never leave her.

"Well, one day as I was writing the dialogue, Little expressed anger over the fact that she didn't like it that I ran away from somebody again because now she doesn't have any friends. I stopped writing for a minute and realized that running away was Outer Child's way of handling my anger. I needed to handle my anger better—Big Me. So I wrote a dialogue between my adult self and my outer self and got Big to tell Outer to stay out of it and let me handle it. After writing about a half hour's worth of the dialogue, Big Me finally felt in control. Then I did the impossible: I called my friend and apologized for disappearing on her and told her, 'It's just that you always pick the restaurant; it makes me feel I have no say.' 'Oh, well,' she said, 'where do you want to eat next time?' and that was that—we're still friends."

In presenting the Outer Child concept, I find that people tend to resist recognizing this aspect of themselves. Who wants to own up to Outer Child's collection of bad personality traits? So before I ask you to identify your own Outer Child, I'm going to take a novel approach and get you to first project it onto someone else. We'll take a look at other people's acting-out behaviors—at their Outer Child.

To do this, I realize I'm asking you to give vent to the most critical, self-righteous side of your own personality. The Critic is one of Outer's least attractive faces. In twelve-step philosophy, focusing on another person's character flaws is known as "taking their inventory," which is something recoverees are discouraged from doing, because it detracts from taking responsibility for their own character defects. My goal here is to use our penchant for criticizing others as a vehicle for ultimately addressing our own behaviors.

Outer Child has many personae: The Critic, The Ostrich, The Enabler, The Complainer…you get the idea. Outer Child has obnoxious personality disorder (OPD), and it takes many forms.

The Critic versus the Heedless

We all know people who are walking exaggerations of our own worst issues. Think about friends who let their desires rule them. Rather than heed their better judgment, they do exactly what they like. They abide by the pleasure principle rather than the reality principle. Since they are heedless of consequences, I call them The Heedless. Since we are critiquing them, let's label ourselves The Critic.

The Heedless act out their desires at the expense of achieving their long-range goals. No doubt they are abandonment survivors like us and have low self-esteem. This is why they succumb to feel-good-now, pay-later behavior in the first place. They gamble money they don't have, drink too much, buy things they can't afford, overeat, risk their health, and get stuck in destructive relationships—you know, the usual. They succumb to the need for immediate gratification, throwing long-term goals by the wayside. They exemplify the intellectual-emotional dichotomy we discussed in chapter 5: "I know I shouldn't do such and such, but I can't stop myself."

Name a friend whose heedlessness brings out The Critic in you.

What about his or her behavior bothers you most?

Interacting with those who seem bent on indulging their impulses can bring out the most intolerant, critical, controlling side of The Critic. Yet The Heedless may not arouse criticism in everyone we know, the way it does The Critic. Others may see The Heedless as doing the best they can, while The Critic (that's us) sees them as emotional eyesores blighting our view of their better qualities.

How does being The Critic make you feel about yourself?

How does it affect your behavior toward others?

How would you like to handle The Critic within?

Popular theory says that when people's faults make you angry, it's probably because they remind you of a quality in yourself you don't like looking at. While this well-known aphorism may be true, there is a less-well-known reason as likely to be true: You become critically fixated on their faults because they are doing something that you would never accept in yourself.[4] They are not abiding by your rule book, flouting your standards of right and wrong, and what's worse, getting away with it. For all of the mayhem their messes create, they don't seem to mind that the sky keeps falling on their heads. They traipse along conspicuously failing to abide by constraints that you impose on yourself for fear of having that very same sky fall on *your* head.

The Heedless are usually caught up in unhealthy relationships. They often bond to alcoholics and become The Enabler, another infamous Outer Child personality. Or they themselves become The Alcoholic, The Shopoholic, or The Abandoholic. As The Heedless indulge their desires and throw caution to the wind, negative consequences do befall them (just as The Critic secretly hopes will happen). But The Heedless thrive on the chaos they create and take pride in self-victimization. Somehow, they manage to pull a rabbit out of a hat just as you thought a really sobering consequence would finally teach them a lesson. And what's most infuriating to The Critic is that The Heedless usually have fifty people lined up willing to bail them out.

Prone to procrastination, The Heedless remain complacent about the so-called minor inconveniences their lives are heir to, like having their car repossessed, the IRS breathing down their necks, or their careers on hold because they postponed completing their college degree indefinitely. That sky keeps falling, and they don't seem to notice.

Okay, we've had enough fun criticizing other people. Now let's see how this helps us deal with our own Outer Child—our Rage nemesis.

Understanding the dynamics of your internal Critic is a boon to self-awareness. By identifying the behaviors in others that disturb you most, you can examine the precepts by which you lead your own life. The tendency to become negatively attracted to other people's faults is another example of false attribution: you presume that someone else's behavior is causing you to feel angry and critical. In fact, our own issues around complying with our own higher expectations are responsible for most of our frustration, anger, and intolerance toward someone else. The point is that catching yourself in The Critic role is always a self-awareness lesson. The lesson may be that you need to ease up on the stringency of your own rule book.[5] Becoming aware of your internal Critic can help you get in touch with the Heedless behavior of your own Outer Child.

Think about The Heedless friend you named earlier.

What alternative behavior would you like to see him perform?

What self-defeating behavior of yours is currently plaguing you?

What alternative behaviors would you like to see in yourself?

What insights and strengths can you use to accomplish this feat?

Gaining Outer Child awareness helps you address the patterns holding you back. To warm you up to the concept, I've given nicknames to some of the outstanding Outer Child types, but there are thousands of varieties residing within all of us,[6] as you will learn when we explore the Outer Child Inventory toward the end of the chapter.

The labels below are not designed to stereotype people but to illustrate that Outer Child defenses fall into patterns.

Outer Child Patterns

THE OSTRICH

The Ostrich looks up from its preoccupation with the sand to see a big predator slowly moving in its direction. How does the Ostrich defend itself? It buries its head in the sand. Hours later, it comes up for air and sees the predator moving even closer, so it sticks its head deeper into the sand.

The most common reason that The Ostrich avoids problems rather than resolves them is that it is overwhelmed by feelings of helplessness and anxiety.

"My mother left us when I was two. My father was so neglectful that the authorities took me away to a foster home where I was abused. Too many bad things happened, too much abandonment, too much anger. I just can't deal. I try to stay in my own world and let whatever happens happen."

THE CONTRARIAN

Outer Child says no to things that are good for you but fails to say no to things that are bad for you. The Contrarian uses self-indulgence as a way of medicating frustration and anger.

"I always seem to be doing the opposite of what I should be doing. I love ice cream, but it makes me fat. So when I'm lonely, angry, or tired—which is a lot lately, a year after Jake left—I eat ice cream by the gallons. I let other things go, too. I take whatever peace or pleasure I can get when I can get it. But all this does is keep me angry and disgusted with myself."

THE CRITIC

Well, if you were able to perform the projection onto The Heedless, then you already have an example of The Critic—you. No further explanations necessary.

THE PROCRASTINATOR

This Outer Child's middle name is avoidance. Its fuel is resistance. Its mode is passivity.

"I always put my term papers off till the last minute. They loom over me every weekend like a dark cloud, turning Sunday nights into a nightmare. Then I go into a rage toward myself to get it done."

QUEEN OF DA NILE

This Outer Child could wake up one morning to find an elephant sitting in the middle of the living room and act as if it were not there. Everyone has to step around it, not mention the elephant, and act like everything is just fine. This denial is a kind of reverse hallucination, where you don't see what you think you see.

"I have a friend whose husband is drunk twenty-four hours a day it seems. I have never seen him without a glass of scotch in his hand, half-crocked. But what gets under my skin is her not him. She works two jobs and he watches television all day. She's a wreck from being constantly abandoned by him, while he just lets her pay all of the bills and take care of everything. She complains about everything else, conveniently avoiding ever mentioning his drinking, creating this awkward gulf of reality standing between us."

THE FOOL FOR LOVE

This Outer Child tends to get caught up in love's whims rather than become master of its creative process. The Fool for Love, a notorious abandoholic, throws caution to the wind and succumbs to patterns of abandonment. He seeks romance instead of relationship—but remains oblivious to the difference. The Fool is able to love for today, heedless of tomorrow's heartbreak.

"All that matters to my Outer Child is whether I'm attracted to the guy. He could be Attila the Hun, but never mind, Outer is hot to trot as long as the guy's cute. She never seems to learn from her mistakes."

The Fool for Love is willing to play the victim and stuff all of the anger that goes with it. Her primary relationships go from intense to nonexistent, creating gaping love wounds and chronic heartache.

THE ACTOR

This Outer's attempts to squelch Little's feelings are not as subtle as it thinks. The Actor tries to cover up his insecurity, but winds up aiming giant suction cups at his prospective lovers—a fearsome sight that scares new lovers away.

"I'm dating a woman I like," says Donovan, "but she's not willing to be exclusive. I get really mad when she's seeing someone else. I try to act like I'm cool with it, that I'm not desperate for her or anything. When I pressure her about it a little bit, all she says is, 'You're emotionally too needy.'"

We all have enough intelligence to establish lasting, quality relationships. We've all seen such relationships succeed in all types of people. Equipped with this intelligence and guided by the examples set by others, we should be able to achieve a fulfilling relationship ourselves, were it not for our Outer Child's self-defeating behaviors. It isn't the feelings that are defeating us, but how we handle them. Outer creates havoc in our love life by trying to defend us from those feelings.

How Did Outer Child Develop?

Outer Child developed within the personality somewhere between the ages of eight and twelve—the age when you no longer took rejection, dismissal, or neglect sitting down. Outer has been gaining power ever since and will continue to do so until you expose its habits.[7]

Outer began acting out during the Rage stage from previous times of loss and abandonment when you felt frustrated, love starved, and angry. The following Qs are designed to give you a picture of your Outer Child by looking at its formative years.

Think of yourself during late elementary school and middle school. Do you remember what your personality was like? What traits stand out most?

Do you remember your usual mood or temperament at that time? Were you usually happy? Worried? Isolated? Angry? Bored? Anxious? Describe.

What family situation contributed to this mood? Put your answer in a Truth Nugget.

Truth Nugget: I felt _____ because my family _____.

Do you remember things that bothered you within your peer group that made you sad, disappointed, angry, or hurt back then? Again, use a Truth Nugget.

Truth Nugget: I felt _____ when others _____.

Who provided you with support when you were hurt or angry?

Who provoked your anger and frustration?

How did you act out your anger?

IQ

Check all that apply.

- ❏ I became hyperactive to avoid feeling sad or angry.
- ❏ I picked on a younger sibling or smaller friend.
- ❏ I overate, overslept, or watched too much television.
- ❏ I sought negative attention from my parents or teachers.
- ❏ I overfocused on schoolwork or projects.
- ❏ I became a control freak.

Add your own behaviors:

Think about who you are today. Is this defensive, needy busybody from your childhood still within you?

If so, do you think you may have just identified a facet of your Outer Child?

How might gaining Outer Child awareness help your recovery?

> People ask: "Is Outer always in control when we're angry? If Big stifles your rage, where does it go?"
>
> I answer: Big doesn't stifle rage; Big transforms it into positive aggression.[8] Anger is a potentially constructive emotion because its energy can lead to action. The key to using it productively is gaining Outer Child awareness. This allows Big You to call the shots, not Outer.

Celebrity Outer Children

Sometimes your adult self, fully in control, chooses to use anger as a way of saving face in public, especially after being dumped. Celebrities provide an excellent example. When they've been abandoned, they show some well-contained anger, managing to keep their tempestuous Outer Child out of the public eye.

Being left is humiliating. Anger is a more dignified public response to it. Celebrities don't sit on talk shows and openly express feeling heartbroken over someone who has rejected them. They don't tell Ellen DeGeneres or Jimmy Fallon how they're up all night crying and yearning for the person who left them. They usually cover up their vulnerable, defeated feelings with an appropriate dose of indignant anger to avoid the appearance of being seen as the loser.

It was known, for example, that Donald Trump left Ivana for another woman. Did she cry in public? Admit to being bested? Bewail the fact that she loved him so much and longed for his return? Certainly she might have felt this way. But she presented none of that publicly. She showed dignified anger, outrage, disgust, entitlement, and became famous for saying, "Don't get mad, get everything."

Donna Hanover likewise demonstrated appropriate righteous indignation and resiliency when she agreed to perform in the *Vagina Monologues* after her husband, New York City Mayor Rudy Giuliani, left her for another woman. She canceled her appearance only when it was announced that Rudy had received a diagnosis of prostate cancer.

Hillary Clinton gained public sympathy because she reacted to her husband's betrayal with grace and dignity, never appearing the victim, always making sure the public could see that she held tremendous power in the situation. She didn't let her Outer Child control her anger, at least not in front of the cameras.

The point is that anger urges you to take actions, but it is up to you to choose positive behavior. Gaining Outer Child awareness is the greatest boon to your success.

AKERU EXERCISE FOUR
Discovering Your Outer Child

This Akeru exercise—Outer Child awareness—works with Rage's outbound energy to empower you with life-changing insight. Rather than squelch your rage, when you are empowered by Outer Child awareness, you work with it to change your life. To help you recognize your Outer Child behaviors along with its many expressions and personalities, I present an excerpt from the "100-Item Outer Child Inventory."[9] The partial list includes recognizable truisms, encapsulated awareness, and little telegrams of insight associated with your Outer Child.*

OUTER CHILD INVENTORY

Please check those items that hold some truth for you. Go back and put a double circle over those that interfere in your relationships. And while you're at it, you can also draw a box around the ones that describe someone you know—your abandoner, perhaps?

❏ Outer Child acts out Little's anger over being left on the rock. Outer encompasses all the outward signs of Little's vulnerability—the scars, the warts, the defenses that show on the outside.

---

*   You can submit an Outer Child Checklist by clicking on the OUTER CHILD HELP button at the abandonment.net Help Center. It will bring you to outerchild.net. Then click on DO YOU HAVE AN OUTER CHILD?, then FILL OUT OUR CHECKLIST.

- ❑ Outer Child is the selfish, controlling, self-centered part of all of us.
- ❑ Outer Child is developmentally between eight and twelve. Self-centeredness is age appropriate for Outer Child.
- ❑ Outer Child wears many disguises, especially in public. Since other people's Outer Child is usually well hidden, we may think we're the only one with an Outer Child.
- ❑ Outer Child is the hidden "Chucky" of the personality. Even the nicest people we know can act like seven-year-olds with full-blown conduct disorders when they feel rejected, dismissed—abandoned.
- ❑ Outer Child has a favorite feeling—anger. In fact, Outer Child's *only* feeling is anger, fueled by being hurt or thwarted.
- ❑ Outer Child is developmentally old enough to have its own little executive ego. It is old enough to forcefully exercise its will, but it is not old enough to understand consequences, let alone the rights and feelings of others. (Little isn't old enough to have its own ego, so Little has to appropriate ours. That's why Little needs Big.)
- ❑ Outer Child steps right in and takes over. Even if we had every intention of handling a particular situation in a mature, adult manner, Outer Child handles things its own way, leaving us holding the bag.
- ❑ Outer Child can really dominate our personalities, especially if we've had a history of repeated abandonments. Many abandonment survivors of childhood are mostly Outer Child.
- ❑ Outer Child throws temper tantrums and goes off in tirades if it feels criticized, rejected, or abandoned. If Outer Child seems emotionally disturbed, it is because of what Little has been through. I don't dare blame Outer—Outer doesn't react well to criticism, even my own.
- ❑ Outer Child blames its faults on my mate. It tries to get me to imagine that my unacceptable traits belong to my mate.
- ❑ Outer Child talks about my friends behind their back.
- ❑ Outer Child thrives on chaos, loves crises, drama.
- ❑ Outer Child is a world-class procrastinator.
- ❑ Outer Child loses things and blames it on others. It can find an excuse for anything.
- ❑ Outer Child is the "yes-but" of the personality.
- ❑ Outer Child can never be wrong. Outer Child hates asking for help—becomes stubborn, ornery, blind, and pigheaded.
- ❑ Outer Child acts like a tyrant but is secretly a coward, unable to appropriately assert its needs in the outside world.
- ❑ Outer Child says, "It's okay," when a friend slights me, but then holds on to the anger for the next twenty years.
- ❑ Outer Child specializes in blame; if it has an uncomfortable feeling, somebody else must be at fault.
- ❑ Outer Child uses crying as a manipulation.
- ❑ Outer Child criticizes others to keep the heat off of itself.
- ❑ Outer Child can't stand waiting, especially when a significant other is expected to call.
- ❑ Outer Child doesn't form relationships—it takes lovers as emotional hostages.

❑ Outer Child will demand, defy, deceive, ignore, balk, manipulate, seduce, pout, whine, and retaliate to get its needs for acceptance and approval met. It doesn't see this as a contradiction.

❑ Outer Child gets right in the middle of things when I try to start a new relationship—it becomes more reactive, more demanding, more needy than ever before.

❑ Outer Child strives for its own self-interest while pretending to protect Little. But Outer wants one thing only—control.

❑ Outer Child is not old enough to care about others (despite its considerable acting skills). Only the adult self can do that.

❑ Outer Child tests new significant others with emotional games. Its favorite is playing hard to get. Outer Child thinks when others are hard to get, it's sexy.

❑ Outer Child can be seductive, funny, charming, full of life, pretending to be interested in the other person's life. Then when Outer succeeds in catching its prey, it suddenly becomes cold, critical, unloving, and sexually withholding. Outer makes me pity the person willing to love me.

❑ Outer Child is the addict, the alcoholic, the one who runs up my credit cards and breaks my diet.

❑ Outer Child seeks all the wrong people—can't resist a lover who won't commit.

❑ Outer Child becomes most powerful when Big and Little are out of alignment.

❑ Outer Child believes laws and ethics are for everybody else.

❑ Outer Child can dish it out but can't take it. Outer Child can be holier than thou.

❑ Outer Child beats up on other people's Little—especially the Little You of a significant other.

❑ Outer Child bullies its own Little.

❑ Outer Child tries to get self-esteem by proxy—that is, by going after someone who has higher social value.

❑ Outer Child can't hide from our closest family members. They get to see it in action. That is what intimacy is all about: the exposure of our Outer Children.

❑ Outer Child can express anger by becoming passive. One of Outer's favorite disguises is compliance. Outer Child uses compliance to confuse others into thinking that it doesn't want to take control. But don't be fooled—Outer Child is a control freak.

❑ Outer Child finds someone to take for granted and treats him badly because it doesn't have to worry about abandonment for a change.

❑ Outer Child refuses to stay on the rock, unlike Little. Outer climbs down and picks up a hatchet and goes on the warpath.

❑ Outer Child doesn't obey the Golden Rule. Outer Child obeys its own "Outer Child Rule": Get others to treat you as you want to be treated, and treat others as you feel like treating them.

❑ Outer Child provokes anger in subtle ways, then accuses the other person of being abusive.

❑ Outer loves to play the indignant injured party. Outer Child is master at making the other person look like the bad guy.*

---

* For additional Outer Child characteristics, see the complete inventory in my *Journey from Abandonment to Healing* (pp. 208–16). Also, see my *Taming Your Outer Child*, or click on the OUTER CHILD HELP button at the abandonment.net Help Center.

How many characteristics did you check? _____
How many did you double circle? _____
How many did you box? _____
What does this tell you about the personality of your own Outer Child?

You may need to take the Outer Child Inventory more than once. You'll pick up new insights each time. Remember Outer Child is unconscious, hidden behind all kinds of rationalizations and disguises (so that it is free to get away with murder). It takes time and effort to get a handle on how Outer Child defenses interfere in your relationships and in your life.

Maintain a diary of daily sightings of Outer Child. This keeps your awareness fresh and allows you to lead from your adult wisdom. Keeping Outer Child in check allows you to maintain a boundary to separate your feelings from your behavior so that your adult self can determine the best course of action, rather than this internal saboteur.

Rage Is Redeemable as Love

During Rage, your task is to harness Outer Child's energy to deepen your connection to yourself and others. Your abandonment experience has underscored the importance of love.

Throughout this workbook, we've laid the groundwork for love. We began by appreciating the miracle of life, which we're accomplishing by using the moment as a source of personal power. We've been engaged in self-love through the Big You / Little You Dialogue. We've restored confidence in reaching our dreams by visualizing the Dream House throughout the day, every day. Now we're taking a next critical step in recovery. Through the vehicle of Outer Child, we're learning to separate feelings from behavior. Gaining Outer Child awareness means learning about our automatic behaviors—the entrenched patterns and old habits we picked up from childhood.

Redirect the aggressive energy that bubbles over the edge during Rage. Divert it in the direction of becoming a self-loving, constructive, caring human being. Let Big take charge of your needs rather than laying them at the feet of Outer or in the lap of your next partner, expecting someone else to feed your emotional hunger. That's your job.

Community Projects

I would like to encourage people to use their Rage energy to become involved in community projects. A special mission of this workbook is to end isolation and loneliness in the world. As a community of abandonment survivors, we bear witness to each person's struggle. I urge you to use your pent-up aggression to reach out to individuals who are alone and isolated—people in prisons, homeless shelters, living on streets, in nursing homes, or isolated somewhere within our communities. Zeroing in on your own abandonment issues helps you connect universally to all humanity. If Big You is looking for productive activity, I can recommend no greater way to employ its time. Through community projects we find ways to stop abandoning each other.

There are other activities on which to spend some of your aggression. You'll see many suggestions in the appendices. You'll learn how to set up abandonment support groups. You'll also gain inspiration from Akeru-to-go—a panoply of activities designed for the weekend and other time voids. It contains ideas for getting out of your head, worries, and wounded spirit and into the moment where you can invest your energy constructively—not only when you are alone, but with a friend, or within a group.

Gaining Outer Child awareness is a first step. Taking action is the next. As your adult self finally rises to power, you get to choose your own behavior rather than get caught in the swirl of Outer's patterns. When you thrust forward to connect, it's not your emotionally driven child acting out, but your self-nurturing adult whose wisdom and love transform your relationships and your life.

The radiating power of love is illustrated in the ninth lesson of the black swan.

SWAN LESSON NINE
Reaching Out to Connect

The little girl had been practicing her idea of love. She was learning to accept others as they are and opening her hand in a gesture of letting go of her fears, anger, and expectations. Yet she continued to feel frustrated among the many people she encountered as she made her way back out into the world. Lonely and at a loss for connection, she returned to the water's edge to seek guidance from the black swan.

"I am angry because no one is my friend," cries the little girl to her beloved swan. *"I don't have anybody."*

"Angry means you want love, and you can create it by bringing your idea of love to others," answers the black swan.

"How can I do that?"

"It takes only two steps. When you're near them, you first create the idea of love within yourself and then get into the moment with them. That's all you do."

"But the moment is when I listen to butterfly wings and things like that," says the little girl.

"The moment also offers a gift for being with others."

"How?"

"It's not difficult, Amanda. You open your senses to those you are with," says the swan. "See them, hear them, and be with them—that's all you have to do."

"How do I be with them?"

"You can just say hello or look at what they are looking at, or you may talk with them."

"No!" cries the little girl. "I am too afraid."

"When you're afraid, you can just remain a quiet presence beside them and think about the love you are creating within," says the swan.

The little girl places her hands upon her heart.

"Can you tell me what your idea of love is about, Amanda?"

She closes her eyes. "Love…" she begins, "is caring if another person is alive," she says softly. "And not being mean," she adds a little louder. "And not leaving them when they don't want you to!" She gazes into the eyes of the swan. "That's about all," she says.

"It's a strong idea, Amanda. It comes from inside your sacred place where no wounders are allowed. Its strength is pure and its warmth is real. And you can use it with others. It's a beginning."

"I don't see how it helps."

"When I first arrived in these waters, I tried to seek refuge among the white swans, but their squawking disturbed me and I was cowered by their scorn. I swam out to the deepest waters to face my separateness. Out there alone, I got away from anger and hurt and I realized how powerful was this force of love. I felt so bereft of love that I wanted it to grow again inside my own heart." The swan dips his long neck in the water and extends it toward the little girl. "I spent many hours creating this idea of love and held on to it, even as the other swans rejected me," he continues. "Soon there was no one to object to the warmth that radiated from me and many wanted to swim within its range, to bask unknowingly in its radiance."

"Then how come I can't see it?" asks the little girl, extending her hand.

"It's very quiet," says the swan, "but powerful." He glides toward the water's edge and looks directly at the outstretched hand of the little girl and then into her eyes. "It is working right now."

In this lesson, the little girl extended an open hand outward in a gesture of reaching out. Try this gesture to help you reflect on your idea of love and its potential impact on others in your life.

What is your idea of love?

Is this idea changing? How?

How would you like it to change?

How does the way you handle love affect the way you feel about yourself?

How can increasing love within your current relationships help you in your everyday life?

Practice getting into the moment with others. Be present. Attend to what is going on in the live action between you and them. Be careful not to leave yourself behind. Stay anchored to your own emotional core. Your personal value is measured in the powerful concept of love you behold—a concept that is constantly growing. Use your Rage energy constructively by reaching out to others and taking actions to improve your life.

 ## THE PARADOX OF RAGE AND LOVE

Check all you agree with.

- ❏ Love converts anger and frustration into connection.
- ❏ Love is a tool for rage—it meets it head-on and overpowers it.
- ❏ Love is a way to heal the source of my anger.
- ❏ Love transcends anger. It uses its thrusting energy to connect to others in a powerful way.
- ❏ Instead of rage, love.
- ❏ I should let love become my way of being with people, and I will find love.

In the next chapter, we will work on rehabilitating your relationships—the ones you already have as well as the ones you expect to form. Toward the end of the workbook, I'll introduce you to the actual steps you can take to make a new connection, called the Five-Point Action Plan. In spite of all of the hurt, turmoil, and anger spilling over the edge during Rage, love uses its jet-propelled energy to build bridges to others.

More Food for Thought

What is the worst thing your Outer Child ever did (at least what you're willing to admit here)?

What has Outer been doing this week?

What's it been up to today?

When you visit your parents, what is Outer doing?

When someone cancels a date, what does Outer do?

When you're afraid of getting caught making a mistake, what does Outer do?

While you are waiting for your date to call you back, what does Outer do?

10 Integrating and Owning

A few months into my breakup, my abandonment wound still tender, I happened upon an unexpected discovery involving the black swan. He was gliding through the harbor, accompanied by a pair of white swans, when a boat pulled up to the pier. Out stepped a man and small boy intent on getting a closer look at the swan. It was not unusual for the black swan to receive a lot of attention from onlookers. The newspapers had been photographing him and featuring articles about his sudden appearance in the harbor. The man and boy shouted and threw bread into the water to entice the swan to come closer. All three swans responded, swimming toward the food, but only the two white swans swam under the dock to get to it. The black swan's efforts to duck under the dock were unsuccessful.

Camera in hand, I ran down to the pier to see what was preventing him. His head was bobbing about rapidly in an apparent display of agitation or anxiety. Observing his predicament, I noticed that he could have swum all the way around the dock, but he did not take that option. He remained behind, his head darting about in distress.

The white swans swooped up the bread in their beaks but soon turned around to see where their compadre was and noticed he was having difficulty on the other side of the dock. They instantly swam back to help him. I watched in amazement as they got on either side of him, and with a few trials showed him how to swim under the dock. Sure enough, he came up on the other side. He instantly swam to the bread, took it in his beak, extended his neck, and swallowed it down. The man and boy boisterously praised his accomplishment. Then he went off by himself, gliding out to the horizon to gain distance from us all.

Observing this spectacle moved me greatly. I remember having the absurd thought, "He's human after all." There was no doubt he was a survivor of some kind of separation. It was clear that he was not at home in this New York harbor and would find no mate here, since he was of a different species.[1] He was isolated. The trauma that separated him from his own flock shone in his distress that day. By revealing his vulnerability, he became more inspirational to me, touching me with a powerful message of humility and courage. I noticed how he maintained his integrity by sustaining himself as a separate being among an alien flock.

I wrote this scene into the story about the little girl and allowed her to react to it in her own way. Watching her beloved swan falter at the docks, the little girl became confused and disillusioned. I present their next meeting in its entirety, as it contains the meaning I ultimately took from the experience.

SWAN LESSON TEN
Integrating and Owning

"I saw you at the water!" challenges the little girl. *"You were afraid, afraid to go under the dock. The other swans had to help you."*

"That is so," says the swan.

"But you are the black swan and you are strong and brave."

"I don't have any special strength and bravery," says the swan. *"No more than I need. No more than you have, Amanda."*

"But you must be stronger and braver than I am!" cries the little girl.

"Why must that be so?" asks the swan.

"Because you know what to do and how to be!"

"I am practicing how to use the moment, just as you are," explains the black swan.

"But I'm not good at it," says the little girl, shaking her head back and forth, *"and I need you to be strong so you can help me."*

"It's not about special strength, Amanda. It's about remembering to favor the moment. We lose the moment because we get distracted by grief and fear—grief over what has passed and fear over what might come. The past and future both have a powerful pull. Grief and fear keep pulling us out of the present. But when we catch that happening, we just take hold and return to the moment so that we can practice what we know."

"But I can't do that by myself! And who are you to give advice?" says the little girl. *"You couldn't even swim under the docks by yourself. You were afraid!"*

The beautiful swan lifts his wings. *"My moment slips away from me just like yours does. That's why I must practice it over and over. You saw me after I took the bread. I swam all the way out to the deepest waters. I went there to regain the moment, face my separateness, and celebrate my lone existence."*

"But I still have too many bad feelings to do that," insists the little girl.

"Life has a way of bringing difficult feelings, Amanda. They are part of its currents. But now you know how to use your tools to find the moment and start fresh each time."

"I keep forgetting to."

"We all keep forgetting the moment, Amanda. But we have our feelings to remind us. When you have a bad feeling, just go back to the moment and practice what you know."

"But I don't know anything!" challenges the little girl.

"Of course you do. You are learning so many things—how to find your center and keep it safe, how to find the moment and accept your separateness, how to face your reality and discover the importance of being alive, and how to treat others with love." The swan swirls in the water.

The little girl feels a strong breeze. She wraps her arms around herself.

"Yes, Amanda. Gather your arms around yourself to gather together all that you know. Then the moment will be yours. You own it. Only you can command it."

I think the body linguists have it wrong. They suggest that when we fold our arms, we're keeping people out. We're not. In holding ourselves, we are performing a gesture of self-acceptance, accepting ourselves as we are now in the moment. Wrapping our arms around ourselves is a way of gathering all that we've learned together with who we are and holding it to heart, embracing our self-wisdom.[2] When such a gesture seems off-putting, it is probably when we use it defensively to protect ourselves from someone whose power seems threatening at the moment.

The swan's vulnerability had significance for me that day because it illustrated that we are ready to gather ourselves together and to take responsibility for our lives before we think we are, even before our recovery is perfect.

Perfectionism

Perfectionism is a trait that runs through the lives of many abandonment survivors. It's a source of self-sabotage because it predicates our success on a false solution, a solution that creates its own set of problems. Perfectionists are always raising the bar on themselves, turning life into a treadmill—despite their efforts, they can never reach satisfaction.

Perfectionism is fueled by Outer Child's penchant for creating vicious circles.

Perfectionism is an attempt to overcompensate for a deficiency we perceive in ourselves. As a defense it doesn't work. It only drives insecurity in deeper. Abandonment survivors are convinced they can never be perfect enough to stave off the rejection or criticism they believe is their due.

Perfectionism creates unrealistic expectations, especially when it comes to recovery. You expect to grow in a straight line and accomplish the healing tasks once and for all—without error. Perfectionists think that to err is a weakness and they fault themselves for slipping back into negative emotions. Perfectionism makes it difficult to appreciate the true nature of achievement. Progress is usually accomplished by taking two steps forward, one step back.

When you lay aside perfectionism, you open the door to change. Release yourself from its rigid hold and take a giant step in reversing the calcified self-doubts you've been harboring.

This chapter is dedicated to overthrowing perfectionism. I'm going to ask you to lay it aside in favor of accepting yourself as you are now. Take responsibility for your present life, even before you've reached that elusive state called perfection,

You are ready now.

That word—*now*—brings us once again to the personal power we contain in the moment. The moment is when you accomplish any difficult task. Not in the future. Not for all time. But now. Gather together all that you know at this point. Don't wait until the conditions are better, until you've perfectly lifted from abandonment. Consider the wisdom you've gained so far.

Realizing you are ready now elevates you to a plateau—an overlook—for the rest of your journey. In Alcoholics Anonymous, this place of personal responsibility is the tenth step. It advises recovering addicts, "Continue taking personal inventory and when you're wrong, promptly admit it."

That is what you're doing here in this tenth chapter—learning to take an inventory of what you've gained so far and make amends to your current situation. The key is to give yourself credit for doing the best you can. Vow to keep doing your best. When you slip, correct yourself and move forward.

If I am going to stand by my principles about maintaining realistic expectations, I hereby expect you to make some mistakes as you progress outward into the world to launch your new life. You will proceed imperfectly, simply because, like me, you are human. Many of the things you'll be doing will be new to you. If you try to be perfect, you will agonize over every one of your backward steps. Becoming realistic allows you to see back steps as part of the gait of progress. Progress is supposed to be slow, steady, and sporadic. When you slip back, rebalance yourself. Learn what you can from the experience, and propel your journey forward.

To celebrate the imperfection of all human beings, I'd like to introduce another boon to recovery: The Correction. Correction is something you do after the fact—after you've said something or done something you later regret, after you've caught your Outer Child acting out, after you've been less than perfect. Perfectionists berate themselves unmercifully for these less-than-perfect deeds. Reformed perfectionists accept them as part of being human. They don't belabor their mistakes, they perform corrections.

The Correction

"I regret that I gave you advice this morning," says Bob. "It wasn't until I was halfway to work that I realized you hadn't asked for my opinion. I appreciate your not getting up in my face about it, even though I certainly harangued you, and I know it's something I agreed not to do. Please let me know when I'm veering out of line next time, in case it doesn't dawn on me."

The Correction is a valuable tool for dealing with little slipups as well as major relapses in your behavior. It's effective in changing deeply ingrained patterns of behavior, the ones you're most likely to fall back into. For example, in my work with counseling couples, I don't expect my clients to change their usual mode of interaction on a permanent basis just because therapy taught them the correct way to communicate. Learning a better way does not prevent them from falling back into their old habits in the heat of the moment. What can couples do? When they catch themselves falling back into old patterns, perform Corrections.

"Everything always revolved around my family," says Margaret. "It wasn't fair to Keith for me to leave him in the lurch whenever my mother or brother went into crisis. Keith claimed it bothered

him a lot. He was the one paying all of the bills, but he felt his needs were never taken into account, only my family's. He resented me being so enmeshed in my family. It was tearing us apart.

"Now when my family pulls at me, I back away a little and disentangle myself enough to consult with Keith. I'm far from perfect with it, but at least I'm learning how to get out before I'm drowning in my family dramas."

So many abandonment survivors become exasperated with themselves for not being able to eradicate unwanted behavior overnight. Habits may die hard, but don't ever give up on yourself. You can't expect to prevent relapsing to old behaviors every time. You can only strengthen your resolve to change, throw yourself into the struggle, and when you err, perform a Correction.

Correction is an effective tool, not only when you've been less than perfect toward someone but when someone has been less than perfect toward you. In the latter case, you correct the fact that you let it happen. To illustrate the magnitude of its application, I'm going to start with one of the most challenging situations facing abandonment survivors, the tendency to get emotionally stuck in a destructive relationship.

Owing to the tendency to repeat themes from childhood, many of you get involved in emotionally toxic relationships and can't seem to get out. First we'll examine the origins of this problem, and then we'll see how to correct it.

Negative Attractions

As I said previously, negative attractions are more compelling than positive ones, and often the most difficult to break.

Why should this be? Why do we get entrapped in relationships that we know are no good for us? For one thing, negative attractions are physiologically addictive.

Fear and pain are powerful reinforcers—powerful enough, in many cases, to transform the strongest among us into Pavlov's dogs who salivate at the sound of a bell. We're conditioned to respond when somebody presses our insecurity button. When a lover arouses our fear of abandonment, a traumatic connection is created.[3] Traumatic bonding is a highly prevalent condition in human relationships, especially among abandonment survivors. It has an addictive biochemistry of its own, examples of which are found throughout the animal kingdom. For example, when a researcher steps on the toe of a duckling (ouch), it follows him (imprints) more closely than before.[4] The hazing ritual involved in joining fraternities creates traumatic bonding, whereby the pain and humiliation inflicted on the new pledges increases their loyalty to the fraternal order. The famous Stockholm study[5] provides another example in which bank hostages became steadfastly loyal and protective toward their captors.

The headline case of Patty Hearst offers a dramatic example of this. She was captured from her family's mansion by the Symbionese Liberation Army and held ransom for her father's celebrated millions. The experience invoked fear to the extent that she quickly entered into emotional bondage with her kidnappers. So emotionally enslaved did she become that as a hostage, she helped them commit crimes for which the court later found her guilty. Her newly acquired criminal behavior appeared voluntary to the court; but, in fact, she had become traumatically bonded to her captors. The fear aroused by the kidnapping helped reinforce her new behaviors as a function of her bondage.

Research into the startle response provides clues as to why this happens. Startling is a response to fear. It has been observed that directly after being startled, people are more prone to obey commands.[6] In certain Malaysian societies, a special term—*latah*—is designated for those who startle easily. It is known that directly after being startled, *latahs* tend to obey commands, even absurd ones. Repeatedly startling people to tease them and get them to follow orders is an acceptable form of social amusement in these cultures. Sometimes the motive can be more sinister. In one example, someone poked a *latah* who was holding a knife, and after startling her, told her to stab the man next to her. She immediately did so and it killed him. When the case went to trial, the judge tested the *latah* to see whether she could be held legally responsible for the murder. He startled her and told her to slap the end of a nail-studded stick. She obeyed instantly and impaled her hand. The verdict: the man who poked her was found guilty, not the *latah*, demonstrating reverse logic to that which was used to convict Hearst.

What this shows is that being frightened can make you more susceptible to falling under someone's domination. You surrender control over your own actions. The fear created by abandonment doesn't occur in a burst; it's not over like it is when you've been startled. It occurs in a continuous flow over an extended period of time (or in pulsating waves). This may account for the loss of personal volition you experience when involved with a partner whose drinking, philandering, or emotional abuses chronically arouse your fear of abandonment.

Feeling "Almost" Accepted

Many abandonment survivors encounter people who dangle the possibility of love in their faces but convey a discouraging message: "You're not quite what I'm looking for." The fear, anger, and insecurity this engenders create perfect laboratory conditions for traumatic bonding. The anxiety of almost being rescued from loneliness serves to reinforce, rather than weaken, your dependence on that person.

> People often ask: "What's wrong with me that I'm involved with someone who treats me poorly?"
>
> I answer: It isn't just so-called hopeless neurotics who are vulnerable to forming negative attachments. Even healthy neurotics like you and me can fall prey to relationships in which the emotional dynamics overrule our better judgment.

We are all capable of becoming traumatically bonded under the right conditions, especially if the person you've grown attached to begins to arouse your deep-set fears about being left. Being in a destructive relationship doesn't prove something is wrong with you but that you've become entrapped in a powerful human dynamic.

Sometimes even when you manage to end the relationship, it's hard to give up the emotional bondage.

"I can't stop obsessing about Lisa even though I was always miserable with her," says Michael. "I found her to be selfish, spoiled, and unreasonable—and that was on a good day. She alienated me from family and friends with her constant demands and criticism. Then things took a turn for the worse when she went on a business trip to Chicago. She started an affair with some guy there and unknowingly came back with a case of herpes. So eventually I wound up catching herpes, and you guessed it, she blamed it on me.

"Then one night I spotted some of her old cell-phone bills and noticed that after her trip, she'd put in all of these late-night calls to a private phone in Chicago. I did some backtracking and found out about her little escapade. She wasn't even apologetic, but I kept hoping she'd declare her love for me. We kept seeing each other off and on for a few more months, but it was holy hell. Then she started living with another guy and I finally called it quits.

"I'm just about out of my mind missing her and can't stop thinking about her, obsessing about what went wrong and how I should have played it differently. I'm dying to call her, but she'll just blow me off again and make me feel worse. My friends are sick and tired of listening to me. They keep telling me she's no good for me. Do you think I don't know that myself? Do you think I'm stupid? Intellectually I know I'm lucky to have her out of my life, but emotionally I can't help myself from wanting her."

Your friends, your family, and your own intellect can chastise you for not being able to say good riddance to your destructive relationship, all to no avail. Until you get a handle on what is driving you to stay connected, fear reinforces your need to hang on emotionally tighter than ever. You remain gripped in the compelling dynamics of traumatic bonding, that is, until you learn how to correct it.

Name someone you know who is embroiled in a similar emotional entrapment.

Have you ever been in a relationship that was no good for you? Explain.

What made it so difficult to break away?

Have you ever become emotionally enslaved by someone else's chronic rejection and unavailability?

What insights can you use to overcome this problem?

Surrendering Your Of

Another aspect of getting stuck in emotionally unsatisfying relationships is the tendency to lose yourself in someone else's power. Considering how common it is for people in our society to get caught in a negative attraction, it helps to have a special term for it. The one I use is Surrendering Your Of and it comes from a colleague, Yvonne Rivers, A.C.S.W., who noted:

> People have a need to dominate and control you out of their own self-centeredness or insecurity, or for whatever reason. The fact that you love them isn't enough. They keep imposing their sense of entitlement over you until they get you to surrender more than just your love, they take your Of. It can be so subtle you don't realize you've lost your own volition until you hit some sort of crisis and discover that somewhere along the line you've lost yourself.
>
> It's the same tactics used in the making of a slave, except less subtle. Slave masters will do whatever it takes to demoralize you with fear, take away your power and control, and convey the message of your unworthiness. They might even pretend to love you; but all the while, they are systematically taking away your Of. To make sure you will be a good slave, they need to destroy your volition.[7]

When your lover takes Your Of, or startles you with his boldness, or overpowers you with his higher sense of entitlement, or arouses your insecurity, he's able to acquire more than his share of power in the relationship.

Sometimes it isn't your lover, but your own self-defeating patterns of people pleasing that cause you to Surrender Your Of. It might be your own need to merge with your partner that causes you to lose yourself.

"I was so willing to have my life revolve around Jay," says Helene. "I was insecure because I knew he'd had affairs on his ex-wife, and what would prevent him from doing the same to me? So, I became over-attentive to his every need. If he seemed to want something, I took it as a command. I became a nonperson around him. I couldn't stand who I'd become."

When the boundary between yourself and your partner becomes blurred, when emotions overrule your better judgment, when it feels more like an addiction than a relationship, the only person who can retrieve Your Of and take back control is you.

Do you know people who have surrendered their power to others?

Has anyone you loved ever stolen Your Of? If so, how did it feel to lose yourself in someone else's power?

Have you ever acquired someone else's Of? If so, how did it feel to have too much power?

What earlier events made you susceptible to losing yourself in a relationship?

Might these dynamics mirror your relationship with your parents when you were a child? If so, how?

Are you still at risk for losing yourself in someone else's needs—Surrendering Your Of?

What insights can you use to overcome this issue?

Correcting Destructive Relationships

Performing a Correction is an act of acknowledgment. You must be willing to come out of denial and see the writing on the wall about your situation. Take responsibility for your side of the equation. Acknowledge that you can do better and put that admission into practice. Remember, practice doesn't mean you have to do it right the first time. It means practice to get it right. By practicing, you are using your own mistakes as mini growth experiences to help you change difficult patterns, one misstep at a time.

To guide the way, here are examples of Corrections performed by clients and members of abandonment support groups.

Correction for Losing Your Power to Someone Else

"I tried to snap out of this worthless position I'd put myself in with Jay, but I kept falling into the trap of wanting to please him," says Helene. "I finally decided to correct this in little bites. I made a commitment to do one small Correction each day. Every day I figured out something I wanted that was independent of what Jay wanted. And that wasn't easy, believe me. Then I put that one little thing on my agenda for the day and I fought for it. I was really fighting myself, because all I really cared about was pleasing him.

"Asserting my sense of self got easier after a while, and I baby-stepped my way out of that horrid nonperson role I'd fallen into. Now I'm building to an equal presence in the relationship."

Correction for Carrying a Torch

"My constant obsessing about Lisa was interfering in a new relationship," says Michael. "I started seeing Beth, someone I really liked and respected. But even this new relationship didn't stop me from thinking about Lisa. The torch I was carrying caused me to pull away a lot. By now I knew better. It was time to move on.

"I handled it by planning little Corrections. Whenever I caught myself thinking about Lisa, I'd get into the moment, center in, take stock of my reality, and remind myself that Lisa was not right for me, that she was not part of my current life. I had to face this simple fact not once, but hundreds of times, especially when I was with Beth, because I kept slipping back.

"I'm finally able to focus my energy on the moment and attend to what's happening now, rather than letting my mind meander to Lisa. She is part of my past. When I catch myself having a stray thought about Lisa, I just do another Correction and dismiss this twang as an addiction to a bad substance. I remind myself that the feeling will pass. I don't let it confuse me or interfere with my feelings about Beth."

Correction for Dangling by a String

"We'd been separated for only a few months and my husband already started living with another woman," says Sarah-Jean. "I wanted him to come back so badly. He kept saying things that gave me hope, like, 'I'm not sure I should be with her,' and 'She's ambivalent about me, too,' and 'Maybe she and I aren't right for each other after all.' This made it impossible for me to let go and also made me want to prove to him that I could correct the problems between us, like my being demanding and controlling. This went on for over eighteen months, with me constantly trying to convince him to take me back."

Like Sarah-Jean, most people find it difficult to break this kind of connection because, as we discussed earlier, attachment is akin to a biochemical addiction. Sarah-Jean was starving for a love fix and her husband was feeding her little crumbs to keep her hooked. He most likely rationalized giving her little glimmers of hope by convincing himself that he was protecting her from the pain of jealousy and loss.

"I knew that by pursuing him I was letting him use me as a security blanket," Sarah-Jean continues. "I was making it possible for him to subsist in a new relationship where he felt insecure. To stop enabling him, I planned a Correction. I meditated on the Swan Lessons every morning, doing the gestures that went with them. Once fully centered and in the moment, I reminded myself that in this moment, I had no control over whether my husband might break up with his new woman tomorrow and come back to me. My life was now. I couldn't prevent myself from wanting him. I could only end the agony of waiting by facing the fact that he wasn't in my life now. For all I knew, tomorrow he might come back. Then again, he might not. The only thing that counted was that right now he wasn't there. Facing this allowed me to start living now."

Correction for Not Letting Go

"After ten years in A.A.," says Keaton, "I find when I'm really struggling, it means I'm trying to be powerful over something I have no power over. So I go back to step one of Alcoholics Anonymous and admit to my powerlessness.[8] Given the fact that I have an addictive personality, I know I can get addicted to anything dead or alive. So when I was going through hell over Gabby, I felt addicted to her and the only Correction for me would be complete abstinence. I couldn't abstain from my feelings about her—because feelings are givens—but I could abstain from my behavior. So I stopped going by her house, stopped calling her answering machine, and stopped isolating from other people. To take these steps I had to be willing to go back out and connect with people and get help."

Correction for a Breakup-Waiting-to-Happen

"My wife says she's leaving me because she doesn't love me anymore," says Bob. "She says I've been too overbearing. I will do anything to get her to stay with me. I'm trying to convince her not to go.

'Please don't do this,' I tell her. I give her a million reasons to stay and work it out. But all she says is, 'See, Bob, you're doing it again—it's always about you.'

"It feels like I'm beating my head against a stone wall, that she's leaving no matter what. Even so, I have to change. I'm a take-charge kind of guy and I need to get out of this self-centered role I've been in. I know she needs to feel safe and comfortable when she's with me and that I have to change things in a hurry or I'll lose her for sure. I'd like to change overnight, but even Superman can't change his costume that fast. So now, I find that the fastest way to change is by making mini Corrections. When I catch myself in the act of being overbearing, I step back and say, 'Barbara, I hear myself. I hear what you've been trying to tell me.' I tell her that the crisis between us is necessary for me because it's helping me wake up and become a better person. To that, she's willing to listen."

Correction for Unfinished Business with Your Ex

Sometimes the Correction is about resolving unfinished business from a relationship gone sour.

"It was almost a year since our divorce and I was still heartbroken that Don had left me, and just as bewildered. But one day it finally came to me. He must have felt he was in a less-than role all of those years—not because he was inadequate, but because the situation was so much more supportive to my self-esteem than to his.

"He'd already started up with a new woman and I didn't know if he'd be willing to talk about this with me, but I approached him with this new sensitivity and found him to be receptive. I laid out my thoughts to him, explaining that I'd begun wondering what it would feel like if our roles had been reversed. What if I had been in a relationship with someone whose career had more notoriety than mine did and had more money attached to it? Would I feel that my world revolved around his? Would I feel relegated to the background? Would I have felt less powerful about myself? I told him, yes, I would have felt less-than, and it would have been demoralizing, and that I couldn't help but wonder if he'd felt any of this.

"Don said it had been difficult to feel important in the marriage and that I seemed to have a greater sense of entitlement than he did, especially when it came to making the big decisions. He felt I'd been oblivious to his feelings about this and that I'd taken his supportiveness for granted. He explained that in his new relationship, he's in a more equal role.

"I told him how painful it was to understand his feelings now that it was too late to make it up to him, but that it helped me. I would grow on it. It was the best communication we'd ever had and it opened up a new door between us. I don't know where it's leading but it feels good to be healing some of our old wounds."

Performing a Psychological Autopsy on the Relationship

Sometimes making a Correction has to do with figuring out how you contributed to the current situation you are in—and then making amends to yourself and your partner. It's important to do this without drama and breast beating. The more responsibility you can take, the greater your sense of control over your future. A member of one of my abandonment support groups said it best:

"When my wife left me for someone else, instead of drowning in sorrow I found it more helpful to step back and see what I could learn about myself. I'm in the medical profession and know that when you do an autopsy on a miscarried fetus you often find a lethal defect, something that would have made it impossible for the baby to survive anyway. I considered that my marriage may have miscarried, and I tried to figure out what the lethal defect might have been. I wasn't looking to blame, just to figure out what had been missing in me so I could find out what I need to change on my end."

Can you find a fatal flaw that might have caused a previous relationship to break up?

What can you learn about yourself from the experience?

How can you use this awareness?

Other Relationships

A Correction can help you strengthen other relationships as well—with your co-workers, friends, and family.

Parents tend to fault themselves for not being able to keep their emotions perfectly contained. Rather than aim toward perfection every time they relate to their kids, they have the option to accept the inevitability of losing their patience sometimes and perform a Correction.[9]

"Just this morning," says Gloria, "I pulled my five-year-old aside and said, 'Remember this morning when Mommy yelled?' He nodded his head. 'I thought about it later and wished I hadn't yelled

at you the way I did. It could frighten you, Nathaniel. It might make you feel bad and I don't want to do that.' I let that sink in for a minute and then added, 'I want to teach you good behavior and I want to use my best behavior too. And when I forget, I make it better as soon as I can, just like I'm doing now.'"

Corrections Are Not a Substitute for Change

Be careful not to use Correction as a substitute for change. Otherwise you are becoming an Apologizer, an Outer Child role often used by abusers to perpetrate repeat behaviors.

"My husband became a genius at apologizing. You never saw anyone say he was sorry more sincerely and convincingly," says Barbara. "He made every time he was abusive toward me sound like it would be the final, ultimate, rock-bottom last. But then within a few months, he'd strike again. Well, I finally planned a Correction of my own. One evening, we went out to dinner, and in the middle of a normal conversation I told him very calmly, 'I need to talk with you about something,' I waited until I was sure I had his full attention and said, 'I realize, Bob, that I have accepted your apologies over the years—and I even believed them. I take full responsibility for this—it was my doing. I know that this gave you the idea that an apology could cancel out the deed. But I was wrong. I have deep resentment, too much water under the bridge. I don't feel love for you like I used to. I'm giving you fair warning that I'm no longer willing to stay in the marriage on these terms. I've got an attorney.' This time he didn't apologize. He went into shock. Things are different, and I'm not sure what the outcome will be."

Wrap your arms around yourself to gather all that you know into the moment—and when you stumble on the path, correct yourself. The result propels your forward, one misstep at a time.

Correcting Your Daily Regimen

The Correction required to set your life on track often involves creating a whole new daily regimen, one that is targeted to your goals. This approach requires self-discipline and commitment.

"I'd come through the worst of it, but I was left feeling this chronic heartache. It was inescapable," says Vicky, "and I'd done every possible Correction I could think up. 'What would it take to come out of this?' I kept asking myself. Finally, I decided to get up an hour early every day and start writing out the exercises. Of course, my Outer Child kept hitting the snooze button and trying to get me to go back to bed. But Big was determined. So I managed to get myself up, writing and writing my way through so many feelings, using the Big You/Little You Dialogue. I would keep writing until Little felt better and she and I had a plan to do something nurturing that day. I also used Back to the

Future to solve problems that came up. I'd imagine that I'd already solved it and then try to figure out what obstacles I'd had to remove and how I removed them and what actions I took. I vowed to take at least one positive action every day. And somehow or other, I took a baby step every day, most of the time, forcing myself through the motions.

"I'm noticing changes, so I'm still following this regimen. I found a new outlet for my Outer Child, which is to get her to do something physical, so I've joined a tennis club. I also started co-facilitating an abandonment support group, and now I'm meeting other people who, like me, are in heartache hell, which is good support—I don't feel so alone.

"I'm Lifting. There is so much self-love going on inside. Little is always by my side, and Big is stronger. On the days when it feels like I'm not getting anywhere, I set my alarm another fifteen minutes earlier and use the extra time to visualize my Dream House and write my way out of the sinkhole. I know I have the tools, the will, and the self-discipline, and this makes me feel good about myself."

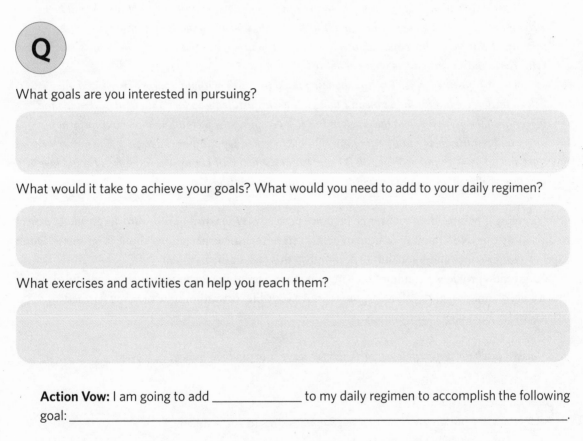

Q

What goals are you interested in pursuing?

What would it take to achieve your goals? What would you need to add to your daily regimen?

What exercises and activities can help you reach them?

Action Vow: I am going to add _____ to my daily regimen to accomplish the following goal: _____.

The Role of Forgiveness

A Correction may involve forgiveness.[10] Forgiveness tends to be one of those easier-said-than-done tasks. One of the things holding you back may be confusion about what forgiveness entails. Forgiving someone's behavior doesn't mean condoning it. It doesn't mean you believe the person's deeds were justified. It doesn't mean to stop defending yourself or to neglect your own needs. By forgiving a painful fact, you are simply accepting that it occurred. At the heart of forgiveness is a simple but difficult act of acceptance. Once you accept that a fellow human being caused you great pain—that the act occurred in reality—you get a glimpse of what unconditional love is all about. This momentary glimpse into a blessed state of forgiving all acts of human beings, holds benefits for you in that it helps you transcend your problems. Forgiveness is the ultimate act of letting go.

"I tried not to argue with Lonny every time we spoke," says Marie, "but he was so cold and aloof. It was just so painful after all those years of loving one another. To have him suddenly turn away from me like that and give all of his devotion to another woman! I got angry every time we had contact, but this only gave him a bigger excuse for what he was doing. I kept vowing to keep my calm, but as soon as he treated me in that disdainful way, I'd lose my temper all over again.

"I decided to plan a Correction. Given my raw emotions, the most foolproof way would be to write a note. Short and sweet, I just told him the truth, that my anger was coming from missing him, that I was feeling hurt and confused about what went wrong, and that he was in my thoughts (which was the biggest understatement of my life).

"Having postured myself in this honest manner—truth without rancor—I realized that it helped me forgive him. It didn't mean I thought he was justified—in fact, I thought he'd made the biggest mistake of his life, and the cruelest. But just accepting the facts allowed me to transform my anger and put my energy into getting my own life together. Up till then, I'd been trying not to feel hurt and angry—an impossible task! If I can accept the fact that Lonny was imperfect, I could love and forgive myself, too—for losing him. It was quite a revelation."

Forgiving a painful deed can never be done perfectly. When you aim toward forgiveness, expect to do so imperfectly in the way of human beings. Have realistic expectations about forgiveness. Don't expect to forgive once and for all but to accomplish this task in the moment.

Forgiveness provides a conduit for channeling the anger of the Rage stage, turning painful emotion into a state of amazing grace, allowing you to move your life forward in spite of being harmed.

Consider Janet's act of forgiveness:

"I asked Jacob for forgiveness—forgiveness for using him to abuse myself."

Think about where you are now. What is the main issue you're looking to correct at this point in your recovery?

What insights and strengths are you using?

> **Action Bullet:** I feel _____ because _____ , and I am ready to work on _____.

Back to the Future

Imagine it's about a year or two from now and you're sitting before your beautiful view feeling extremely peaceful and happy because you're no longer mired in uncomfortable feelings.

Q

What problem did you solve?

What obstacle was in the way? (What Outer Child resistance did you encounter?)

How did you overcome it?

Use this space to name an unresolved conflict in your current life and plan a Correction:

Action Vow: I will undertake the following Correction: _____

Stay Committed

Preparing to make Corrections may come naturally to you in a lot of instances, but when you're faced with a truly challenging conflict, it helps to gather all of your recovery tools and summon your grit and strength.

Check the items you are incorporating in your recovery.

I'M COMMITTED TO...

- ❏ Integrate all the awareness I've gained so far.
- ❏ Own responsibility for where my life is now.
- ❏ Use my ability to exercise self-control.
- ❏ Strengthen my resolve.
- ❏ Be determined to resolve this issue.

Will you resolve it perfectly? Most likely not. You'll move forward in fits and starts. When you fall off the wagon, get back on and right your wheels. The change required to set your life straight is not going to happen on its own. You have to make it happen.

You are ready now.

More Food for Thought

Name three people in your life on your not-yet-forgiven list.

Does being unforgiving affect the quality of your life? How?

What are your feelings about forgiveness?

Can forgiveness benefit your life in any way?

What might you have done to contribute to the ending of your relationship?

What can you learn from owning up to your part?

What strengths do you have for resolving these issues with your ex or with yourself?

11 Transcending

Become Larger Than Your Problem

I have coached many people through the stages of abandonment, offering every known technique and self-help tool. I have found abandonment survivors to be cooperative and highly motivated to do whatever it takes to come out of the debilitating grief. After availing themselves of all the exercises and taking every positive action, they turn to me during the final leg of the journey and ask: "But what do I do about my unhappiness? I'm still alone."

Don't throw your arms up in exasperation. There is one more growth level to push for. It is called Lifting. Lifting is about gaining altitude above your problems so you can create a higher purpose for them.

During this final stage of abandonment, life pulls you back unto itself.

Like so many sublime states, Lifting does not occur once and for all, but occurs in ever-increasing intervals. We experience moments of Lifting many times as we swirl through the various stages. Over time, the tornado weakens and we arrive at a place of calm and perspective. Gaining altitude over the process, we can see where we've been to appreciate how far we've come. We recognize the impact abandonment has had on our lives and how our spirit has grown.

Once again, Marie offers an example:

"I felt so shattered when Lonny left, it totally destroyed me. It forced me to start from scratch and grow a whole new me. It wasn't until the Lifting stage that I realized I liked the new person I was becoming better than the old one."

Akeru energy has helped you turn heartbreak's energy to your own advantage. Akeru reminds us that "to pierce a hole in" is to create a new opening. Feeling emotionally destroyed turned out to offer an opportunity to build a self. Let's review what we've gained so far. In the empty space created by abandonment, we've inculcated the Four Cornerstones of Self: Accepting Your Separateness, Beholding the Importance of Your Existence, Accepting Your Reality, and Increasing Your Capacity for Love. These four principles are based not on narcissistic notions about our relative attributes, but on our capacity to transcend rejection and loss.

We take pride in who we're becoming because we directed this growth ourselves. The tools of abandonment recovery empowered us to take back control of our lives and use our adult wisdom to navigate the journey. We nourish this growth by remaining open to our feelings. Lifting is a time to honor the feelings. They are gifts of the child within.

The metaphoric language of the wound describes what you've been through. During Shattering you felt the piercing pain as abandonment's knife to the heart severed the tender tissues of your attachment. During Withdrawal your laceration remained open, raw, and festering, tormenting you with the nagging, pulling, and aching of love deprivation. During Internalizing, the wound became susceptible to infection, threatening to leave permanent scars on your self-esteem. During Rage, you felt burning agitation as the tender, taut tissues tried to mend over the wound. And now, during Lifting, your wound seals over, protecting the self from further injury. The danger is that calluses can form, causing numbing and sensitivity to the area, sealing in your self-doubt and sealing you off from your feelings once again.

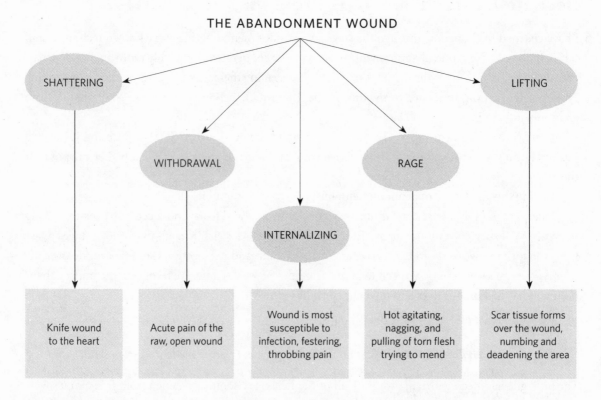

How you handle residual feelings of abandonment—the insecurity, self-doubt, and depression—determines why some of you will be positively transformed, and others will become remote, detached, and less likely to reconnect than before.[1]

The task of this final stage is to transform your abandonment into a higher purpose for your life. One abandonment survivor writing to abandonment.net put it this way:

"The saying 'That which doesn't kill you makes you stronger' is so trite to me now. If I have to hear that one more time, I'll literally spew. There is a quote by Albert Einstein that I much prefer. He said, 'The significant problems we face cannot be solved at the same level of thinking we were at when we created them.' In other words, the very purpose of our problems—their gift to us—is to trick us into outgrowing them. I realize that we never stop learning, but I'm hoping I've graduated from this level of hell without any more classes."

During Lifting you take pride in your separateness as a human being. No longer a terrifying prospect, you see aloneness as purposeful, as part of life's journey, a blessing to your spiritual and personal growth.

Abandonment has taught you that inside our skin we are each alone. The hackneyed phrase about coming into the world as a separate human being and exiting the same way now rings with personal truth. You know that, whether you're married or single, madly in love or going through heartbreak, we are each existentially alone.

Abandonment has poignantly shown us that we can never truly know another person completely. We may try to reveal ourselves to those we trust, but we always remain on the outside of the other. No one can see inside us to know exactly what we feel, think, and need. Others remain external to us also, even as we try to peer into their souls to grasp their essence. Even in the height of intimacy we remain separate individuals. The sense we have of another is a matter of perception, colored by our needs, anxieties, and values. We construct subjective pictures in our minds to represent the other, but the idea of truly knowing another is an illusion.

Most of us have experienced how painful this illusion can be. We believed our partners would never leave us, and yet they did. The fact that people do things that surprise and disappoint us proves the point: We never completely know another human being. We cannot exercise control over any person other than ourselves. And even though we need one another, abandonment has taught us that we don't need any one person to find love and fulfillment. We need people, possibility, and hope. When we stay connected to our feelings, the possibility for emotional fulfillment is always present.

The task for Lifting is to seek a greater purpose, to grow larger than our problems. Such is the next Swan Lesson.

SWAN LESSON ELEVEN
Transcending

The little girl had been gathering together all of the healing wisdom she gained from her contact with the black swan. Wrapping her arms around herself, she gained the strength to finally face the trauma she suffered at the hands of her father. She was shaken by the memory, but knew that her beloved swan was there to guide her. She told him about her torment and awaited his response.

"Your reality is difficult, to be sure, Amanda," says the swan. "By accepting its challenges, you grow bigger—a bigger sense of yourself. You grow so big that your problems become just a small part of you. Then they can't harm you as much."

"How do I do that?"

"It involves using your imagination, as always. It means you must set aside a special time every day to practice looking out at the universe to grasp its infinite possibilities."

"What does the universe have to do with it?"

"The universe is bigger than you and your problems combined, Amanda. Letting your mind expand all the way out to infinity increases your sense of wonder and guides you to greater purpose for your life."

"How?"

"It takes imagining."

The little girl looks at the swan and shrugs her shoulders.

"I'll show you how. Think about how wide and vast the universe is and what it means to be alive within it. Pretend that your every need and desire is possible to attain, that it's all just waiting for you to find it."

"Pretending doesn't make it true," the little girl argues.

"It doesn't have to be true," replies the swan. "Pretending brings pleasure to your mind—a special gift sent to you from your imagination. Imagining helps your mind expand to a place that makes all things possible and helps your reality to grow."

"But I don't believe it!" insists the little girl.

"You don't have to believe anything that isn't true or that you can't see right in front of you. Use your imagination to help you enjoy a bigger picture of life. The universe goes on forever, just as your imagination does. They are alike in many ways, each composed of energy and endless possibility. Think of the infinite universe and imagine that you are its grateful child. Imagine that what you ask for is possible, if not now, later. Be grateful for the hope this thought brings."

"How can I do this?"

"Spend your special time each day thinking about the largest reality you can imagine. Let your mind expand all the way out to infinity and back. Know that all is possible. All you need is just waiting for you to find it. Imagine that if you ask reality to open itself to you, you will receive many gifts."

"Can I ask for anything I want?"

"As long as what you imagine doesn't rely on someone else changing but on what is possible for you to find for yourself."

"It works just by imagining?" asks the little girl, gazing skyward.

"What you desire comes in its own way and time. Some things involve a lot of work; some, great patience; others, luck. Whether or not you get all that you imagine, Amanda, the important *thing to remember is that it is always possible. But you must spend every day seeking your higher purpose in a universe of possibilities."*

Notice that as the little girl practices this new idea, she gazes skyward—a common gesture I have noticed people perform when they attempt to grasp the greater meaning of their lives.

Do you know someone whose problems provide a purpose for her life? Describe.

Do you know someone whose problems are large but whose life's mission is so much larger that his problems shrink by comparison? Describe.

Think about your current problems. What larger purpose might they serve in your life?

A Word of Caution

Lifting out of abandonment into a greater meaning and purpose is a desirable outcome of this final stage, but it's not without its downfalls.[2] Many people make the mistake of Lifting above their feelings. They are anxious to forget the pain, and they run from emotional wounds that remain unresolved, forsaking Little You once again. Lifting does not mean to close up shop emotionally; it means to experience intervals of freedom from your pain and administer to your feelings as they arise. The message of abandonment recovery is to stay in tune with your feelings, especially your vulnerable and needy feelings. Don't lift above them just because you're Lifting out of grief. In Lifting to your higher purpose, don't forsake your emotions. Stay integrated with your emotional core.

Without proper direction, people surviving abandonment tend to overdefend themselves and let calluses form over their wounds, making it more difficult for others to get close. To prevent these calluses, remember that when you lift, take your feelings with you. They hold the key to meaningful connections to others. If you bury your emotions, those who try to connect to you are confronted with your outer shell, rather than your warm emotional center.

Think about your friends or former lovers who have gone through painful heartbreaks and losses. Name someone who seems more closed off than before.

What about the effect of your past losses on you? Do you feel you've accumulated emotional scar tissue of your own?

Do you believe you are at risk for developing new calluses from your heartbreak?

If so, how does this numbing affect your ability to connect to self and others?

What insights and tools can you use to overcome this?

The following IQ helps you identify some of the characteristics people develop when they overlift (or lift above) their feelings. Consider any calluses you may have acquired from having gone through childhood hurts and disconnections.

Check all that seem familiar.

IN CHILDHOOD…

❏ I tried to hide uncomfortable feelings around my friends.
❏ I tried to remain invisible at home or school.
❏ I was ashamed of my feelings.

IN ADOLESCENCE…

❏ I tried to cover up when I felt embarrassed or humiliated. Sometimes I used diversionary tactics, such as becoming the class clown.
❏ I was emotionally stoic, refusing to cry when I felt hurt or unfairly punished.

IN ADULTHOOD…

❏ I hide my insecurity from my friends or lovers.
❏ I tend to wear a jovial mask in public, even when feeling disappointed in myself or uncertain about my life.
❏ Other people seem to feel more deeply than me.
❏ My friends prefer to share their feelings with others rather than with me.
❏ I isolate from people when I'm upset.
❏ I am sometimes more a "human doing" than a human being—always on the go, a taskmaster, workaholic, or escape artist.
❏ I tend to live in my head—preoccupied with myself—to avoid dealing with unresolved emotions.
❏ I go into an emotional haze and become numb to what is going on around me, by oversleeping, zoning out in front of the TV, or burying myself in a book.
❏ I avoid expressing important feelings directly to loved ones, even positive feelings, because I'm afraid my voice will shake or that I might cry.
❏ Others find me remote, difficult to relate to.
❏ I wake up with an emotional hangover from having had an intense experience, unable to identify the source of my feelings.
❏ I have trouble naming my feelings and identifying their source.
❏ There is a lack of intimacy in my primary relationships.
❏ I have difficulty showing affection, tenderness, sexuality.
❏ My partner is detached, hard to connect with emotionally. My partner's behaviors may reflect my own tendency toward Lifting.
❏ My best friends are hard to reach emotionally. I may be letting the people in my life do my Lifting for me.

Name someone you know whom any of these characteristics remind you of. Explain.

Do any of these items pertain to you? If so, what earlier events might have caused you to develop emotional calluses?

What gets in your way when you express your feelings?

What strengths do you have for staying emotionally connected to yourself and others?

During Lifting, we prepare to love again. We begin to feel warmth rising from within, not only because we've been working on expanding our capacity for love but because we realize how much love and support others extended to us. We're grateful to be relieved of the constant grief that gripped our life for so long, grateful for the independence and emotional growth we've gained by surviving the experience.

In spite of all these gains, most of us still have problems as we emerge from abandonment. The challenge of Lifting is to become larger than those problems. The ultimate gift of abandonment is the opportunity to increase our capacity for love. Abandonment taught us that love is the primary focus of a meaningful life. During this final stage, we discover a wellspring of purpose in our human need for love.

The energy we use to connect to others is the procreative life force. Attachment energy binds people to one another. During Rage, the drive for connection moved your energy back out into the world. During Lifting, you feel its centrifugal force pulling you back into life, urging you to connect to something outside yourself.

Andrew Solomon writes, "Grief is profoundly important to the human condition....If we did not suffer enough loss to fear it, we would not love intensely."[3] Anyone who has endured serious heartbreak and learned to love again knows how true this statement is.

Soon we'll be discussing Akeru Exercise Five, designed to work with the centrifugal force of the Lifting stage to help you connect to others with love.

Lingering Uncertainty

For most people coming out of abandonment grief, love remains a primary unresolved issue.

"I'm doing okay, in fact, great—considering what I've been through. But I'm still not at rest. I'm searching. My life is missing its centerpiece. I need to find someone to love."

The ongoing craving for a relationship is the kingpin of abandonment grief, a need that is not as intense for people grieving a death. When your loved one dies, you know that it does not reflect on your worthiness or desirability as a man or woman. But when someone chooses not to be with you, the rejection creates a narcissistic injury—a stinging hurt that goes beyond grief and insults the self. The wound is painful and persistent. You question your own lovability and worthiness indefinitely.

"When Yvette left me," says Steve, "it made me feel bad about myself. I need to find someone to love and want me again, but I feel condemned to being alone."

As we've discussed, at some level we all worry that there might be something wrong with us. Abandonment reinforces this fear, convincing you that your own lackings and imperfections caused someone to dispose of you. Since it was someone's leaving you that created your self-doubt, it is only natural to want to find someone else who can reassure you that you are acceptable and desirable.

It is important to understand that your desperate need to find love stems not just from loss, but from the narcissistic injury you sustained. Abandonment survivors seek human salve for this deeply personal affront to their sense of worth. Rejection caused you to feel disqualified and you're desperate to find someone to validate you.

"I feel good about my career," says Alice. "I'm proud of my accomplishments and think I'm a good person. But I need someone to want me so I can feel desirable again as a woman. Otherwise I feel lonely, unattractive, and unworthy."

Understanding the reason you crave love as intensely as you do is an important step in recovery. The message here is not to give up on your dreams to find someone but to not wait till you find Mr. Right to be happy. Fulfillment is now. Your task is two pronged: One, use the tools of abandonment recovery to heal your injured sense of self. This is your wound. You are the physician. Diagnose the source of the problem and administer to your wound.

Two, open yourself to a new level of love. When you don't have the love you want, create a higher purpose for love to serve in your life. This means broadening your concept of love. It can be much bigger than you currently think. We discussed how to increase your capacity to love in chapter 7. Now we're talking about developing a higher purpose for this need for connection, one that centers on an expanded concept of love. When loneliness bothers you, use it as motivation to administer to your injuries and transcend to love's higher purpose.

> Clients complain: "But I don't have anyone to love."
>
> I answer: Yes, you do. You have yourself—
>
> They interrupt: "Don't give me that love yourself crap. I want somebody special to love and for them to love me back."
>
> My answer: Loving yourself comes first. But you're right. It does not end there. It must extend to others.

You may be single and have nobody special, but you can begin loving right where you are now. In the next chapter, I present the Five-Point Action Plan for Making a New Connection, a program that offers a framework to find that special someone.

AKERU EXERCISE FIVE
INCREASING YOUR CAPACITY FOR LOVE

Akeru Exercise Five prepares you to make connections by seeking the meaning and purpose of love in the larger scheme of your life. This requires a stretch. A leap. A creative effort. Each person comes to it in a unique way, but most of us have to be determined to get there and willing to apply consistent effort. One effective way is to spend quiet time every day journaling or meditating on a larger context for love. Open yourself to its higher purpose and soon your life brims with hope and opportunity.

COMMUNITY PROJECTS

One of the goals of abandonment recovery is to create a people-to-people movement to outreach to members of our communities who are in need. As I noted in chapter 9, after what you've been through, you're in a position to understand the despair and anxiety behind each person's struggle. Your compassion can make a big difference in people's lives. As you progress through recovery, this important option remains open: again I invite you individually or as part of a group to develop Community Projects. The aim is to reach individuals who are alone and isolated. In most cases, you don't have to look hard to find them. They are languishing within prisons, in shelters, on streets, in hospitals, in nursing homes, in lonely apartments, or in bus stations. There are millions of people in your midst who can benefit by your connection and support. Community Projects can become the focus of your abandonment support groups as well.*

Have you noticed people within your environment who could use some human kindness? Who are they?

Â

What are their apparent problems?

Â

What aspect of their difficulties arouses your sympathy, caring, or concern?

Â

Why are you sensitive to this particular issue?

Â

Has it ever occurred to you that you could do something to help people in need? What form might this take?**

Â

How would it make you feel if you expressed your caring to others through kind deeds?

Â

---

* See Appendix A for instructions for support groups, or go to the Group Center at abandonment.net.

** Go to abandonment.net and click CONTACT US to tell us about your efforts to help other people.

Action Bullet: I feel _____ because _____, and I'd like to _____
_____.

An essential ingredient in fomenting this momentous development in your life—creating a higher purpose for love—is to increase the power of love in your life on a daily basis. You can best facilitate this by weaving love into the lessons and exercises we've discussed. The mechanism for accomplishing this is already contained within their structures, ready and waiting to take on this new love mission.

I'm going to show you how to incorporate love into each of the *Akeru* exercises. Love serves as a substrate to integrate the exercises into one unified life plan.

ADDING LOVE TO THE AKERU EXERCISES

I. When you get into the moment, bring other people with you

II. Administer to Little's need for love when you perform the Big You / Little You dialogues

III. Build your need for love into your Dream House

IV. Correct Outer Child's interference in your relationships

V. Take an action every day to increase opportunities for love

I: When You Get into the Moment, Bring Other People with You

Getting into the moment brings you in touch with the bounty of life's sensations, an infinite universe of possibility, which includes the human need for love. When you center in, attend closely not only to the sights, smells, and sounds of your environment but also to the people in your midst. Make a conscious effort to be fully present with other people. Even with a relative stranger, it is possible to practice the art of being in love's presence.

"I made a personal commitment to practice getting into the moment with at least one person each day," says Roberta. "So time having run out on the day, my one remaining chance was to practice this with the woman at the dry cleaners. I centered into the moment and gave her my full attention—making good eye contact and asking how her day had gone. She gave me a stock response. So, I proceeded to tell her that my day seemed long and I was anxious to go home and collapse. I told her that this was my last stop. It was the truth. Sure enough, at the recognition of sincerity, she said, 'I know what you mean. I've only got one hour to go and then I'm calling it a day.' I've been on friendly terms with her ever since. Nothing intense. Just smiles and nods of recognition and learning each other's first names, etc. In fact, I'm on first-name basis with a lot of people lately."

"I decided to do a Community Project," says Steve. "I visit an old high-school buddy at a V.A. hospital once a week. At first it felt like a mistake. He didn't recognize me and couldn't care less that I'd come. I don't know what I was expecting, considering his disabling condition and how long it had been, but I decided to get into the moment and give him my undivided attention whether it mattered to him or not. It meant just hanging out with him in the day hall. It was very moving for me to see how limited his range of activity was.

"By about the fifth visit, I'd become familiar with a whole group of guys there and we didn't do much but hang next to my old friend. I wouldn't miss these visits for anything. It's become a sacrament of the moment where I get far more out of it than they do."

Practice the art of being mindful with others and watch your love capacity expand in concentric circles, generating positive feelings to more and more people. Eventually your warmth will radiate outward and envelop significant others in your midst.

II. Administer to Little's Need for Love When You Perform the Big You / Little You Dialogues

The issue of love becomes grist for powerful dialogues between Big and Little and keeps you motivated to take positive action every day in the direction of love. All it takes is to ask Little You what he needs by way of love.

Here are samples of questions Big can ask to get Little to open up on the subject. Take a moment to answer the Qs, but plan to incorporate the sentiments into your next dialogue.

What do you need from other people in your life, Little?

Do you have enough love?

What can I do, Little, to bring more love into your life?

What would it feel like to have someone special?

What type of loving person would help you feel more secure?

What could you and I do, Little, to love other people who need help to make you feel good?

Remember, Little thrives on being appreciated, accepted, desired, and nurtured by you, as well as by the special people you bring into your life. In other words, Little needs love. Little's greatest fear is being abandoned again—especially by you. Make a pact that you will do everything within your power to meet Little's needs for love. Reassure Little that you will always be there and never leave him alone again. Don't expect Little to trust you right away. Being patient and persistent in your dialoguing leads to a breakthrough that can change your life.

> *"Little Bob got pissed off when I promised I wouldn't abandon him again. He said I wasn't capable of loving him. According to Little Bob, all I knew how to do was chase skirts and make Barbara angry. I thought I was being quite sincere when I reassured my little guy that I'd always be there for him. But he told me off big-time. It took me at least six more dialogues—I used up a whole legal pad—to break through Little Bob's mistrust and rage. It was actually a turning point in my life to realize how out of touch with myself I'd been. When Barbara fell out of love with me, I was forced to realize how sacred love was. It helped me find myself—and I hadn't even realized I was lost."*

III. Build Your Need for Love into Your Dream House

Imagine that you construct your Dream House in a way that is so well suited to your hopes and dreams that, just by living within its beautiful environment, you become increasingly more capable of love. In this love-inspired house, imagine that the anger and hurt you feel about your present abandonment have been completely forgiven, corrected, and released. Imagine that living within this house, you and Little are finally at peace because you now have all of the components of love you ever hoped for.

Check items you can imagine.

- ❏ Commitment
- ❏ Security
- ❏ Intimacy
- ❏ Sexuality
- ❏ Mutuality
- ❏ Affection
- ❏ Generosity
- ❏ Tenderness
- ❏ Companionship
- ❏ Openness
- ❏ Respect
- ❏ Trust
- ❏ Admiration
- ❏ Compatibility
- ❏ (add your own) _____

Think about the features that you need to add to your Dream House to promote this kind of growth.

Q

Describe your renovations in the design, furnishings, ambience, location, etc., that would lead to increased love capacity.

Back to the Future

Imagine that it's a year or two from now and you're sitting before your beautiful view, feeling good about the quality of love in your life. You feel good about yourself because you made the necessary changes to achieve this love. You did it through your own determination and wisdom. Imagine the personal changes you made between now and this future time in order to feel this contented.

Q

What internal obstacles did you have to overcome?

How did you remove them?

Describe the observable behaviors you committed to achieve these goals.

> **Action Vow:** Within the next twenty-four hours, I will take the following tiny step in the direction of love: _____.

IV. Correct Outer Child's Interference in Your Relationships

Outer Child is the nemesis of love, the internal saboteur of your relationships. In chapter 9 you double-circled items in the Outer Child Inventory that represented Outer's attempt to interfere in your relationships. If you're still not in touch with Outer Child, just wait until you're trying to establish a new relationship. Taking a chance on love is likely to reawaken your old doubts and anxieties, and Outer will gladly emerge just as you're feeling your most vulnerable and insecure. Outer tests new relationships to the max.

Outer becomes especially pesky when you're trying to change patterns of abandonment. For example, when your newfound wisdom prompts you to finally choose an emotionally responsible person, Outer is liable to stage an emotional or sexual sit-down. Outer resists your efforts to be in a secure, loving relationship by treating your partner like dirt and trying to nudge you back into the pattern of seeking unavailable partners.

Don't get discouraged when Outer causes you to relapse into old behaviors. When you catch yourself, perform a Correction and move forward.

A good way to keep Outer in check is to share your growing awareness with your friends, therapists, members of your abandonment support groups, and even prospective lovers. You can also work on your Outer Child defenses at home by maintaining a daily journal in which you keep tabs on what Outer is up to and how you're overruling her. Update your daily Outer Child Inventory. Keep Outer in your sights. Strengthen your ability to pursue healthy relationships and fulfill your higher purpose.

V. Take an Action Every Day to Increase Opportunities for Love

Many people continue to focus their love efforts on making a connection with a significant other. This kind of connection is one of many ways to achieve greater life and love, but it is one of the most popular pursuits of abandonment survivors—finding someone special. If you are determined to find greater love, it helps to devote special time every day to center yourself in this goal. The Daily Goals Chart exercise below is designed to help you formulate a daily plan. It takes more than a few stabs at a half-baked effort. To be successful, create a new daily regimen and follow it. Your task is to integrate the exercises around your need for love.

By weaving the element of love into all of the lessons and exercises, you give them a unified purpose. You enhance your capacity for love on many different levels: through your ability to experience the moment, by increasing your connection to your own emotional core (Little), by visualizing your ultimate goals, by gaining control over Outer's patterns, and by taking positive actions to achieve connection.

Combining the exercises into a daily regimen propels you toward your higher purpose. As you go about your everyday activities, your actions are channeled toward your goal. With consistent, focused effort, fulfillment is inevitable.

Make copies of the Daily Goals Chart and use a fresh one each day as a way of staying on target.

AKERU EXERCISE

ADD LOVE TO YOUR DAILY EXERCISE REGIMEN

DAILY GOALS CHART

1. Describe how you plan to get into the moment with at least one person today.

2. Perform your Big You / Little You Dialogue and describe how you plan to attend to Little's requests for love today.

3. Visualize your Dream House and describe renovations that will inspire your ability to increase your love capacity—just by living there.

4. Think about what Outer Child is up to. Does Outer tend to procrastinate when it comes to tasks that might otherwise help you find greater life or love? Describe today's plan to overrule Outer's attempt to sabotage your love efforts.

5. Plan one activity for today that will increase your opportunity to connect with others and learn more about who you are becoming.*

---

*   See the Five-Point Action Plan in chapter 12 (page 295) for ideas.

Lifting to Perspective

Gaining altitude over your abandonment experience allows you to grasp where you are within a vast universe of possibilities. At each stage you've gained emotional wisdom with which to guide you on a path of lifelong recovery and created a higher purpose for love to serve in your life.

Let's see how far you've gone. In the IQ, check the gains you feel you've been making while swirling through the stages. The benefits of this process are cumulative. As you grow, your capacity for love grows with you.

 SWIRLING THROUGH THE STAGES

GOING THROUGH SHATTERING

❏ I'm gaining self-reliance from surviving the experience of being separated and alone.

❏ I'm learning about my patterns of abandonment and how they have kept me outside of love.

❏ I'm facing the fears that keep me stuck in old patterns.

❏ I'm administering to primal feelings reawakened from my lost childhood, through Little Me.

❏ I'm learning how to center in as a beginning point of recovery.

❏ I'm using my senses to get into the moment.

❏ I'm using the moment's power to deal with life's most uncomfortable emotions.

❏ I'm learning to cleanse my abandonment wound of negative messages left over from previous rejections and hurts.

❏ I'm creating a sacred space within—a beginning point of renewal and healing.

GOING THROUGH WITHDRAWAL

❏ I'm gaining emotional wisdom by discovering my oldest and most important feelings and needs.

❏ I'm identifying emotional baggage from past wounds.

❏ I'm learning how to work through feelings, through Little Me.

❏ I'm learning about my control issues and how they make it difficult to let go.

❏ I'm learning how to interpret the longing and yearning I feel toward my abandoner, not as proof of how special he is but as evidence of my need for self-love.

❏ I'm getting in touch with the source of my emotional hunger, identifying times of deprivation in childhood and adult relationships.

❏ I'm learning to put my emotional wisdom to work by creating a daily dialogue with my inner feelings.

❏ I'm addressing my most basic emotional needs directly, rather than medicating them with substances, people, obsessive thoughts, and other compulsive behaviors.

❏ I'm learning to resolve the conflict between what I know intellectually and what I want emotionally.

❏ I'm learning to accept my separateness as a human being.

❏ I'm learning to honor the importance of my existence.

282 The Abandonment Recovery Workbook

GOING THROUGH INTERNALIZING

❏ I'm developing integrity by facing my core emotional truths.

❏ I'm reevaluating my deeply held aspirations, values, and goals.

❏ I'm learning how to resolve insecurity created during times when my sense of self was injured.

❏ I'm identifying the emotional blockades holding me back.

❏ I'm learning to accept life on life's terms by facing my reality in one gulp.

❏ I'm learning how not to falsely attribute my feelings to the wrong cause.

❏ I'm letting go of my need to have others fill my emotional void.

❏ I'm discovering an internal resource for healing—my imagination.

❏ I'm using my imagination to increase my sense of entitlement and establish a new foundation of principles in my life.

❏ I'm using my imagination to build self-esteem, expand my vision, and target new goals.

❏ I'm learning to identify whether I or someone I know might be love challenged.

❏ I'm discovering the creative process of love.

❏ I'm learning to delay gratification to achieve long-range goals.

❏ I'm reviving lost hopes and dreams, including my dreams of love.

❏ I'm learning how to use *love* as an action verb.

GOING THROUGH RAGE

❏ I'm learning to redirect my anger into healthy aggression.

❏ I'm identifying anger and resentment bottled up from past rejections and losses.

❏ I'm gaining insight into the Outer Child behaviors that interfere in my relationships.

❏ I'm learning to lay aside perfectionism.

❏ I'm learning to perform corrections as a way of practicing positive change.

❏ I'm letting others be who they are, learning to love unconditionally.

❏ I'm letting go of the need to control others.

❏ I'm learning the rewards of self-discipline.

❏ I'm asserting my needs with greater control of my attitudes and behavior.

❏ I'm learning to take responsibility for where my life is now.

GOING THROUGH LIFTING

❏ I'm learning to reach out for a higher level of love.

❏ I'm identifying the emotional calluses that may have formed over my old wounds.

❏ By filing away old calluses, I'm finding my way back to my soft emotional center.

❏ I'm learning to remain open to my vulnerability.

❏ I'm reestablishing emotional contact with myself, discovering that I'm more able to connect with love to others.

❏ I'm learning to create a higher purpose for love to serve in my life.

❏ I'm learning to integrate the tools of abandonment recovery into a life plan for increasing this capacity for love on a daily basis.

❏ I'm learning how to reach out to others in my community who need my support.

❏ I'm learning how to participate in a person-to-person effort to end isolation and loneliness in the world.

❏ I'm adding my voice to a collective forum of abandonment survivors whose wisdom can enhance recovery around the world.

❏ I'm about to learn about the Five-Point Action Plan for Making a New Connection.

❏ I will learn how to take actions in the direction of making a new connection.

❏ I will learn how to join (or start) abandonment support groups.

In short, you're swirling through the stages of abandonment—Shattering, Withdrawal, Internalizing, Rage, and Lifting—and emerging from its funnel-shaped cloud with greater Strength, Wisdom, Integrity, Redirection, and Love than before.

You may well be looking love in the face at this very moment. Your task is to recognize its presence. The kind of love you are seeking was most likely invisible to you in the past. Some of you may have already found a love relationship, while others are still looking. Whatever the case, you can increase love and rise to its greater purpose in your life.

I've outlined twenty-five points in Advice for the Love Challenged in chapter 7, but many of you are still seeking a context in which to practice them. Never fear, in chapter 12 you'll find dos and don'ts for making a new connection.

More Food for Thought

Abandonment survivors' spiritual perspectives run the gamut.[4] Some have a concept of God, others tend more toward the existential. Some belong to traditional religious sects, others create an individual path of oneness with the universe. Describe your current spiritual perspective and how it serves your need to gain a sense of purpose and meaning in your life.

How does this purpose relate to your need for love?

What insights and tools can you use to attain this?

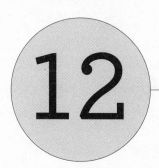

12 Connecting

SWAN LESSON TWELVE

Connecting with Others

The little girl was living in a home for children and began a friendship with a boy named Jonathan, who lived in an adjoining building. He was upset and she went to the black swan for advice on his behalf. What unfolded revealed the meaning of her journey—a lifelong path of growth, recovery, and connection.

The swan is already waiting, turning gracefully in the water to face the little girl. "How is your practicing, Amanda?" asks her beautiful swan.

"Every day I take special time," she reports proudly, "and I think about how big life is."

"How big is it?" asks the swan.

"Bigger than me," says the little girl. "But I have a question. What do we do about Jonathan? He got mad on visitor's day and broke the window. Now he's in lots of trouble, and he's crying all the time."

The swan swoops close to the little girl and gently touches her outstretched hand with the brilliant red of his beak. "Why not share what you've learned with him, Amanda?"

"Me?" asks the little girl, her eyes brightening at the unexpected touch of the swan. "But the boy is so upset and crying all the time," she explains.

"He's not alone in his pain, Amanda, just as you were not alone in yours. There are always people who suffer torment and hurt. But we are here to help each other."

"I don't know how to help Jonathan," says the little girl.

"Begin at the beginning. Let him see how you find your center and keep it safe inside," suggests the swan. "Show him the path."

"I still have bad feelings of my own," says the little girl. *"I can't help somebody else. I was hoping you would talk to him for me."*

"You can help him yourself, Amanda. Show him the steps you're taking."

"How?"

"Begin at the beginning. Let him know he is not alone. Just as you are not alone in learning how to experience life. It is a great gift. But it is not yours to take; it is yours to give. It is the moment. Help others find it. And love them, Amanda, as you are learning to love life."

"What if I do help Jonathan? I'm afraid he will be mean to me someday. He will throw me away."

"You cannot be thrown away. You can only give yourself away, Amanda. And even if you do, you can always return to your center and find yourself and create love all over again."

"I still need someone to love me," implores the little girl to her friend.

"Of course you do. And if you spend special time every day expanding your mind and imagining all that's possible, you will have what you want—including someone special. You will have other loving people as well—all the love you need—if you just keep imagining. But remember that you are a source of love yourself, Amanda. Feel its warmth and let it shine outward. Give yourself fully to the moment and each moment will be love. It will be a journey, always in the present," says the swan. *"As you find it, share it with others. You have the whole universe to explore, within and without."*

The little girl stands up and opens her arms to the swan. "I have to go now," she says. *"I don't want to keep Jonathan waiting. He might be worried."* She turns and runs back up the slope.

In opening her arms upon receiving the swan's lesson, the little girl completed the cycle of gestures involved in surviving a great loss. Let's review them.

In Lesson One, the little girl went inside to find her center. *She placed her hands on her chest*, a simple, familiar gesture of self-contemplation.

Turning inside, she encountered powerful feelings. Most often our pain is about another person or not having a person in our lives. The little girl had been very hurt and needed to get to the very center of herself—a place that isn't about other people—a sacred place of her own. It is where her separate self resides, her healing self. In Lesson Two, the little girl cleared this space, *turning her palms outward* in a cleansing gesture to push away the hurtful feelings, so that they could evaporate into the vast forgiving universe.

In Lesson Three she learned that getting into the moment is a powerful way to deal with emotional pain. When you're in grief or panic, this takes a great effort. The little girl learned to use her senses as tools to help her get into the moment and away from her sadness and fear. She tilted her head to the side as she listened intently to the background noises. When she is able to hear the fluttering of distant seagull wings, in that moment she is no longer in her painful thoughts. *Tilting her head to the side*, she signified that she attended to the sensations of the moment.

Learning how to use the moment as nature's refuge from pain prepared the little girl for Lesson

Four, which is to accept the fact that she is a separate person, something that can be accomplished only one moment at a time. We are all separate—alone inside—whether we have been left on a rock or are blissfully coupled. She accepted this basic fact of human life by *raising her face* to connect to the vast universe we all share.

Lesson Five is to realize the importance of being alive. As the little girl received this lesson, she *lifted her chest* in an almost imperceivable gesture of self-validation. When people recognize their importance on an egotistical level, this gesture looks arrogant. When it comes from recognizing the importance of their existence, the impetus comes from gratitude. In this instance, this strengthening of one's posture— this lifting—appears dignified rather than pompous.

In Lesson Six, having realized that she could experience the importance of her own separate existence, the little girl was ready to face life on life's terms—a critical step in healing. In one deep breath, she confronted the reality she faced. Hers is a difficult reality, to be sure, but it is her reality. With this gesture—*taking a deep breath*—she faced it back, performing the universal gasp of recognition. Reality must be gulped whole for healing to continue.

Facing the powerful truth that she was left on a rock to die, hurt in her heart. Releasing her breath, she *pressed the warmth of her palms down into her heart*. Thus she practiced Lesson Seven, recognizing that she had the capacity to increase her own love from within. No matter what other people do or don't do, she can generate her own warmth and love all by herself. This gesture is the turning point in her recovery.

Able to generate her own love from within, she was ready for Lesson Eight—to let others be who they are, releasing them from her needs and expectations. As she let go of her need to control, she *opened her hand*.

Now that she began learning how to accept people as they are, she received Lesson Nine, which is to extend the love that she generates from within. She *extended her open hand* in a gesture of giving.

In Lesson Ten, she recognized that she had all the tools she needed to help herself in this life. She *placed her arms around herself*, gathering these insights together, owning and embracing responsibility for herself. It is a gesture of self-recovery and self-love. The body linguists have misinterpreted this gesture. They tell us that when we fold our arms, we are closing ourselves off from others. In fact, we are embracing our emotional wisdom, which includes reaching out to others with unconditional love.

But there is still more to healing.

Lesson Eleven is the recognition of our higher purpose—becoming aware of the miracle of existence. The little girl *gazed skyward* to fathom the vastness and mystery of infinity, to recognize her oneness with the universe and all of the possibilities it holds.

Finally she came to Lesson Twelve, when she learned that the gift of recovery is not hers to keep but hers to give. She *opened her arms* as she moved forward to share her journey with others and embrace the world with love.

These gestures flow into one another and create the wordless signature of healing[1]— from placing your hands on your chest for centering yourself, to pushing your palms outward for cleansing your wound, to tilting your head for getting into the moment, to lifting your face for accepting your separateness, to raising your chest for honoring your existence, to taking a deep breath for accepting your reality, to pressing your palms against your heart for recognizing your ability to create love, to opening your hand for letting others be who they are, to extending your hand in a gesture of reaching out with love, to wrapping your arms around yourself for embracing your awareness, to gazing skyward for seeking your higher purpose, to opening your arms for connecting to others.

My clients and workshop attendees find it helpful to perform the gestures as part of a daily routine, contemplating each lesson's application in real life. In directing movement choirs of people performing these gestures, I have observed that each person's signature has its own contour and personality.

Take a moment to practice them yourself, one after another in succession, and then combine them into one fluid movement. Make your own unique signature of healing.

Centering: cross your hands on your chest.
Cleansing: push your hands away from your chest.
Attending: tilt your head to the side.
Separating: lift your face.
Beholding: lift your chest.
Accepting: take a deep breath.
Increasing Love: press the warmth of your palms into your heart.
Letting: open your hand.
Reaching Out: extend your hand.
Integrating and Owning: wrap your arms around yourself.
Transcending: gaze skyward.
Connecting: open your arms.

Swan Lessons are designed for discovery. They are brief and cryptic—presented in story form—to inspire you to take a leap of insight. Each person makes discovery in her own unique way, contemplating how personally to apply the lessons. In contrast, the five Akeru Exercises come with detailed instruction. They are designed not for contemplation, but for doing. They guide you step by step through a hands-on program of healing.

The Swan Lessons and Akeru Exercises complement one another. Akeru Exercise One—Staying in the Moment—reinforces the swan's message about the importance of staying in the now. Akeru Exercise Two—the Big You / Little You Dialogue—provides a practical way to administer to Little You on the rock: Big to Little. Akeru Exercise Three—Building a Dream House—puts the swan's teachings about the power of your imagination into practice. Akeru Exercise Four—Discovering Your Outer Child—addresses a developmental stage beyond the little girl (Little You) in the story. Your Outer Child is older and more willful than Little You. Outer won't stay put on the rock for a second, but wants to climb down and go on a rampage to avenge Little's wound—probably taking it out on innocent bystanders, including you. Akeru Exercise Five—Increasing Your Capacity for Love—creates a daily regimen to implement the swan's message about the transforming power of love. Together, the tools of abandonment recovery empower you to move forward to lifelong growth and connection.

By bringing the Swan Lessons and Akeru Exercises into daily practice, you are able to integrate insight with action. Action without insight is Outer Child. Action with insight is the emerging adult.

Abandonment Recovery Leads to Connection

Mental health and well-being are all about connection.

Heartbreak is the antithesis because it is all about disconnection. Earlier, we talked about how when your relationship is torn, the wires get pulled apart and go off sparking. You feel the painful disconnect at every level—from yourself, from your emotions, from your hopes and dreams, from your adult control of your behavior, and from love. Abandonment recovery provides the tools to reconnect the wiring and restore balance.

I'd like to present the case of someone who has yet to make these all-important connections.

I met Alma in college. When she was a child, her parents were divorced, and she lost touch with her father. On campus, she was known as the Blond Bombshell. She had a radiant personality, big heart, and great wit; and like so many of us, she had trouble in her relationships.

After graduating, we moved two hundred miles away from each other but managed to get together every few years to catch up.

About ten years ago, Alma told me that she'd fallen out of love with her husband and was itching to end her marriage. "Tim is a nice guy, good provider—doesn't drink, smoke, abuse women, or anything like that—but he doesn't have any oomph."

She said she needed to get out on her own, didn't want to be married anymore. She felt flat. I tried to play devil's advocate, but she insisted that there was no fixing her marriage. "We are inherently incompatible," she asserted. "The relationship has no passion and never did."

"I remember when you were crazy about Tim."

"It didn't last long," she retorted.

"When people lose their love feelings, sometimes it's hard to remember ever having had them," I said. "When you fall out of love, you get emotional amnesia and think you never loved the person. You rewrite the history, having deleted the love that really was there."

"But I was never really in love with Tim," she insisted. She was nonnegotiable about wanting out.

Three years later, Alma and Tim had been divorced for about a year, but Alma was miserable because she was hung up on another guy—Brendan.

"Brendan and I were a hot item for over a year—that final year of my marriage," she said. "In fact, Brendan was the incentive I needed to finally break it off with Tim. We saw each other every chance we got, but I got tired of the sneaking around. Wanting to be with Brendan broke the suction that held me in my marriage."

"What happened with Brendan?"

"The usual," she said. "The whole time I was trying to leave Tim, Brendan was totally in love with me. Then, soon after I got separated, he started singing a whole new tune. He suddenly wanted to just be friends. It ended like that."

Two years later, Alma described a series of romantic misfires—relationships that were pretty intense in the beginning but all ended the same—with her partners going back to their estranged wives or girlfriends.

"I'm beginning to feel desperate because I know I'm doing something wrong but I don't know how to stop myself. All the guys I've been with become unavailable and wind up leaving in the end. Will I ever find love?"

I stepped into my therapist's role a little bit and played back what she said about her choices in unavailable men. She was open to getting some feedback, so I explained what abandoholic meant. "It's when you get emotionally hooked on someone because he's hard to get. The insecurity hooks you. And then you have the opposite response toward the available types. If you don't feel that conquest fever, you have no interest. Does this sound like you?"

She laughed again and said, "If that's an abandoholic, then I'm the poster child." She grew thoughtful for a moment. "Actually, I don't know if that's really true. I've never met anybody to test that last part on, because no one's ever available."

"What about Tim?" I asked. "Wasn't he madly in love with you and willing to stick it out?"

"He doesn't count. I wasn't in love with him. But tell me more about how I get hooked on the unavailable types."

I explained, "If you've got this problem, available men remain invisible to you. You simply don't feel any chemistry toward them. You wouldn't be attracted to them even if they were just right for you in every other way. The only guys you notice are the ones who get your dander up—the ones you have to reach for."

"The ones who keep me begging," she agreed.

Two years later, Alma was involved with a new person, Edmund. She still wasn't content, reciting a litany of complaints about him. Edmund, it seems, was always putting her off, never wanted to stay overnight, always had something important to do on weekends other than be with her—play golf, get together with a friend, fix his boat, or all three. He saw her on an average of once a week. And even at that, when they'd go to a public place, his eyes roved to other women. Or if he ran into people he knew, he'd leave her alone for hours while he went off to socialize. He usually didn't call if he was going to be late, even though she repeatedly asked him for this simple courtesy. He was more than an hour late for most of their dates and rarely offered an explanation. He insisted Alma was his one and only, that they were exclusive, but he didn't seem to want the relationship to move forward. It had gone on like that for over two years.

I responded by saying that in spite of Edmund's apparent neglect and insensitivity, he seemed like the most available of the unavailable men she'd been with so far.

Alma laughed. "He insists he loves me. He says that he just doesn't have time to get together more. He never runs out of excuses. When I tell him I need more from him, he feels pressured. I can't seem to break this vicious circle we're in together. It drives me nuts."

I referred Alma and Edmund to a couple's counselor I knew in her area.

Three months later, Alma reported that she managed to drag Edmund to one session. He'd sat on the opposite side of the sofa with his coat on, and when the therapist attempted to draw him out, he gave one-word answers or went off on tangents about his business, his child-support payments, rather than focus on his relationship with her. When Alma confronted him about his lack of interest in the session, he blamed it on a migraine he'd picked up that morning, to which Alma rolled her eyes.

A year later, Alma was still determined to get Edmund to love her, and he'd been pulling away more and more. After telling me about her more recent trials, she said, "Ironically, the only man who ever wanted to stay with me forever—who ever professed undying love—was my husband."

"How did that feel," I asked, "to have someone love you and be willing to stick it out?"

"It didn't feel like anything because, with Tim, I didn't love him back. My friends used to envy me because he was a good-looking guy, loved to keep the house up nice, and was devoted to our kids. But they didn't know the real Tim like I did. I couldn't base a whole relationship on him being a nice guy and the fact that maybe he liked to cook dinner every night. There has to be love."

"What caused you to shut down?"

"His neediness turned me off."

"Could his neediness have been caused by the fact that you'd stopped loving him?" I asked.

"Yeah, he drove me crazy with it. That's the main reason I had to get out."

I asked her how Tim reacted when she left him.

"He begged and pleaded—and in typical Tim fashion, said he'd never love anyone but me, putting on this whole scene to make me feel guilty. It didn't work." Then she added, "Well, maybe I felt bad for a while, but I knew I was doing the right thing."

Alma went on to describe how Tim acted after the breakup. Reading between the lines of Alma's descriptions, it sounded like he went through intense abandonment grief for over a year—to which Alma seemed oblivious. I attributed her tendency to minimize Tim's pain to the fact that in this relationship, Alma was in the abandoner role.*

"What's Tim doing these days?" I asked.

"He started going with someone about a year after we broke up, and they're going strong, in fact—still married."

This was a test.

I did not share most of my own thought process about Alma's love trials, because I was hoping that the issues might seem obvious to you, now that you're becoming a pro. Here are some Qs to help you garner your insight and express your enlightened perspective.

What issues do you think led to Alma's wanting to end her marriage?

---

* To gain insight on the Profile of an Abandoner go to abandonment.net and click on the ABANDONMENT HELP tab, and then click on the button on the pinwheel that says PROFILE AN ABANDONER.

Do you feel Tim was at fault? Why? Why not?

What do you make of Alma's tendency to minimize Tim's pain? What allows her to remain oblivious to his abandonment grief?

In leaving Tim, was Alma acting out or acting on her own behalf?

Do you think she would have been able to break her secure connection with Tim without overlapping into an emotionally intense affair with a third party—Brendan?

Did her plan backfire? If so, why?

Does Alma seem to have insight into these dynamics?

Circle those you think might be love challenged: Alma, Tim, Brendan, Edmund. What was there about Edmund's personality that hooked Alma?

What do you think Brendan and Edmund might have in common?

What do you think Alma had in common with either or both of them?

Do you think Alma has enough insight to be able to overcome her abandoholism?

If Alma has a problem with adjusting to the emotional responsibilities of a long-term relationship, do you think she's aware of it?

What kind of insight would it take for Alma to reverse her problems?

What about Brendan? Do you think he's abandoholic?

What about Edmund? Without abandonment recovery, do you think he will overcome his love barriers? Why?

What would it take for him to develop "constancy"—the ability to sustain a long-term emotional connection?

How could abandonment recovery help him?

Do you think Tim could have picked up self-doubts and insecurities from going through abandonment over Alma?

How might reading this workbook benefit him?

If you were able to respond to any of these questions, give yourself an A+ for the insight you've gained. You deserve a diploma for graduating from abandonment recovery. Always keep the concept of graduating in the gerund tense: "-ing." The milestone you've achieved is not something you finish once and for all. Graduat*ing* means you're equipped with tools and insights to embark on a lifelong journey of connection.

Graduating from abandonment recovery is all about connection. It doesn't mean just reconnecting old wires to old functions but creating new ones. That is what the Akeru Exercises are designed for. Through gaining access to the moment, you create a deeper connection to life by intensifying your experience in the moment—just by tuning in to your senses. Through the Big You / Little You Dialogue, you create an empowering connection to your emotional core. Through Building your Dream House, you create a new connection to your hopes and dreams. Through Outer Child awareness, you create a new connection to your adult self, gaining the insight you need to overcome entrenched behavior patterns. Through the Daily Action Plan, you create a new connection to your higher purpose—Increasing Your Capacity for Love.

Graduating with these tools in hand does not spell ultimate relief for everyone. For many, the process remains incomplete—too many sparking wires have yet to be connected. If you are alone not by choice, making a connection to a higher purpose is particularly important, because you don't have a relationship to medicate the pain coming from those unhooked wires. The tools of abandonment recovery are adequate to the task, but you may need more time to practice them on a daily basis. Six months to a year is probably a minimum for most people who are deeply entrenched in patterns of abandonment.

> *"I understand that I have to connect to something important in myself and in my life— so that I can feel passionate about something that really matters,"* says Jennifer. *"But I still want a relationship. I want to be with somebody."*

My message is, don't let your need for a mate overtake your primary mission—to make a significant connection to life and to yourself.

I can hear a chorus of abandonment survivors in the background as I write this, crying out to me: "You're not hearing us," they chant. "We want a love connection."

Yes, I'm hearing you. The lingering grief of abandonment makes us feel unloved. This crushing feeling creates an urgent need to find a significant other.

Meeting someone involves luck, timing, and circumstances. What follows is a program to maximize your chances. And I include it here by popular demand.

The Five-Point Action Plan for Making a New Connection*

Action One: Step Outside of Your Usual Circle of Friends and Activities to Explore New Interests

By getting involved with people outside of your usual circle of friends and activities, you get to explore new interests, strengths, and capabilities you may not have experienced before. Extending beyond your usual boundaries has a twofold purpose: One is to learn more about yourself. The other is to increase your exposure to potential partners. Making little changes in your daily routine leads to new discoveries. Connecting with people beyond your usual social set helps you discover who you are capable of becoming and what new kinds of relationships you are capable of forming. Every day, make a commitment to engage in new experiences.

Some of my clients, caught up in the process of exploration, find it helpful to move to a new location or find a new job. This allows the changes they're making on the inside to take root in fresh soil.

As you're exploring new territory, be sure to give each experience time to reveal its hidden benefits.

Action Two: Initiate New Contacts with at Least Ten New People to Explore Your Alter-Ego States

Initiating contacts with a wider range of people allows you to explore your alter-ego states. Alter egos are various facets of your personality that may not have found expression before. At this stage, it is too soon to be concerned about finding that special someone. These ten new people are supposed to be human connections, not romantic ones. Connect to people of both genders.

Be yourself, but be open to responding to new people in new ways. You most likely have talents you haven't recognized and interests as yet undeveloped. There may be many unlived lives squirming within you to finally gain expression. Now is the time to expose yourself to people, places, and things that bring them to the surface. Relating to a variety of people increases your exposure to a wider world within and without.

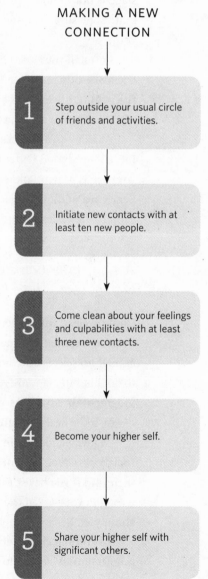

MAKING A NEW CONNECTION

1 Step outside your usual circle of friends and activities.

2 Initiate new contacts with at least ten new people.

3 Come clean about your feelings and culpabilities with at least three new contacts.

4 Become your higher self.

5 Share your higher self with significant others.

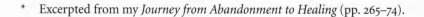

*   Excerpted from my *Journey from Abandonment to Healing* (pp. 265–74).

How to make these new contacts? Maybe you'll take up a group sport like volleyball or join (or start) an abandonment support group. Maybe you'll attend a weekly function at a religious center; register for a course at the university or adult education center; or join a library club, political organization, dating service, or bicycle club. Maybe you'll encounter someone by getting involved in Community Projects. Be open to chance encounters and make a special point to connect on a new level with people you know.

Take advantage of opportunities that present themselves by being open, in the moment, and out-reaching. Suggest going for coffee with a new acquaintance. Where appropriate, explain your quest—that you're following the prescriptions outlined in this workbook.

Do not dismiss someone just because you're not physically attracted to him or her. Your goal at this stage is not to find a primary relationship but to reinforce your emerging interests, talents, and capabilities. Be sure to connect with those who share your interests as well as those whose interests extend yours.

Forestall your need for romance until you've made connections on a variety of levels. Reach out to friends, group mates, co-workers, extended family, and one-time encounters. When you reach out, you risk rebuff, of course. Be courageous. Don't take people's closed attitudes personally. Don't let Outer Child get you to avoid taking risks out of fear of getting hurt.

At all costs, avoid clamping on to the first person you meet—especially during this exploring stage. Little is needy and Outer is bent on acting out, but be strong. Now is not the time to clamp on. Think of yourself as Marco Polo exploring the Orient, rather than someone looking to take up permanent residence in an ultimate relationship. Making contact with at least ten people increases your opportunity to explore the variety of hidden alter egos and discover your higher self.

Action Three: Come Clean about Your Feelings and Culpabilities with at Least Three New Contacts

Coming clean with others about how you may have contributed to the failure of your last relationship helps to cleanse the wound. Finding those you can be open with involves getting to know people well enough to select someone who can listen without judging or criticizing you. Not everyone is equipped to do this, but many are receptive once you explain what you need. Ask someone to listen to you without judgment or advice. As you practice a new level of emotional honesty with at least three people, you discover the healing power of human acceptance.

Many abandonment survivors have difficulty finding people to trust. Depending on your current social opportunities, you may be right. Hard doesn't mean impossible. There are trustworthy people out there and if you haven't met them, your job is to keep searching until you do. Maybe that's what's been wrong in your life in the first place—you weren't associating with solid people. Consider what this says about you. Reliable people are out there. Go find them.

In coming clean you're taking responsibility for the part you played in life's conflicts and disappointments. At first, you can come clean with an old friend or practice coming clean with the person you're dating, if you think there's enough depth and compassion to support it. If you're dating someone worthy of you, there should be. It goes against the rules in the dating books to talk about the problems in your past relationships, but it's a matter of timing. Sharing the depth of your experiences—good and bad—helps you break through the shame barrier and builds intimacy.

Share your Outer Child Inventory with others. It offers a nonthreatening way to share your culpabilities. Get others to reciprocate in the process. You might even have them complete the Outer Child Inventory so you can have fun exchanging insights.

When someone comes clean to you, feel honored to be chosen as an empathic, nonjudgmental, caring recipient of such sacred information (even if your friend shares it in the lighthearted spirit of the Outer Child Inventory). Another excellent place to cleanse your abandonment wound is within your abandonment support groups, although it is important to open up to people in the natural setting of everyday life as well. It's important to transfer what you are learning in your support groups to your relationships in the real world.

Why share with more than one person? A minimum of three ensures an opportunity to reveal different levels of your capacity for honesty and receive a wider range of responses. If you single out only one person to come clean to, you can easily dismiss the response as just one person's opinion. Human acceptance is not the exception to the rule. It is always available. Human acceptance is there to embrace you, waiting for you to reach out for it. Coming clean allows you to see that we are all imperfect human beings—that you, like everyone else, are worthy of love and acceptance.

Action Four: Incorporate Your Alter Ego into Your Ego—Become Your Higher Self

As you practice new activities and engage honestly with people, you slowly discover your higher self. Watch your values change and your possibilities expand. Your higher self is capable of greater empathy and emotional openness.

Treat others as you would like to be treated. Put yourself in their shoes. For example, as part of your Community Project,* you may visit a homeless shelter and find that the residents are not willing to discuss their problems with you. Set realistic expectations for yourself and for those you are trying to help. Maybe they just need to know you care by being there. Maybe you can help in some concrete way to relieve the burden, such as read a book to their children or help with their homework, or help with the laundry. At all times, listen without commentary, advice, or attempting to fix it. Your task is to be fully attentive and in the moment with them. Come from your higher self in your thoughts, words, and deeds.

Action Five: Share Your Higher Self with Significant Others

Find those who bring out the best in you—those who can relate to your higher self. Share your journey of recovery, extending your emotional wisdom to them. Connect your higher self to the higher selves of those you've selected to be in your world. If you haven't met enough people with whom to share your emerging self, double up on your efforts for Actions One through Four.

---

*   To share your Community Projects, contact us at abandonment.net.

It's important to avoid people who push your old emotional buttons, setting off the old cycles. When seeking a new relationship, rather than looking for someone with the right chemistry, be alert to mixed signals your body sends out. Beware of the abandoholic in you. Remain suspicious of those to whom you feel intensely attracted, as they may be emotionally toxic (or intoxicating) for you. Instead, seek people who are emotionally responsible, capable of commitment. They often have a track record to prove it. Share your relationship histories reciprocally to find out how their previous relationships ended. Is this person an abandoholic? An abandoner? A reformed abandoner? As your values change, you learn to appreciate honesty, trustworthiness, and a person's ability to communicate feelings above all of his other attributes.

Don't overdefend yourself from your feelings of vulnerability and neediness, as these are a source of deep personal sharing and connection to others. Your insecurity, self-doubt, and feelings of shame are as much a part of your personal truth as are your talents and accomplishments.

Think of love as an action rather than an overblown feeling that's supposed to medicate you from your anxiety and emotional hunger. If you meet someone who seems right but doesn't arouse your love feelings, before you walk away, review all of the steps in the Advice for the Love Challenged in chapter 7.

Let's catch up with Alma to see if she finally makes a connection:

"I realized I'd never feel comfortable with Edmund," says Alma. "In fact, I felt emotionally starved with him. I met another man about a year ago, not my usual type. For one thing, he is warm and giving, and this is hard to get used to. But we manage to stick together and I feel happier than I've felt in years. What changed in me? Joining an abandonment support group and listening to the other members who had similar problems to mine. Half of them had the same pattern of pursuing unavailable people. Hearing about their cycles of abandonment was like catching a glimpse of myself in the mirror on my worst day.

"I'd hit my bottom with my constant heartache over Edmund. It was time to stop banging my head against that stone wall. I had to give up the old ways. I stayed alone for a long time—no Edmund, no anybody. I put all of my energy into making being alone work. It was the biggest challenge of my life. But eventually I met Don. I had taken myself to the movies one Sunday afternoon, and there he was getting popcorn. We went out for coffee. He started calling me after that, and finally I said, 'What the hell, what have I got to lose?' Now all I have to do is get over my squeamishness about having someone lavish attention on me. I find visualizing a future scene where I am happy and at peace helps me overcome my barriers and keeps me living in the now."

Testimonies

Consider the testimonies of others along the journey to connection.

"I thought I'd never get over the depression I had after Lonny walked out on me," says Marie. "For a long time, I was going through the motions of life, nursing a painful wound. I tried to do constructive things for myself, but I still felt awful. I lived every day by the motto 'Fake it till you make it,' but

I had trouble making it. So I started a daily regimen of writing the Big You/Little You Dialogue and filled out my Daily Action Plan. It helped me do something special every day for Little. Every day I practiced getting into the moment to really experience a vignette of life, giving it my full attention. I visualized my Dream House on the way to work, during lunch, and going home. The House really kept me going, because I started to see changes in my life. I also did the healing gestures and concentrated on each lesson. At first, the lesson on cleansing was my favorite. I'd really push the wounder out of my center. After a while I began favoring the lesson about filling your chest with your name. When I'd feel low, I'd lift my chest and imagine bursting with my own essence and identity. Now, I'm concentrating most on 'letting others be who they are,' and I practice opening my hand as a reminder to let go, especially when I have contact with my ex.

"In the meantime, I discovered something: sailing. I never expected to fall in love with sailing. I met Phillip, who took me for my first sailing lesson. I hate to admit it, but at first I liked sailing a lot more than I liked him. I probably wouldn't have seen him a second time were it not for my desire to go sailing again. Well, now we're into our second year, and going strong. Phillip, me, and the sailboat we're living on."

"Barbara and I are still married," says Bob. "I got wise to what I was doing to destroy my marriage and fixed it. Well, not all at once. She left me for about six months, even though I was trying to change. That was hard. I was the most heartbroken man in the universe, with the added torture of knowing I was the one who destroyed it. But I managed to keep a dialogue going with Barbara, and I was able to slowly win back her trust. I'd slip back into my domineering, selfish behavior a lot, but I got good at catching myself and performing Corrections. Barbara didn't want to hear any more apologies. She had to see change, and that's what I gave her. I put Outer Child on a short leash and corrected my actions and owned up to them before she even noticed that I'd committed one. All of this showed her that I was finally hearing her—finally becoming the caring, sensitive human being she could love. I'm still changing and have a long way to go, but I cherish having Barbara's support."

"I have a lot of fears when I'm in a relationship," says Keaton. "What helped me most was the day I accepted that fact. I gave up trying to change it. I applied the Serenity Prayer to this problem: 'God grant me the Serenity to accept the things I cannot change, Courage to change the things I can, and Wisdom to know the difference.' I began using the gesture of the little girl on the rock—taking a deep breath—every time I had to face something difficult about myself. Doing the Big You/Little You Dialogue really cinched it. It got me to stop trying to squelch my fears. Little Keaton didn't like it when I tried to hide my fears and he yelled at me during the dialogues. He wanted to be accepted as he was, fears and all.

"When I dated someone, I stopped putting on the act that I was secure when I wasn't. I got honest with people. I didn't ask my girlfriends to feel sorry for me or give me any special treatment or anything like that. I used the expression, 'This is about me, not about you,' to convey to them and to myself (I needed to remind myself constantly) that I am 100 percent responsible for meeting my own emotional needs.

"Then I met Holly. It was a slow beginning. We were both insecure. The fears we had caused us

to shadowbox for a while. Now we kick back and enjoy a rare commodity: security—except when she's late coming home from work. Then I freak out. Not as bad as before. Since we're both sensitive to each other's abandonment fears, we're good about calling in if we're going to be late."

"My marriage was on the rocks for so long," says Jill, "I didn't know if I'd ever recover from my husband's affair. The trust was drastically damaged. I wrote my Big You / Little You Dialogue like mad and became really self-protective. Little's feelings became sacraments to be honored and cherished. I started to detach more and more from my husband. He sensed it and tried to pull me back in.

"Now, Barton says he's completely over the other woman. My head believes him, but my stomach still goes into a knot when he leaves the house. The marriage may be shaky, but I'm not. I'm stronger than ever. I keep visualizing my Dream House and focusing on my own achievements. I've become involved in a Community Project in which I help plant vegetables and herbs with some of the people from the homeless shelter in town. Interacting with them is a joy and I've become active on the board."

"I had so much trouble feeling anything for my new partner," says William. "I was still pining away for my ex and it seemed to go on forever. I finally realized that I was love challenged—not a pretty thing to admit to yourself, but it helped me realize some important problems in my life. Love is not pursuit. Love is caring. I've been applying the twenty-five pointers for the love challenged. I'm learning how sublime love can be when you make it an action."

"It felt like it was too late to start over again," says Cynthia. "I was in overwhelming despair when my husband left me for a newer model after forty years of marriage. I felt all washed up. Life was over. Who wants a woman in her sixties? Men look for younger women. I find younger men attractive too, but the feeling isn't reciprocated.

"I found out someone was there for me, and it was me. I never had much of a relationship with me. I'd always been wrapped up in taking care of my family. It wasn't until I did the Big You / Little You exercise that I found out how much I'd neglected my own needs. Now I feel really connected. I have lots of new friends and I've started a business. I'm going full steam ahead."

"I had too many suction cups for anyone to want to stay with me," says Aimee. "My insecurity caused me to act like the Co-Dependent from Hell. I kept putting myself in the one-down position. It turned all the guys off. I realized I needed to give up relationships for a while. It was time to learn how to become emotionally self-reliant. I turned being on my own—unattached—into a major project. I knew it was going to be tough to stay out of a relationship. I also knew being alone was no picnic—that it could be a lonely road. But I decided I'd just need to be prepared—and be determined to rise to the task. It was trial by fire and I'm making it.

"Now I'm not sure I want to go back out there into the realm of intense relationships, at least not for a while. I have too much to gain by conquering this new territory—independence and self-respect. There's a lot I enjoy about being on my own."

"I had given up on love," says Nick. "The only thing I ever wanted was to find someone, and here I was forty and still alone. Looking back, I still don't know what my problem was all those years. All I know is that I had an abandonment history—I was adopted—and somehow became an adult who was blocked from love. I followed the Five-Point Action Plan and got involved in all kinds of things. I kept sharing myself openly, making deeper and deeper connections to more and more people. Now I'm in love and it's mutual. We call each other every day. It was well worth the wait."

Whether you're alone or coupled, the message I want to leave you with is that life is Now and tomorrow holds endless possibility. Be forever graduating to greater and greater connection.

Check all the principles you intend to live by.

❏ Be guided by my broader definition of love.
❏ Surrender my losses of the past.
❏ Accept myself as I am.
❏ Consider the importance of my own unique constellation of feelings.
❏ Be grateful for my special endowments.
❏ Don't take criticism personally but invite feedback to expand my self-awareness.
❏ Bring my capacity to increase love into each experience.
❏ Share myself openly.
❏ Engage people with my human warmth.
❏ Lay aside perfectionism.
❏ Overthrow old notions of who's a great catch.
❏ Don't be put off by someone's looks; love comes wrapped in many surprising packages.
❏ Value a person's essence above his status.
❏ Forgo the temptation to get emotionally high from pursuing hard-to-get lovers.
❏ Seek those who engender a sense of trust and comfort.
❏ Beware of those who try to get me to Surrender My Of; honor my autonomy.
❏ Don't seek self-esteem by proxy; be my own person.
❏ Adjust my expectations of myself and others realistically.
❏ Find people with whom to wear my vulnerability openly; if they take advantage of it, accept this as feedback about them not as an indication of my own weaknesses.
❏ Remain open to people's fears, needs, and vulnerabilities as well.
❏ Strengthen my connection to myself; it's the bridge I need to connect with others.
❏ Be vigilant of the fact that love is within and all around me waiting to be consummated in action.

Abandonment is a unifying experience, linking people to one another, creating a connection that transcends age, social status, spiritual belief, education, sexual orientation, culture, and ethnicity. Abandonment does not discriminate and neither should we when we reach out to connect. Abandonment recovery asks that we don't abandon each other. Its path remains open to everyone.

The next step in connecting for many of you will be learning how to join or set up abandonment support groups; instructions can be found in Appendix A.

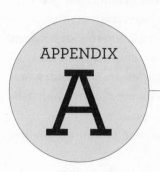

How to Set Up
Abandonment Support Groups

Soon after writing the twelfth lesson of the black swan, a light bulb went off in my head. Why not develop a format for abandonment support groups? Not only had I experienced my own personal abandonment as profound and difficult as any suffered by my clients but I had spent over twenty years of my career developing and running groups in every possible setting—in psychiatric hospitals, day treatment centers, school systems, professional organizations, and private offices; groups of every possible type and composition—group therapy, bereavement groups, divorce groups, addiction recovery groups, creative arts groups, children's groups, parenting education workshops, clinical supervision seminars, training groups.

So, I decided that my Community Project would be to create a program that could be run on a self-help basis by people surviving abandonment and to create a group protocol for mental health professionals to use.

So I set out to test various formats in the abandonment recovery workshops I was running in Manhattan and elsewhere. I am especially indebted to the members—very special people recovering from painful abandonment wounds past and present—who showed their interest and concern for others by providing input to the development of this program. Their generous feedback helped me hone the final group format, a format now in use throughout the country and world.

Abandonment support groups are designed to meet multiple needs of diverse people surviving abandonment, especially the need to be heard, understood, and validated. Abandonment is a crisis of disconnection and the connections you form in group are crucial to restoring well-being. Group members offer each other support and camaraderie to help supplant some of the nurturance you're missing. The group puts person-to-person healing into practice. It gets old-fashioned competitiveness to work in your favor, motivating you to summon the extra strength it takes to scale your wall of pain. These groups promote positive peer pressure, goading you into taking superhuman strides because you see others doing it. The powerful dynamics of the group spur you on to achieve your goals and find greater love than before.

One of the most important tenets of abandonment support groups is the prohibition against giving advice. It's a great relief to express yourself without someone trying to fix it or minimize the gravity of your situation. Members listen to one another and provide sacred space for your feelings.

Why go it alone when there are so many others living within your community who are suffering through the same grief? Lending your ear to give caring attention to the others enhances your own and everyone else's healing. Sharing your feelings with people in the trenches with you normalizes your experience, lifts you out of isolation, and generates hope. You bear witness to one another's heartache within a safe healing environment, gaining self-esteem and confidence in the process.

It's easy to set up abandonment support groups. This appendix is dedicated to showing you just that. I will guide you through the process, beginning with the self-help format.

The support group model is designed to be run by its own members—on a peer basis. Peer organizers show the other members how to follow written guidelines. The format is so simple it can be written on a three-by-five card and followed like a recipe for baking a cake. It does not require a professional leader because the members read directions about what is supposed to happen first, next, and last. The basic format consists of an opening round, during which you give yourself a positive stroke for this week's accomplishments; a discussion round for exploring an in-depth topic related to abandonment; and a closing round, in which you share your weekly resolution and receive positive feedback from the group. The support group format is designed to create safety and cohesion within a group. The proviso is that people must be willing to strictly adhere to its guidelines.

RECIPE FOR ABANDONMENT SUPPORT GROUPS

Opening Round: give yourself a positive stroke.
Discussion Round: this week's topic question.
Closing round: weekly resolution.

How to Start

You may choose to open a chapter of abandonment recovery in your community as your Community Project. There is no fee or charter necessary for opening a chapter. You simply gather together a group of people going through abandonment, find a meeting place, and agree to follow the guidelines. Forming the group immediately connects you to person-to-person support.

It's important that group organizers as well as all prospective members read this appendix to get the whole picture of how the group functions. This will help everyone understand that responsibility for the group is shared equally among the members. The group follows a leaderless format and does not require a professional leader, providing all members adhere to the format and guidelines. When professionals are available, they can enhance this process, however. Professionals have the option of using the more advanced format described later. *

---

* Mental health professionals looking to start abandonment groups can go to the abandonment.net Professional Page to access training information.

What Do Organizers Do?

You reach out to people going through abandonment through meetup.com or by contacting people within your social networks. In many cases abandonment.net can make referrals to your group, depending on your area code, as a lot of people contact the website requesting abandonment support groups. Library bulletin boards, social agencies' fliers, or local newspapers' calendars of events often post these groups.

Once you've found prospective joiners, organizers take everyone's schedules into account to coordinate a time and location for the group. Groups meet in a variety of places, such as people's homes, community or religious centers, and libraries.

The task of setting up a group is not as daunting as it sounds, because the onus is on all of the members equally—not just the organizers—to abide by the guidelines and strive to make the group successful.

Have Two Organizers Per Group

Getting a program started means finding a co-organizer—another person going through heartbreak. Then you have each other to share the effort. If you can't initially find anyone to co-organize, you may choose to start the group by yourself and then tell prospective members that you need a volunteer to help you coordinate. Once joiners have an opportunity to read this appendix, they'll understand that becoming a co-organizer does not mean being responsible for running a group, because all members pitch in to keep the group running. Co-organizers encourage participants to read the additional books related to abandonment to deepen their understanding of the issue and to help them better participate in the healing process.

The Circle

Co-organizers set the tone and structure for the group by arriving early for the first session to set the chairs in a circle. The circle ensures that all members are equidistant from the center, which reinforces a message of equal responsibility and worth of each member. Ensure that each person is able to see the others without having to crane necks or block one another. If one member's chair is too far forward, it will block someone else's view of at least one other member, creating a disconnection. After the first group, all of the members help create the circle, making sure the chairs are carefully lined up in a circle to maintain visible connection between each and every member.

The center of the circle needs to be open, which means, if possible, avoid having large coffee tables in the center. Large objects between people tend to interfere with intimacy developing in the group. Consider the nonintimate tone of business meetings that take place around conference tables. Abandonment support groups are not board meetings or coffee klatches, but an assemblage of people seeking to support one another's recovery by following a structured format that promotes open sharing and connection.

Organizers' Script

The co-organizers make sure written guidelines, a list of topic questions, and Name Wheels are available to all members on the first night.

The organizers sit across from each other in the circle and explain their roles—that they are equal members who join the recovery process as participants in the same manner as the other members. Organizers have the option to read or paraphrase the following script:

> ## SCRIPT FOR ORGANIZERS
>
> We helped to get this group started, but were not group leaders. We don't have answers or give advice. It is the group members—all of us—who are responsible for using the written materials in a meaningful way—and for following the format and guidelines.
>
> You'll notice that, per the written guidelines, we set the chairs in a circle so that everyone can see everyone else equally.
>
> Please keep enlarging the circle as people arrive to make sure there is equal room for them in the circle and that everyone can still see each other without craning.
>
> We need a volunteer to read the first item on the format.

If Members Disagree with the Rules

Get prospective members to read this appendix and review the guidelines. This way, if they have disagreements, they can express them to the organizers before attending a group. This helps avoid arguments during the group.

If arguments should arise, the onus is not on the organizers to resolve the dispute, but on all of the members equally. Most likely, there won't be any arguments because if the format is adhered to, its structure automatically preempts disagreement and confusion. For instance, there is no cross-talking in the group—people take turns speaking, one at a time, in a circle.

Self-Help Format

The format is easy to follow. Through years of working with groups, I've learned through trial and error what works and, even more important, what doesn't work. This format has been ordained by decades of personal, professional, and clinical experience—not just mine, but that of many professionals who have worked on it to iron out the kinks. Follow the recipe, and your cake will rise. Follow it and each person will transform his life.

It is essential that every participant abide by the guidelines to ensure emotional comfort and emotional safety. It is understood that any group calling itself an abandonment support group is following the format outlined in this appendix and that all members are adhering to the guidelines. The structure of the format is designed to safely contain your experience and ensure positive direction.

The guidelines prevent the group from breaking down into chaos and destructive dynamics. Since there is usually no professional present, people tend to remain on their own recognizance, rather than overexpose themselves emotionally and expect a trained psychotherapist to close their wounds. The group promotes structured sharing, using the format of going in a circle.

Topic Qs

You'll notice that most of the Qs on the Topic Question List (see page 327), as well as those found throughout the workbook, are broken down into subquestions, so that each Q is really a cluster of items related to a topic. These itemized Qs are designed to draw you into the various layers of self-discovery and give you a sense of the depth required for healing.

Here is a sample weekly topic Q used in the discussion round:

What am I insecure about? When did it develop? Did my parents have anything to do with it? Explain. How has insecurity interfered in my relationships? In meeting my potential? Did it crop up in my most recent relationship? What strengths do I use in overcoming it?

In preparing to share your response to one of the itemized Qs, you can silently glance over its subquestions to get the gist of what it's looking for, but only answer the part that jumps out at you. *You do not need to answer all of its subquestions.*

Group Composition

Groups work very well with a mixture of diverse ages, sexual orientations, genders, and ethnicities. There are also successful homogeneous abandonment support groups running throughout the country, such as gay and lesbian abandonment groups, abandonment groups for people going through divorce, and women's abandonment groups.

It is no surprise that more women than men join abandonment support groups, even though abandonment is not exclusively a woman's issue. Men need this kind of support as badly as women do but don't have as many socially sanctioned outlets for addressing their feelings. So it is helpful for your abandonment group to remain open to both men and women, even if this means the majority who attend will probably be women. We hope, over time, the demographics will change, and groups will become more gender balanced.

When men and women are in the same group, things can get challenging sometimes. Although I'm not a fan of gender stereotyping, it is both clinically and personally evident that the politics of the man-woman relationship can give rise to power struggles, especially in peer-led groups. Men and women tend to have disparate levels of entitlement to power, aggression, and dominance skills. Whether gender is a deciding factor or not, groups' favorite power struggles involve the format. For example, without understanding the rationale for the mandate about going in a circle and no cross-talking, some feel it's okay to dispense with the round's rigid strictures. To those who have no problem asserting themselves in a crowd, the round seems restrictive and artificial.

LET'S NOT GO IN A CIRCLE, LET'S JUST TALK OPENLY

Indeed, the round is an artifice designed to create safety, comfort, and fairness. But it's important for all members to understand that going in a circle provides everyone with sacrosanct time and space in which to respond—regardless of one's ability to be assertive.

WHY DO POWER STRUGGLES OCCUR?

People have a tendency to disagree with something they don't understand, and resist following rules they had no part in creating. Since your group is leaderless, newcomers who fail to see anyone big and powerful in charge may think it's incumbent on them to take control and try to improve the rules. This instantly puts you and the other members in a double bind where you're forced to act like a dictator just to enforce the egalitarian format—a tricky paradox to find yourself in.

This is why it's important for all prospective members to read this material and commit to follow the guidelines *before* joining.

Rule for Latecomers

Another rule that creates disagreement is the one about latecomers. As you will see in the guidelines, when people arrive late, everybody is asked to move their chairs outward to make room for them in the circle. Members are asked to expand the circle no matter how great the effort, even if everyone has to get up and move the furniture. This is so that latecomers can sit equally within the circle.

It's common to hear people suggest that the group create a double circle.

Here are two reasons for keeping a single expanding circle. First, if it were not a written rule, the members who are the polite, don't-want-to-inconvenience-anybody type would insist on not bothering the group. "Oh, it's my fault I'm late, so I'll just sit over here in the corner—don't worry about me." So rather than leave the decision up to the latecomer, I've written the expand-the-circle rule into the guidelines. Second, and even more important, is making sure nobody sits outside of the group. Inviting people inside the circle sends a message to all the members that each person is integral and important to the group. There are no observers, leaders, or outsiders, only equal participants. Furthermore, the single circle ensures eye-level connection with each and every member.

If you want to make alterations to the guidelines, please go to abandonment.net and contact us with your issue. I participate in this process.

Rationale for Avoiding an Unstructured Discussion

Most of us prefer an open discussion where we can freely interact, rather than stick to a format where we have to take turns in a circle. But even when an unstructured discussion remains orderly, things can happen that break the sense of trust and safety for some. For example, in the spirit of free interaction, someone might inadvertently give you unsolicited advice. Although you realize the advice was most likely well intended, you come away feeling that the advice giver must have perceived you as emotionally inept in handling your problems.

Or what if someone were to interrupt during *your* turn? This can make you feel that the interrupter didn't think you were as important or interesting as the other members. People are sensitive to the implicit criticism contained in interruptions and unsolicited advice, especially when they've been chafed by abandonment.

Please note: If there are extenuating circumstances requiring an unstructured discussion, before dispensing with the round, please read "If You Must Have an Open Discussion" on page 326.

WHY DO OPEN DISCUSSIONS BREAK DOWN?

There is a profoundly disparate level of assertiveness among individuals. If you've got a lot of natural aggression, you probably have no problem negotiating your way through an unstructured discussion. But not everybody has the same dominance skills as everybody else. During abandonment, your stress hormones, namely the glucocorticoids we talked about in chapter 6,[1] are elevated and your ability to assert yourself is lowered. With or without surging stress hormones, there are those who impose a strict doctrine of politeness on their behavior, one that prohibits them from interrupting when someone else is speaking. It doesn't matter if everybody else is jumping in at random, they continue waiting for the right moment, a moment that never seems to arrive. With other people chiming in and interrupting each other all over the place, these well-contained folks remain silent and often leave the group feeling disregarded and invisible.

Not surprisingly, the least assertive members in the group are the least likely to complain about not getting an equal share. What's worse, they may blame themselves for being too timid and insignificant, a painful outcome for someone seeking relief from the demoralizing pain of abandonment. Many just drop out, and the more assertive members usually fail to guess why.

Abandonment Support Groups Are Not Group Therapy

Group therapy is run by a psychotherapist. Support groups are run not by professionals, but by peer members. When a professional is in charge of things, the dynamics of an open discussion are less likely to get out of hand. Group therapy, for instance, thrives on spontaneous expression, because it brings people's conflicts to the fore, providing clinicians with grist for therapeutic intervention. Interactive groups are more competitive, lively, and challenging than groups run according to the highly structured format I suggest. But abandonment is about real pain. People are in a real crisis. In the absence of a trained professional, taking turns and going in a circle are necessary to create a sense of safety, equality, and support.

Like other self-help groups, abandonment support groups are not equipped to assume responsibility for members' emotional health; rather they provide listening space and camaraderie, connecting you to your peers for the purpose of sharing the common threads of your life.

A Special Name for Your Group

When opening a chapter of abandonment recovery in your community, you can adopt a specific name for your group like Akeru Workshop, or SWIRL Group, or People in Transition. Just make sure that whatever the name, people identify with the issue of abandonment.

Size of Groups

Abandonment support groups can begin with as few as five or six people (including the co-organizers) and can get as large as ten or twelve. Above twelve, it's difficult to ensure that people have ample time to express themselves and listen to each other—both critical aspects of recovery.

Commitment

Ideally your group should continue for about a year. It can meet once a week or every other week. The question list has fifty sequential Qs to keep you going weekly for a full year. There are also twenty-five Group Recipes designed for professionals that provide a progression of tightly structured groups.* In addition, there are enough Qs sprinkled throughout this workbook to keep your group moving forward with new material every week.

It is essential to the integrity of the group that new members commit to at least ten sessions before joining. Be careful that your group doesn't take long breaks between sessions, as members tend to use the hiatus as a natural cutoff point to discontinue their attendance. Groups that take long breaks can lose momentum.

Open versus Closed Enrollment

Some groups begin and end with the same members—these are closed groups. If the group doesn't grow beyond a manageable size, however, you have the option to receive new members. The group doesn't need to make a final decision about this. It can negotiate at any time to take in new members; this involves a circle discussion with a vote. Just make sure that each new member familiarizes herself with this appendix and agrees to follow the guidelines.

---

*   For professionals to use, available through the Member Center at abandonment.net.

IS THERE ANYBODY WHO SHOULDN'T BE IN THE GROUP?

Abandonment casts a wide net and encompasses many different types of disconnections. The most likely candidates for the group will be those who are going through a breakup, having a crisis in their current relationship, or having trouble finding a relationship.

WHAT ABOUT PEOPLE WHO ARE HAPPILY MARRIED BUT WHO HAVE ABANDONMENT ISSUES?

Some people may want to join, for example, because their childhood issues of abandonment are impinging on the quality of their present lives, even though they have a long-term, satisfying relationship. It is possible that these folks will find it difficult to relate to the level of pain and desperation of the other members. But perhaps not. It helps to have a little blurb handy to be read to prospective members. Here's one taken from an abandonment support group bulletin:

> Abandonment support groups are designed for people seeking to overcome the breakup of a past or present relationship or experiencing insecurity or love loss in their current relationship. They may be in acute pain or be caught up in chronic patterns of abandonment. Or they may be alone due to wounds from previous abandonments and have difficulty finding and keeping a relationship.

WHAT ABOUT PEOPLE WHO ARE EMOTIONALLY DISTRESSED?

If a person's emotional crisis places her at risk, she should seek psychiatric help at once. People in acute phases of heartbreak tend to be pretty torn up, prone to feeling their lives are over, as we have discussed. Timing can be a factor: when the abandonment wound is too fresh, a candidate may not feel ready to share feelings and may decide to postpone participation. Responsibility for emotional well-being is up to each participant. Prospective members need to read this appendix before joining so they can understand that the group offers peer support and does not substitute for professional mental health services.

Absenteeism and the Phone Chain

Exchange phone numbers. Members create a phone chain to notify each other of scheduling changes and to let someone know if they anticipate being late or absent. Announcements about who's going to be absent or late are made at the beginning of the session.

When someone is a no-show, group members need to acknowledge this absence during the group. Someone volunteers to call him to catch him up and let him know his absence was felt. This conveys the message to all present that everyone is important to the group and would be missed if absent.

WHAT DO NO-SHOWS MEAN?

If your group doesn't have committed members, there will be a lot of abandonment happening right in the group. When people don't show up, it triggers self-depreciating feelings in the other members, sending members into a mild form of S.W.I.R.L., even though they may not register it consciously.

"Maybe it's something I said or didn't say."

"Maybe we lack engaging personalities."

"Maybe our group isn't dynamic enough."

One of the most prevalent reasons for dropouts has to do not with the quality of the group but with people's unrealistic expectations toward the group. They might not admit this even to themselves, but many sign up in hopes of meeting that special someone. They show up for the first session, look around, don't see anyone who looks enticing, and never come back. The purpose of the group is not to meet someone. Abandonment recovery has a much higher purpose—to enter a new consciousness, increase your awareness, and gain greater life and love than before—as you can see from the Group Goals below. The group offers a working laboratory where you practice communication skills and other tools with which to change your life; it doesn't serve as a singles meeting place. The format helps you meet people both inside and outside of the group, because it promotes positive risk taking and guides the way toward making new connections within your world. But these benefits take time.

ABANDONMENT SUPPORT GROUP GOALS

To end isolation and loneliness.
To provide a safe, comfortable, equal environment where each person's feelings are honored.
To enter a new consciousness and increase your awareness.
To promote personal growth and positive change.
To raise self-esteem, restore sense of security, and build confidence.
To provide a person-to-person program of caring and sharing.
To transform abandonment into a life-changing experience.
To practice increasing your capacity for love.

Timekeeping

Each week someone other than the co-organizers volunteers to be the timekeeper. Timekeepers play a critical role in helping groups get off to the right start. They ensure that everybody gets equal time to respond to the topic Qs. Members figure out how much time they can allocate for each round. That time is then divided by the number of participants to determine how long each person gets to speak for that round. Let's say your group runs for two hours. So, you allocate thirty minutes for the first round, an hour for the discussion round, and thirty minutes for the closing round. If ten members are present, each person gets a little under three minutes for the first round, a little under six minutes for the discussion round, and a little under three for the final round. Timekeepers may use a timer to help members stick to the designated time.

TIME ALLOTMENTS FOR THE BASIC FORMAT

Times are based on a hypothetical two-hour group of ten people

Opening Round:	Positive Stroke	30 minutes	just under 3 minutes/person
Discussion Round:	Topic Question	60 minutes	just under 6 minutes/person
Closing Round:	Weekly Resolution	30 minutes	just under 3 minutes/person

Depending on the size of the group and the nature of the round, a person's speaking time can range from thirty seconds to ten minutes. Believe it or not, in large groups, one minute is enough time to express your issues and listen to all of your group mates without getting bored. For smaller groups of five or fewer people, more time is available, and it's not unusual for each person's turn to exceed ten minutes.

Strict timekeeping is one of the things members come to believe they can do without. Before dispensing the equal time rule, though, here's a hypothetical situation to consider: What happens when someone is in so much pain, he needs extra time from the group? When the timer goes off, everybody suggests, "Oh, just let him finish."

While giving extra time may be okay in some instances, here's why it doesn't always work. Suppose there is someone sitting right next to that person who is in just as much pain, but not as outspoken. She doesn't have as big a sense of entitlement as the speaker does, so her needs go unmet as the group's sympathy and extra time are spent on him. She may leave the group feeling invisible or blame herself for not being assertive enough.

When people are in crisis there are other ways, besides giving them extra time, to address their needs. They can ask for a volunteer to talk with during an off-group time (which is one of the reasons to exchange telephone numbers). For serious cases, members can urge a person in crisis to seek professional mental health services. Support groups are not equipped to provide professional assessment and referral services, but members can help and encourage a member to find a therapist.

ANOTHER REASON TIMEKEEPING IS SO IMPORTANT

Another reason for timekeeping is that some people are more loquacious than others and don't realize they are hogging the time. Rather than have to cut them short and create resentments all around, using a timer helps everybody act like equal parts of a whole. For self-centered people, this restriction promotes growth.

Another reason timekeeping is critical is that abandonment recovery addresses trauma. Trauma means you will release adrenaline as you verbally revisit the experience.[2] Adrenaline creates a tendency to go overboard and compels you to give a blow-by-blow account of the whole story. The nature of abandonment trauma and the type of neurochemistry involved make it difficult to leave out the details of your traumatic experience. They also cloud your judgment about the impact on the listener.

This is one of the reasons I presented Truth Nuggets throughout the chapters. They help you get out of the details—the "story"—of your abandonment scenario and into the most important part to share—your feelings. Incidentally, Truth Nuggets make excellent warm-up exercises for the opening round.

If someone is driven to go into detail, one option is to write out the complete story at home. She can opt to share it with one of the members during an off-group time. She can also highlight the five most important sentences with a highlighter—to share with the larger group during her turn during the round.

Timers

When I am acting as timekeeper, I use a large-faced digital timer. It's easy to read and I can hit the start button without losing eye contact with the person speaking. Timekeepers equipped with just the right timer can give a ten-second warning to help the speaker wrap up. After a few sessions, depending on your group composition, as members get the hang of the group format, timekeepers might be able to dispense with timers. Once the group devolves into overtalking, however, you always have the option to take out your timer once again.

Timers with a bell help people stick to the allotted time without causing the timekeepers to lose eye contact with the person speaking. Timekeeping is hard work, so it's a good idea to rotate this role each week.

How Long Should the Group Be?

Groups can range from ninety minutes to three hours, depending on people's schedules. Whatever time you allot, running past the time can be a problem for those who are paying a babysitter, working two jobs, or driving a great distance to attend. Try to make the group length fit everybody's needs. If certain people have to leave early each week, they will be cheated, feel cheated, be cheating themselves, and most likely will be acting out a deprivation pattern that's been the story of their lives. To avoid having time-deprived members, adjust the length of the group to give everyone equal opportunity to participate fully.

Fairness Minders

Each week someone can volunteer to be the fairness minder—another role that rotates among members. If you have an unruly group with alpha members[3] bent on trying to change the format or you have people who cross-talk during the round, the fairness minder's role is to gently remind the group to stick to the guidelines. "Let's not break the round tonight," the fairness minder can suggest at the beginning of the group. "Let's avoid cross-talking and keep to the circle." Or "Let's review the guidelines to ensure that everyone gets equal time."

Please note: When your group has trouble sticking to the format, another option is to go online to abandonment.net to get troubleshooting help. I participate in this process. Fairness minders can suggest rereading the rules and the format. Or they might suggest following topic questions *sequentially* to keep the group on track.

Fairness minders set an example by looking out for the well-being of all members. For example, they encourage volunteers to call the absent members.

Rotating Roles

The fairness minder and timekeeper work together as unobtrusive helpers for that group. They sit across from each other so that they can co-ordinate their efforts. They prompt the group to figure out the time allotments and help the group keep to the schedule, all the while participating in the group as equal members. These roles rotate to allow each member the opportunity to have responsibility within the group and to alleviate the burden from the co-organizers.

What Remaining Roles Do Co-Organizers Have?

Very little. They continue to play an overseer role. In a smoothly running group with everyone pitching in to take responsibility for the group, co-organizers can enjoy the luxury of participating equally, volunteering to be timekeeper or fairness minder from time to time. They may help recruit new members and take care of other administrative aspects of the group, such as making and distributing copies of the guidelines and other written materials.

Fees for Abandonment Groups

Abandonment support groups are free. Members may have to chip in to cover room-rental fees, timers, training or materials fees; but these costs are nominal and should be evenly distributed. If you have professionals involved in running your group, they may charge fees to compensate their time and resources. In groups run by mental health professionals, medical insurance often reimburses per-session costs to clients.

Role of Mental Health Professionals

Mental health professionals frequently write to abandonment.net requesting training to set up abandonment recovery groups. Many of them were asked to set up groups by their clients; others have taken initiative on their own. Professionals can develop their own format or can follow one of the two struc-tured formats—the basic or advanced format. Professionals target their groups to abandonment issues, focusing on the Twelve Swan Lessons, the S.W.I.R.L. Process, the Akeru Exercises, the Five-Point Action Plan, the Five Steps to Emotional Self-Reliance, and the Four Cornerstones of Self. Depending on their skills and training, mental health professionals may opt to create an unstructured, interactive format for the groups. Let's return to the self-help model—the format organized and run by peers.

> Through the Group Center at abandonment.net, people can request training for two types of groups:
>   Abandonment support groups run by peers
>   Abandonment recovery groups run by mental health professionals

How Peer Organizers Run the First Session

Co-organizers should plan for the first session to be at least two hours long to allow members to orient themselves to the format and get to know each other. Here is a recipe for the first session.

First Session Recipe

Co-organizers make sure chairs are set in a circle so everyone can see each other. Everyone should have copies of the written materials.

ORIENTATION (15 MINUTES)

Co-organizers briefly introduce themselves. They can read or paraphrase the Script for Organizers (page 306). They invite the rest of the group to introduce themselves in a round. They encourage members to write down each other's names on their Name Wheels.

If your group starts with more than five or six people who are unknown to each other, co-organizers can opt to use the Name Game (page 319). You begin this warm-up activity by asking a volunteer to read the Name Game directions. Afterward someone volunteers to begin the game. This exercise instantly puts everyone at ease and on a first-name basis.

After names, co-organizers ask someone to start the review of the guidelines (page 320). Members take turns going in a circle to read each item.

Co-organizers ask for a volunteer to be timekeeper and hand over the timer.

OPENING ROUND (15 MINUTES)

All members: Create a Truth Nugget by thinking about your abandonment scenario and how it makes you feel. Think of a feeling word—one word—that describes this feeling and complete the sentence with a *brief* phrase that explains the situation creating the feeling.

Truth Nugget: I feel _____ because

_____.

Someone volunteers to be the first to share, after whom the person to his right or left takes a turn, thus setting the direction for this round.

Members are encouraged to write brief notes on the

Name Wheel about what each person reveals, with an eye for making positive comments at the end.

Note: Timers aren't necessary for this round because each person shares only one sentence.

DISCUSSION ROUND (60 MINUTES)

Someone volunteers to start today's Discussion Round, in which you share your abandonment situation in greater depth (approximately five minutes per person).

Q What brings me here? What is my abandonment scenario and how am I coping? What am I hoping to get out of the group?

If the timekeeper uses one of those easy-to-read digital timers, she can give people a sixty-second warning before their time is up without losing eye contact with the person who's speaking.

CLOSING ROUND (30 MINUTES)

Self-esteem-building activity: Write one positive word (one word only) in the Name Wheel about each person, depicting a positive quality that jumps out at you. Try to aim at the essence of each person's personality.

Someone volunteers to go first, reciting a resolution:

Weekly Resolution: This week, the positive step I'm going to take is _____.

After each person's resolution, she receives the positive words called out at random from the entire group.* Next Week's Topic Q is announced. If you're following the Topic Question List in sequence, your next topic would be Childhood Feelings.

---

*   For further instructions, see Self-Esteem-Building Activities on page 321.

Name Wheel

© Susan Anderson, abandonment.net

Write your name at the bottom (6:00) and everyone else's name relative to your position in the circle—that is, who is sitting at 12:00, who is at 3:00, etc. When a new member arrives, just add a line emanating from the center with her name. As you listen to each person, jot down brief notes (without losing eye contact) to help you remember important aspects of his situation. This information is used later in the self-esteem-building activity.

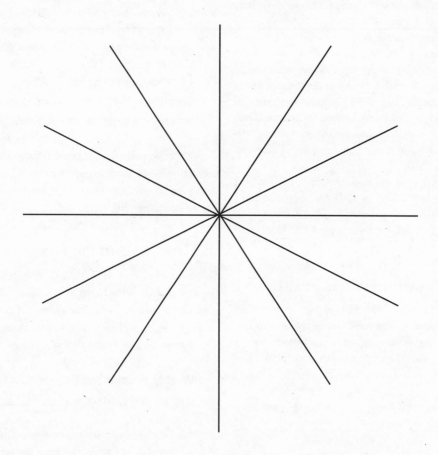

How to Use the Name Wheel

You can photocopy the Name Wheel or make your own on a blank sheet of paper each week. Each session begins with a fresh wheel. Follow the instructions above.

THE NAME GAME

The Name Game is an optional activity for newly forming groups of five or more members.

After the group goes in a circle to share their first names (and writes them in the Name Wheel), someone volunteers to see if he can remember at least five of the names (without peeking at *his* Name Wheel). When he comes to someone whose name he can't recall, other members help out by calling out the name, or the specific person may do so. Then another member volunteers to see if she can remember at least five names. Then another volunteer tries it, and so on, until everyone in the group can remember everyone else's name. This activity is fun and instantly creates positive feelings and intimacy.

How to Review the Guidelines During Session One

It is important that each person read and agree to abide by the guidelines before joining the group to ensure safety and comfort with the group process. The list of Guidelines for Abandonment Support Groups (page 320) is distributed to each member and read aloud during the first session. Each member takes a turn, going in a circle, reading the items, one at a time.

Guidelines for Abandonment Support Groups

How do we promote each other's sense of self-esteem and personal growth?

We offer confidentiality. What's said in the group stays in the group.*

We offer freedom from judgment, advice, and criticism.

We don't rely on the organizers to govern the success of the group. We understand that this is a leaderless format. We are all responsible for following the guidelines and making the group successful.

We agree to practice good mental health hygiene while participating in this group, which means that each member is responsible for seeking professional mental health services if necessary to ensure his or her stability and well-being.

We arrange the chairs in a circle, making sure each person has equal position and visibility to one another. We arrange our circle in an open space where no large tables intrude between us.

We agree to follow the format of the round in which we share one at a time in a circle.

We offer each other sacrosanct time and space to speak, by sticking to the format of the round.

We agree to stick to the time allotments to make sure everybody gets equal time.

We agree to maintain an unbroken round. We refrain from interrupting, cross-talking, asking questions, or making commentary during the round.

We commit to one another and to the group. Each member commits to at least ten sessions. We agree to keep this chapter of abandonment recovery running as long as possible—as long as members continue to need support.

We are peers to one another. We don't give each other counsel or advice—no matter how much we're tempted.

We make "I" statements about our own issues, rather than make commentary about each other's.

We understand that this is not a therapy group but a group of peers who can offer support, camaraderie, and equality—a powerful growth vehicle in itself.

We listen intently and give unbroken eye contact to the person speaking to show the depth of our interest and concern.

We avoid getting out of our seat (to get coffee or use the bathroom) during someone's turn. We don't want to give anyone the impression that what she has to say is less important than the person before or after her. If necessary, we stop the round to let someone take care of an emergency.

We see each person as equally important and entitled to our undivided attention. We realize that some people are adept at sustaining attention; others are not as outreaching. Regardless, we provide equal time and attention, making sure that each member emerges as an equal piece of the pie.

If someone arrives late, we expand the circle to make room for her, even if it means moving furniture.

If we expect to be late or absent, we use the phone chain to notify someone in the group so that it can be announced at the beginning of the session.

When someone is absent, we mention his absence during the group. Afterward, one of us volunteers to call to let him know his absence was noticed.

If size permits, we consider taking in new members and help orient them in the ways of the group (optional).

We understand that topic Qs are presented to stimulate self-discovery and depth of sharing and not intended to imply that every feeling, situation, or problem is true for each person. We honor diversity and individual difference.

We support each other's Community Projects. We have the option to reach out together as a group or individually to isolated people within our communities.

When possible, we offer to do Akeru-to-Go Exercises with other members who need some additional support during empty weekends and other off-group times.

We cooperate as a group to make sure there's enough time to complete the Self-Esteem-Building Activity at the end of each session. This involves group willpower and is well worth the effort.

At all times we demonstrate respect, caring, and love.

---

*   It is understood that confidentiality is requested but can never be completely guaranteed. Each member takes this into account when disclosing personal information.

How to Use the Self-Esteem-Building Activities

As each person takes a turn during each of the three rounds, every member of the group directs positive thoughts and feelings to that person. Focus only on the good—not only her attributes but her essence of personality. Jot down brief notes on your Name Wheel to help you remember positive things about her. Then, during the Closing Round, you put your positive thoughts into a few words and deliver them equally to her during the Self-Esteem-Building Activity. There are three options: Round of Compliments, Round of Interest, and Round of Positive Words. As abandonment has caused injury to our sense of self, we use our person-to-person power to help each other rebuild it.

Self-Esteem-Building Activities

ROUND OF COMPLIMENTS

In preparation for Round of Compliments, review the notes you've taken on your Name Wheel to help you come up with positive comments about each person. Be sure your comments are free of any implicit advice or criticism.

As each person shares his weekly resolution, he receives positive comments from three and only three other members. Members with comments raise their hands so that he can call on them. The fairness minder's role is to make sure people who raise their hands are not repeatedly overlooked. Very important!

It is important for everyone to work hard to think of positive comments for each person. Imagine if it were your turn to receive your three compliments, and the members hesitated in coming up with positive things to say about you. It might not feel very good. Owing to differences in personality, it is easy to think of complimentary words for some people, and not so easy for others. Coming up with positive comments for each person is hard but important work. By sharing positive feedback, we serve as a Hall of Mirrors for one another, reflecting back positive light. Riding in on positive energy, we get right into each other's healing core.

ROUND OF INTEREST

Same as Round of Compliments, except instead of compliments, you let each member know what moved you or aroused your interest. You might say something like: "I was very moved when you mentioned your mother moving out of the house."

It is understood that these comments are not questions that expect answers, as time wouldn't permit. They let members know of your regard for them.

ROUND OF POSITIVE WORDS

In preparation for this activity, write down one word on your Name Wheel to describe a positive quality about each person. It is okay to come up with the same word for more than one person, since originality isn't the issue, as long as the word you select describes a certain quality that jumps out at you about the person—something you feel—the essence of her personality.

Be sure to share one word—and one word only—for each person, to avoid the inevitable problem of some people getting a bigger collection of words than others. As each member takes a turn to recite his weekly resolution, he receives all of the one-word compliments from the other members. The words can be called out at random.

Round of Positive Words:
Example from a Hypothetical Group

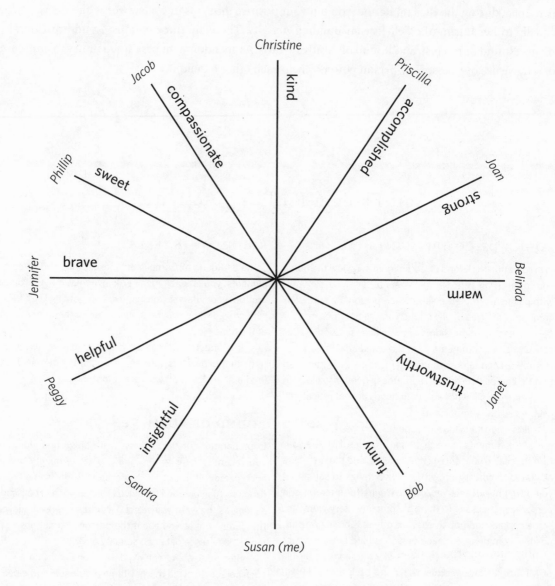

How to Make the Rounds Flow Smoothly

Fairness minders can suggest having a volunteer read the Guidelines for Rounds (p. 323) aloud at the beginning of each group (until the format becomes second nature). When a well-established group begins to lose its structure, to safeguard group safety, the fairness minder, organizers, or other group members can suggest reviewing the Guidelines for Rounds.

GUIDELINES FOR ROUNDS

All other rules and guidelines apply.

Someone volunteers to go first.

The person either on his right or left goes next, and so on, to start the round.

Everyone agrees to keep to the allotted time.

Going one at a time, each person gets equal uninterrupted time.

The round remains unbroken—that is, no one cross-talks, interrupts, comments, or asks questions before, during, or after each person speaks.

Everyone maintains eye contact with each person speaking.

No one gets out of her seat during someone's turn. If necessary, stop the round to allow someone to go to the bathroom.

Members may postpone their turn. The fairness minder or other group members can ask them at the end of the round if they'd like to take their turn. No one is forgotten.

By the same token, no one is pressured.

Every word of every person is important and attentively listened to by all members.

Each Round Has a Purpose

The Opening Round starts the group on an upbeat note. It gives you a chance to give yourself a positive stroke for any changes or new awareness you've noticed recently. For the sake of new members, very briefly restate your abandonment situation to help them participate in your recovery.

The Discussion Round is the longest round and addresses that week's in-depth topic taken from the Topic Question List (see Appendix B, page 327). Groups are encouraged to follow the questions sequentially, taking up one question each week. Groups also have the option to choose one of the Qs sprinkled throughout this workbook.

The Closing Round ends the group on a positive note. The Weekly Resolution is designed to help you formulate what you gained from today's group and what concrete steps you will take this week to fulfill your goals. Members can jot down each other's goals on their Name Wheels to help track and support one another's progress. This round includes the Self-Esteem-Building Activity: as each member shares his Weekly Resolution, he receives positive words or comments from the group.

Timekeepers and fairness minders seek volunteers at the end of each session to take over their roles. Someone volunteers to call absent members. Next week's topic Q from the question list is reviewed.

Subsequent Group Sessions

Here is a recipe for the three-round group to use in all subsequent groups. It is based on a typical two-hour group.

Recipe for Three-Round Group

© Susan Anderson, abandonment.net

RULES

Confidentiality.
Commit to at least ten sessions; commit to each other.
Call someone if you're going to be late or absent.
Avoid cross-talking during round.
Each person's space is sacrosanct.
Avoid getting up during someone's turn.
No advice or commentary; instead speak from "I."
All members cooperate to ensure that the final Self-Esteem-Building Activity is completed.
Write brief notes about each person on your Name Wheel with an eye for making positive comments at the end.

OPENING ROUND: POSITIVE STROKE (APPROX. 30 MINUTES)

Give a brief update of your situation, and give yourself a positive stroke for any recent changes you've noticed. Mention what, if any, steps you took toward your goals (or toward your Community Project).

DISCUSSION ROUND: WEEKLY TOPIC QUESTION (APPROX. 60 MINUTES)

Topic Qs are chosen from the Topic Question List or from the Qs sprinkled throughout the workbook. This is your opportunity to explore an issue in depth.

LIFTING ROUND: WEEKLY RESOLUTION (APPROX. 30 MINUTES)

Weekly Resolution: The positive action I'm going to take this week is _____.

SELF-ESTEEM-BUILDING ACTIVITY

Option 1: Round of Compliments
Option 2: Round of Positive Words
Option 3: Round of Interest

ANNOUNCE NEXT WEEK'S TOPIC

Professionally Run Abandonment Workshops

Advanced Format

To intensify the change process within abandonment groups, you can add the visualization exercise for Building a Dream House and Back to the Future to the format. Adding additional activities creates greater complexity in keeping the group on track and requires additional training. Professionals are best equipped to administer the more complex format.

The complex format involves not three but *five* rounds. It requires rigorous timekeeping and real cooperation from each member to adhere to the format—even when professionals are facilitating this process.

Here is the skeleton of the more complex format, ideally facilitated by mental health professionals. The format assumes you have two hours.

ADVANCED FIVE-ROUND FORMAT IN BRIEF*

Opening Round (15 minutes): Give yourself a positive stroke this week.
Discussion Round (30 minutes): Discuss this week's topic question in depth.
Akeru Exercise (30 minutes): Visualize your Dream House during group and then share your renovations.
Back to the Future (15 minutes): Jot down your answers and then share how you solved your problem.
Closing Round (30 minutes): Share Weekly Resolution and do Self-Esteem-Building Activity.

In closing this appendix, I'd like to present guidelines for having an open discussion. When your group is professionally run, open discussions tend to run smoothly.** If, on the other hand, you're part of a leaderless self-help group, and if there are extenuating circumstances for which you absolutely must break the round and have an open discussion, I encourage you to follow the guidelines below to ensure safety and to prevent the discussion from breaking down into power struggles and unfair dynamics. Review these guidelines by having a volunteer read them aloud.

---

*   Available through the Member Center at abandonment.net.
** Open discussions are best facilitated by professionals or trained facilitators. For training opportunities, go to the Professional Page at abandonment.net, then click on TRAINING IN ABANDONMENT.

IF YOU MUST HAVE AN OPEN DISCUSSION

During an open discussion, all members agree to become a unified mind of equal parts, acting as a leaderless group to create fairness in the open discussion.

All of the guidelines apply (except for the one for going in a circle): *No judgment *Speak from "I" *No advice *No interrupting *No leading *No directing *No controlling *No overtalking *Confidentiality

The timekeeper and all group members work to keep to the established time period.

Two fairness minders are chosen. They sit opposite each other in the circle.

Someone opens the discussion—about, for example, whether to invite new members or whether to go out of sequence to select a topic question. Others can then respond at random.

Despite the lively interaction of an open discussion, all members need to be mindful that some may not have had a chance to speak. Fairness minders or other members can draw these members out by asking respectful questions.

At all times, each and every member is shown equal concern. No one is abandoned or ignored—not even the quietest member. By the same token, no one is pressured.

When people overtalk, rather than correct them, the timekeeper can simply mention to the whole group how much time is remaining and that some people haven't spoken yet. This information usually helps the more loquacious members wrap up without embarrassing them. The purpose is to give everyone a chance to speak.

To allow time for closure, the timekeeper gives a five-minute warning for the end of the session.

During the last five minutes, members cooperate to tie up the discussion (rather than looking to a leader to do it), by commenting on common threads or group themes. The timekeeper warns when there is one minute left.

When time is up, time is up. This is only fair to those members who have obligations and can't stay late.

Topic Questions

Topic Question List: 50 Weekly Questions

This Topic Question List serves as the "leader" for a Discussion Round. Everyone should have a copy. Someone can volunteer to read the day's question aloud.

Most of the Qs have subquestions. Members don't need to answer every part—just the parts that jump out at them. The idea is to answer the Q whole without looking at the page.

The group can follow the Qs in sequence or choose at random from the list. Or make up its own.*

Topic questions are designed to promote self-discovery and sharing and are not intended to imply that every issue referred to holds true for every member.

Week 1: Introducing My Situation. Describe the abandonment situation that brings me here. Explain what was so shattering about it. What am I hoping to gain from the group?

Week 2: Childhood Feelings. Thinking about my abandonment situation, what is my earliest memory of feeling this way? Who was this feeling about? Mother, father, sibling? Who? Was this similar to my current situation in any way? How? Is it related to where I am stuck? How am I handling these feelings: How would I like to handle them?

Week 3: Stuckness. What stage of abandonment—Shattering, Withdrawal, Internalizing, Rage, or Lifting—am I struggling with the most? How does it feel? Describe an earlier experience that caused me to feel stuck in these feelings. How am I currently stuck? How would becoming unstuck benefit my goals?

Week 4: Aloneness. Describe my current living status. Am I coupled or single, living alone or with a roommate, friend, or family? Am I emotionally alone? Is my aloneness by choice? Do I

---

* If you'd like to add to the collection of Qs, contact us at abandonment.net.

feel isolated? Growing up, did I believe that living alone was undesirable? Who influenced my belief? How do I feel about the single lifestyle now? How would I like to feel about it?

Week 5: My Breakup. Describe what led to my breakup. Explain my ex's point of view about it. My own. How well am I handling the aftermath of the conflict? What do I regret? What do I feel good about?

Week 6: Who Is My Abandoner? Describe how my abandoner treated me during the breakup. What about after the breakup? Was he sensitive to my feelings? Is my abandoner a repeat abandoner? How was my abandoner's behavior similar to another member's ex? How do I currently react to my abandoner? How would I like to?

Week 7: Transforming. Shattering means hitting an emotional bottom—a transforming bottom. Describe how this bottom helps me transform my life. What am I discovering about myself? How has my abandonment motivated positive change? In what direction does this change seem to be taking me?

Week 8: Neediness. Losing someone's love is a trauma powerful enough to activate fears and dependencies left over from childhood, causing us to need our lovers most when we feel abandoned by them. Describe my struggle in this area. How does it make me feel about myself to be needy and desperate for a love fix from my abandoner? Am I ashamed of these feelings? Which is more destructive to me—being ashamed of my neediness or the neediness itself? What would it take to manage my dependency?

Week 9: Pulling Out the Splinters from Previous Shatterings. Name an earlier breakup or loss that caused me to pick up self-doubts, fears, and insecurities. What bits and particles of my shattered self are working their way to the surface of my awareness now? How do these feelings affect my recovery?

Week 10: Dealing with My Primal Feelings. Thanks to abandonment, our oldest needs and feelings have resurfaced and we can finally administer to them, now as capable adults. How is Big Me handling this task? Is she strong enough? How about Little Me? Is she too needy and overwhelming? Describe how Big Me handles my primal feelings. What positive strides is Big Me taking in this area? How does Little Me feel about me this week?

Week 11: Goals. How wide is the gap between my current life and the life I want? Identify my goals. Am I already doing all I can to reach my goals, or am I remiss in some way? Am I on the right path? Sidetracked? Moving in the right direction? Stuck? What goal am I targeting as we speak? What plans do I have for achieving it?

Week 12: Emotional Hunger. Our parents couldn't possibly meet all of our needs. Describe what they left me needing and not getting enough of as a child. What situation created my emotional hunger? Do old feelings of longing and neediness haunt my adult life? How do

I self-medicate my chronic feelings of deprivation—shopping, food, people, alcohol, drugs, sleep, watching too much television? Which of my quick fixes are most likely to defeat my long-range goals? How am I changing this?

Week 13: Security. The world is divided into two camps—those who have a background object and those who don't. In my opinion, which camp has it easier? What has losing my background object been like for me? Describe the special challenges it created in my life. What are the advantages to having my security ripped away? How would I like to handle having no background object for security?

Week 14: Parents. When we were children, our primary relationship was to a parent. Describe the connection I had to my mother or father. Was it a secure or insecure attachment? A weak or strong connection? Were my parents calming? Anger provoking? Supportive? Ego deflating? Empowering? Emotionally toxic? What impact did the quality of these attachments have on my ability to form secure primary relationships in adulthood?

Week 15: Always and Never. Going through heartbreak tends to throw us into catastrophic always-and-never thinking. Describe the always and nevers I've been struggling with since my breakup. What do I fear will *never* happen in my life—that I'll *never* be able to do? What do I fear is *always* going to happen—that will *always* be a problem in my life? How do I handle my fears and worries? How would I like to?

Week 16: Unlived Life. Life is a series of splits in the road. Each path we choose takes us in one direction, excluding another. Life has taken us to one particular twig on the branch of a branch, on the limb of a limb of a tree within a whole forest of unclimbed possibilities. What are some of my regrets about my unchosen paths? Describe something about me—an interest perhaps—that even my friends would be surprised to learn about. What part of me have I yet to express—a skill, a gift, a personal responsiveness to something—an aspect of my essence that never got picked up by my parents, nor perhaps by myself—something that lay dormant and undeveloped. How do I feel about this unlived life? What would I like to do about it?

Week 17: Little Me. What was I like as a young child? What did I look like at about four or five years old? What was my situation at the time? How did I feel about myself in relationship to my family? What activities did I enjoy the most? What didn't I like to do? What made me angry? What made me sad? What made me afraid? What made me bored? Who gave me emotional support? Who withheld it? What mood was I in most of the time? Describe the main conflict of my childhood. What part of my childhood personality is still with me today?

Week 18: Old Wounds. Paradoxically, Little is the oldest part of the personality. What are Little Me's greatest needs? Deepest fears? Describe the main event that caused these fears. How do I take care of the feelings rising out of this old wound? How does Big Me need to change to be better able to care for Little?

Week 19: Insecurity. Describe the earliest time I felt insecure. Did my parents have anything to do with it? Has it held me back from reaching my potential? How would being secure within myself—Big to Little—help me with my goals?

Week 20: My Role in the Family. Describe my role in my family. Was I the middle child? Oldest? Youngest? Favorite? Scapegoat? Star? Princess? Hero? Was it my job to keep everybody happy? Was I expected to be invisible—seen but not heard? Or did I act mischievous, annoying, or cute to keep my parents distracted from a more pressing problem (for example, their depression, mourning, illness, anxiety disorder, or alcoholism)? What impact has my family role had on my personality? On my confidence? How would I like to change these patterns?

Week 21: Triangles. What triangles have I been in? Was there a triangle involving mother, father, and me? Sister, mother, and me? Father, uncle, and me? Spouse, mother-in-law, and me? My lover, his old girlfriend, and me? What was the earliest triangle I can remember being involved in? Describe some triangles in my adult relationships. How do I avoid getting triangulated? How would I like to handle the triangles in my life?

Week 22: Personal Inventory. Explain what my greatest impediment (besides insecurity) is. Is it my rigidity? Lack of insight? Fear? Self-deceit? Low expectation? Denial? Tendency to avoid uncomfortable feelings? Failure to take positive risks? Am I too hard on myself for all of the wrong reasons? Too easy on myself in regard to my real character defects? How could I be a better parent to myself? How could acknowledging my character defects benefit my life?

Week 23: Self-Esteem. Describe how my last breakup affected my self-esteem. How did I feel about myself before the breakup? During the relationship? After we broke up? How is my self-esteem now? Name something I currently like about myself and something I don't. What can I do to feel better about myself?

Week 24: Your Teenage Self-Image. If I could have changed an attribute about myself in high school, what would it have been? Was it a physical attribute? Personality attribute? Intellectual attribute? How did this attribute affect the way my peers responded to me? How did it affect the way I felt about myself? How do I currently feel about this attribute? Do any of these past issues remain unresolved? How would resolving them help me today?

Week 25: Psychic Limp. Psychic limp refers to the impact past abandonments and losses have had on our ability to perform in life. Describe a situation that caused my "psychic limp" to develop. What kind of situation causes me to limp the most? How would overcoming my limp benefit my life? How does this limp help me?

Week 26: Positive Change. How am I growing and developing as an adult? Am I still working on the same issues I had as a child or teenager? What are they? Explain what causes me to get stuck in self-doubt. What specific issue do I find most difficult to overcome? How am I changing it?

Week 27: Disappointment. Describe my greatest disappointment. Was I disappointed in someone else (a family member, friend, etc.) or in myself? Is my current abandonment an example of being disappointed in myself, in my partner, or both? Do I tend to overreact to disappointment? How would I like to handle the setbacks of life?

Week 28: Becoming My Own Worst Enemy. Am I sometimes my own worst enemy? Name an instance. In what situations am I most likely to get in my own way? Is this my most vulnerable area? How would my life improve if I got out of my way? What would I have to change?

Week 29: Peeling the Layers, One at a Time. Working through the internalizing process is like peeling an onion one layer at a time. We make our way through layer upon layer of defenses—deeply entrenched beliefs we have about others and ourselves. Each time we peel back another layer, it causes a little "tissue breakdown." The uncomfortable feelings are part of recovery. Do I hold back from personal change to avoid the little breakdowns? Describe my process of self-discovery. Why am I resistant to change? What strengths can I use to surmount the uncomfortable feelings of growth?

Week 30: Love. How do I feel about the quality of love in my life? Do I feel loved enough? Do I have enough self-love? Are the two related? Describe the greatest love I've ever known. Who was it with? What were the circumstances? What became of this love? What did it give to me? What did it take from me? What are my current love needs?

Week 31: Transition. Abandonment is a time of transition. What is my transition leading to? What positive benefits am I aspiring to? What strengths do I have for converting the unwanted change of heartbreak into a positive change?

Week 32: Who Rescued Me? Did anyone ever come along—a teacher, an aunt, a neighbor—at a crucial moment in my life and help me feel good about myself? Describe what he did to help me. Did I let his positive messages in? Am I receiving a positive message from this experience today? When this group gives me positive feedback, do I let your messages in? What makes it difficult to receive people's love and support? How do I deflect it? Why do I? How can I better use positive feedback from people who care about me?

Week 33: Reaching Out? When have I made a difference in someone else's life? Describe the first time I reached out to help someone else. Describe the last time. How does reaching out feel? How might this relate to developing a new career for myself or becoming involved in a Community Project?

Week 34: Community Projects. Which people in my community (or in society) arouse my greatest sympathy? Explain what about them I identify with the most. What does this say about me? How would I like to help them? What Community Project could I become involved in (or create) to reach out to people in my world?

Week 35: Unresolved Anger from Childhood. What was the strongest rage I ever remember feeling? What triggered it? Is this anger a theme in my life? Do similar things make me angry today? How does anger affect my behavior? Does it interfere in my goals? How could I better manage anger?

Week 36: Love Rage. Does my struggle to feel loved get me frustrated? How do my partners experience my anger? Do I displace my anger on them? On myself? On innocent bystanders? Explain where my anger from past breakups and losses went. Did it dissipate? Did I stuff it? Swallow it? Let Outer Child act it out? Has anger interfered in my adult relationships? If I could use my anger as a source of constructive energy, how would I reinvest it?

Week 37: Anger Control. Abandonment survivors are famous for getting too angry in some situations, and not angry enough in others. What usually causes me to underreact? In which situations do I usually overreact? How would I like to use my anger in the future?

Week 38: Nobody Listened. Does it ever feel sometimes as if nobody were listening? Who understood my feelings as a child? Who took care of me when I was afraid, hurt, or angry? Who listens to my feelings today? What about my abandoner? Did she care about my feelings during the relationship? How about during the breakup? How does it feel when the group listens to my feelings? Who else listens today?

Week 39: Unsolicited Advice. When I tell my friends what I'm going through, do they try to fix it instead of listen? Do they give me unsolicited advice? How does it make me feel? What would I like them to understand about my situation? Am I assertive about my needs in this issue? Do I give unsolicited advice? Has my abandonment taught me a better way to relate to others in need?

Week 40: Abandonment Trauma. Abandonment is trauma. One of its posttraumatic stress symptoms is the tendency to freak out, especially when our lovers are late showing up for dates or when they neglect to return our phone calls. Describe a situation that causes me to freak out. Is my overreaction related to trauma from previous abandonments? When I'm overwrought, do I lose emotional control? How would I like to better handle intense emotion?

Week 41: Shame. Our Outer Child has been acting out since we were about seven—and is still trying to control our behavior today. Thinking back, what was the worst thing Outer Child ever did (at least what I'm willing to admit here)? Has Outer ever gotten me into trouble? Made me ashamed? Describe a recent Outer Child event. Name a specific area of my life that would improve if I gained control of my Outer Child behavior.

Week 42: Outer Child Patterns. What is Outer Child's biggest pattern? Explain how it developed. How has this pattern interfered in my goals? In my relationships? What was Outer up to this week? How would my life be different if I overcame this pattern?

Week 43: Rewounding. Abandonment leaves us vulnerable to rewounding. As we move forward, things inevitably happen to temporarily pull us back into the muck. For example, when we have contact with our exes, the encounter can hurt even more than the original breakup. Likewise, when we try to make a new romantic connection and it doesn't work out, this new failure can hurt even more than the original breakup. Describe the last incident that created a setback. Did it send me right back into abandonment grief? How did I handle it? How would I like to handle future sinkholes?

Week 44: Abandoholism. A common bind for many abandonment survivors is the tendency to pursue emotionally unavailable partners. The flip side: when someone comes along who is available, abandoholics get turned off. Describe a time when I was attracted to an unavailable partner. What happened? What did I expect to happen? Have I ever been involved with a serial abandoner? Have I ever pushed someone away because she didn't have the right chemistry, even though she seemed right for me in every other aspect? Was there ever a time when love showed up and I wasn't ready to recognize it? What can I do to overcome my cycles of abandonment?

Week 45: Am I a Loving Person? Is there someone in my life receptive to me when I'm being loving and nurturing? Do others see me as a loving person? How do I show others my increasing capacity for love? What can I do to increase my expression of love on a daily basis?

Week 46: Lifting. Describe the last time I lifted above my worries and concerns and enjoyed the moment. What elements were in place that allowed me to let go? What blocks me from feeling this way all the time? What can I do to increase my ability to lift? What activities help me most when I want to get into the moment? Does this suggest a new life goal?

Week 47: Personality. Who (parents, friends, teachers, lovers) had the greatest impact on my development? What do I believe to be most compelling about my personality? What is least so? What type of person or situation brings out the best in me? The worst? How can this awareness help me? How would I like my personality to evolve?

Week 48: Self-Image. Self-image refers to how we believe we come across to other people. The enemy of having a positive self-image is rejection because it instills self-doubt. It makes us feel self-conscious, inhibited, and less-than. Describe a recent event that injured my self-image and caused me to doubt myself. How am I overcoming it?

Week 49: Next Plateau. Abandonment challenges us to grow bigger than our problems. Describe the next plateau I'm reaching. How did my abandonment derail my dreams and goals? What about the reverse: How did my abandonment help me seek higher ground? What emotional baggage did I pick up from my abandonment? What emotional strength did I pick up? So far, does my abandonment add up to a net gain or a net loss? How can I improve my balance sheet?

Week 50: Life Direction. What lessons have I learned from going through abandonment? Am I discovering my higher self? What higher purpose does my abandonment serve? What higher purpose would I like it to serve? Describe the direction in which I'm moving my life and how my abandonment has helped.

Please note: Additional topic questions can be taken from Qs in the workbook or generated from issues that arise in the group members' lives.

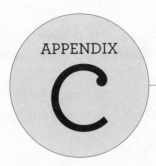

Akeru-to-Go Exercises

Inspired by Celeste Carlin

There are many books on meditation, power of prayer, and other spiritual pursuits to help you along your journey. Akeru-to-Go Exercises are designed to take you beyond these contemplative and solitary realms to activities not quite as sedate or reverent—activities that nourish your spirit by doing.

Akeru-to-Go activities were inspired by psychotherapist Celeste Carlin, who helped me explore the data sent to abandonment.net from abandonment survivors from all over the world. After reading the many personal stories and responding to people's requests, she wanted to contribute some ideas of her own to supplement the program of abandonment recovery—things to do to get out of your head, out of your wounded spirit, and into the moment.

Here are some of the recipes, rituals, and enchantments she offered to momentarily call you back from the abyss.

Alone or with a friend, the Akeru-to-Go Exercises suggest taking Outer Child by the hand, rather than be controlled by inner forces. Invest your energy constructively by letting one of these suggestions inspire you. As you discover your own activities, send them to abandonment.net to share the wealth with others surviving abandonment.

On the worst days you need major repairs—lots of self-nurturing, lots of positive activity. The problem is that when we feel really down, most of us don't feel like doing much. Self-nurturing doesn't mean self-indulging your desire to keep the covers over your head.

One suggestion is to hat up and go for a ride—somewhere in the opposite direction of your ex. Decide the purpose for your destination along the way. Continue questing until you feel hungry, tired, or satiated or you reach a point of interest—or until it feels like the right moment to return home.

When your whole day seems like too long a period of time to conceive of—the pain is just too excruciating—the idea is to get up and do.

Just take it one minute at a time and accomplish something small.

Clean out one dresser drawer.

Call one friend you haven't talked to in a while and suggest a future lunch plan.

Buy a plant to nurture in your home or garden. Make a commitment to that plant—you won't abandon it the way you've been abandoned.

What if you find yourself reverberating through Shattering again—just as you were sure you were done with this stage? Maybe you've just talked to your ex and you feel the agony of rewounding. He bumped into your tender sore and sent you reeling.

It feels like it sent you right back to the beginning, but it didn't. You're revisiting the pain, not moving in permanently. You'll get through the feelings much more quickly this time. You're more experienced at pain management than before.

"I know I'm alive because I feel incredible pain."

Even on good days it's sometimes hard to feed the soul and indulge in your senses.
We're here to say, make the effort. Try one of these activities.

Rituals and Offerings

On fifty slips of paper write different words that describe the person you are getting over. In an outdoor fireplace or a barbecue (make sure it's safe, now—we're not kidding), burn the slips of paper, one at a time. Imagine that you are offering up your greatest prized possession to the universe for the opportunity to live more fully and wholly. When the ashes have cooled, gather them. Place them in a cherished vessel. Someday, when you are ready, take the ashes to a special place, the sea, a mountain, the woods. Let the ashes fly and say good-bye.

Because closure is such a problem with abandonment, if you can't say good-bye, say so long.

Take one item that either belonged to your beloved or that your beloved gave to you—an article of clothing, a picture frame that held your favorite picture of him. Whatever it is, make sure it's something a little hard to let go of—but you *can* let go of this one thing. Donate this item to a thrift shop. As you are coming home, imagine that someone who really needs the item will come in after you leave and pay $1.00 for it. Or give it to someone in need. Whatever, imagine that she feels lucky to have found just what she truly needed in that moment.

Build a burial mound of rocks in your home, in your garden, in the nearby woods. Visit the mound as often as you need to. Leave an offering with the intention that with each offering you set onto the rocks, you are giving up more of your grief and getting more of your life back.

When you're bored, antsy, feeling out of sorts, lonesome, in a daze, or just plain worn down by the grind of the day…rent the movie *Castaway* and see how, on the brink of oblivion, Tom Hanks's character creates a new life.

Find a metaphor that works for you…what about when it feels as if your whole body were made of lead and every little task, no matter how small, takes every bit of energy you can muster? (There's good news here; we're not asking you to write anything this time!)

Begin by getting into an activity of the mind. Imagine you are stuck on a mountain, a plane or train wreck, You're lost. Frozen or parched…maybe in a desert…barely a breath left. Imagine the glorious feeling of coming out a victor.

Then get up and take one tiny step in a positive direction. Empty the dishwasher. Go out and buy a newspaper. Take a walk around the block.

Call up a college or an adult education program and ask for a catalog. Fantasize beginning a new career from scratch or enlightening yourself with an old interest.

Go to a car show and fantasize about your car of the future (to park in the driveway of your Dream House).

Go online and find out about the least expensive vacation deals—even if you have no intention of taking a trip at this point. Fantasize. If your head is still nailed to your pillow and you can't move forward on your own, call a therapist, call a spiritual guide, call a power animal, call a friend. The idea is to find someone who can help you get active, until you're ready to move out of the ICU into a regular room.

Heartwarmings*

Friends help you get involved in being outside of yourself—outside of the pain.

> *"The only time I wasn't feeling the desire to shoot myself,"* says Roberta, *"was when I was telling my closest friend how badly I wanted to shoot myself. The heartbreak wouldn't hurt as badly while I was in the throes of ranting and raving and crying tears about it. It was only when she tried to take a turn to speak that my heartache would come back to me full force. It seemed that the only thing that helped was to do all of the talking. She had to do all of the listening. But is this fair? Do I have a right to expect my friends to turn into ears?"*

Besides turning your friends into *ears*, here are other things to do with them. Maybe you'll find someone else going through a rough time.

How about doing a project together?
How about journaling on a topic and exchanging responses?
How about exchanging self-portraits of where you want your life to go?

Or do an exercise where the two of you surrender to the pain in the joint acknowledgment that "what does not kill you heals you." Or make a promise or a commitment to walk with a friend for one half hour in silence and in "witness" to one another. Practice mindful breathing, and at the end of the walk just talk about what you heard.

Get together for an outing, a self-indulgence, a distraction. Agree to spend a designated period of time (one hour each, perhaps) speaking about your painful situations. Then agree to spend the rest of

---

*   Friendship connections were suggested by psychotherapist Donna Carson.

the time trying to get distracted by the day's activities. Be sure to have realistic expectations. You can never guarantee pure bliss or ongoing peacefulness. Why? Because the pain of heartache has a tendency to bleed through. So, as you try to get involved in the distractions of the day, approach it as you would a grueling workout at the gym or as an experiment. Be prepared to strain.

Take out your recovery tool kit with a friend…exchange those things you have in duplicate. Work together to make each of your kits better.

Notice to Friends

You can be lifelines, saviors, guardian angels—real flesh-and-blood angels. Your heartbroken buddy doesn't have to conjure you up by her imagination or faith. You're an angel without wings just by caring. Your friendship makes a difference. All you have to do is listen and be there. The connection takes care of the rest. You will be cherished forever.

Notice to Abandonment Survivors

You'll probably need more than one friend. Better consider also reaching out for family members. And, come to think of it, ministers, rabbis, priests. This is so that after you've worn out your first friend, you can go to a spare while the first one is recuperating. (Friends, stop complaining: That's what friends are for. God forbid something like this should ever happen to you, you've already built your equity.)

What if none of your friends are home?

Get a recording of "I Will Survive" sung by Gloria Gaynor. Play it over again until you can sing it out loud at the top of your lungs.

Blast "Respect Yourself" by Aretha Franklin or Beethoven's *Ninth Symphony*.

When they are pining for their ex, some people sing along to "Change the Locks" by Lucinda Williams.

What about those down days when you don't feel like moving, but you've taken the last nap you can possibly take? You know it's time to do something, but inertia wins out.

Well, propel yourself out of the chair and create a purpose for your lethargy.

Go plant a tree or a seed.

Go into the woods or find a local tree. Hug it so tightly you can feel its rough skin against your chest. Try to push it over and appreciate how strong it is. Bark out loud.

Even when you're just forcing yourself to go through the motions, you can still bring yourself to feel something. Smile to yourself. By taking a single action, you've earned the right for one more nap.

You feel wistful, empty, out of sorts. What to do? Create a purpose for your malaise.

Get a balsawood airplane…let it catch the breeze.

Put sand in a shallow box and play with it. Use a fork as a rake.

Go to the beach and use your fingers and toes as rakes.

After a rain, you're still feeling cloudy inside?

Go find a small twig and put it in the rain gutter at the edge of the street and follow it on its journey …imagine you're on the twig.

One woman writing in to abandonment.net suggested, "Go bush walking in the Tasmanian wilderness." Yeah, try that.

Primal Food

On a lonely day, think of feeding your spirit. Create a purpose for your loneliness. Discover your capacity to be self-nurturing.

Imagine that whatever season it is right now, whatever climate your corner of the world is experiencing, decide if you want warm or cold on your insides and on your outside.

Will warm coddle your insides? Melt the frigid fear?

Will cool be refreshing and soothe the tired aches and chafed pride?

Which feels better on your skin?

Which feels better on your tongue as it slips down your throat?

Can you feel it as it washes down past your heart?

Do you want ice cold? Or barely warm? How about burning hot? Gentle cool?

If you don't know, experiment. Quench with iced tea or warm broth. Immerse yourself in a warm bath or a cool lake. Go for it. Experiment.

Sensualities

Go dip your toes into a pot of cold water, the ocean, a river, a brook, a hot tub.

Hold a rock in your hand until it grows warm from your energy.

Build a fire.

Toast marshmallows.

Massage warmed oil into your feet.

Cover your eyes with cool cucumbers and imagine they are sinking deeper and deeper into a cooling pool of water.

Cover your eyes with warm chamomile tea bags.

Cover your feet with the thickest socks you can find, or the silkiest, thinnest, softest.

Take a bath—warm or cool—then climb into bed sans clothes between freshly cleaned sheets, and put mounds of pillows on top of you.

Pay attention. What soothes you most, what captures your aliveness and brings you to the present? Indulge.

It may be hard to think about food at a time like this. Either way, think soup. If you thought it was just a remedy for colds, think again.

Now, we're not saying that you need to make soup. You may not be in the mood. Right now, consider what an imaginary bowl of soup would need to contain to soothe or nourish you—soup for the ICU days.

If you've decided that cool feels better than hot, there are infinite chilled varieties to dream up. Find the ideal soup-of-the-mind or of your tummy's desire that satisfies like mother's milk for her baby.

As for real soup, maybe you'll heat some up or you'll stop at a local eatery on your way home and take out their soup du jour. Turn your tongue into a highly discriminatory soup critic.

The moment is not a time for thinking; it is a time for experiencing.

Ever think to ask someone close to you to make you some soup? For many of us, this would be a big step forward—asking someone for what we want.

Are we suggesting comfort food? Absolutely. Especially for those days when you can hardly keep anything down. If only a peanut butter and jelly sandwich seems palatable, don't be shy. The idea is to get enough nourishment to survive another day. As psychotherapist Carole Ann Price once put it, "The goal is to outlive the pain."[2]

Make a pot of tomato sauce. Watch everything disintegrate into the simmering pot. Consider the transience of life.

Make meatballs, feel them in your hands taking form. Cook them until tender—tender as your heart—and then share them with a special friend.

Remember those Community Projects? How about nurturing a hungry family?

What about the bad days, critical ICU days that call for *Intravenous TLC*? Do something to make you sweat.

Prune your trees.

Hammer some nails.

Chop wood.

Do it, damn it. With what seems like your last breath, endure long enough to see if you can find a purpose for the feeling. That purpose? To discover your own strength. Recover one more piece of yourself to discover the mysterious surprises hidden in life's most uncomfortable moments.

What activities over the past months helped pull you out of your heartache and into the moment?

What things have you done most recently that gave you a tiny little respite from the pain?

What helped you get through a difficult hour?

A lonely evening?

A whole day?

If you could inspire others to walk in your footsteps, what have you accomplished that you'd like to share with others?

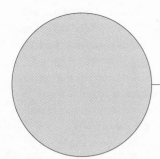

Endnotes

Introduction: Where the Healing Begins

1. Drugs offer immediate and powerful relief, even if the "benefit" is short lived and laden with side effects (such as addiction). According to Roy Wise (1988), drugs like alcohol and heroin activate brain mechanisms responsible for positive reinforcement with "greater intensity than can ever be summoned by environmental stimuli like food, water, or the reinforcing beauty of nature, art, or music" (p. 127). William McKinney (1985) found that alcohol ameliorated the despair response in rhesus monkeys (however, in higher doses, it exacerbated this condition).

    Some people are more susceptible to substance abuse than others. Some of the physiological underpinnings have been identified. Jamie Talan (2002) reported that gene therapy curbed alcohol consumption in rodents. Chronic drinkers are known to have far fewer dopamine receptors in the nucleus accumbens where the dopamine serves as a pleasure switch.

2. Suicidal feelings are part and parcel of the intense emotional crisis of abandonment. Mental health professionals sometimes have difficulty distinguishing "danger to self and others" from merely having destructive feelings. The newspapers frequently report murder/suicides at the hands of jilted lovers. There has been an attempt to curtail publication of these events so as not to sensationalize them and create copycat incidences. Educators and mental health professionals should note that Jim Mercy, a researcher at the Centers for Disease Control and Prevention, found (contrary to expectations) that friends and acquaintances of those who committed suicide were less likely to take their own lives (reported by Paul Simao, 2001). This has implications for primary prevention programs.

3. Loss of a primary attachment creates high-risk conditions in which expressions of rage and violence are commonplace. As an example, Virginia Colin (1996) cited a study of sixty white middle-class subjects going through divorce. She noted a high incidence of aggressive impulsivity: "Subjects attacked former spouses through burglaries, poisoning pets, kidnapping and brandishing weapons" (p. 340).

4. Carole Ann Price, A.C.S.W., friend and colleague, compassionately offered this term to me as I tried to go about my normal routine during my own abandonment.

5. Paraphrased from an enlightened statement by my friend Zachary Studenroth in 1994.

6. I am indebted to Nancy Hume, yoga teacher and mind-body healer, for the opportunity she gave me to direct movement choirs in performing the twelve gestures.

7. As reported by Ellen Barohn (2002), according to a study by James Pennebaker, writing helps people assimilate trauma. Follow-up research conducted by Alan Kael and Arthur Stone at Stony Brook's School of Medicine found that writing (as a method for coping) reduced rheumatoid arthritis and asthma. Barohn said, "Researchers don't know why it reduces disease severity, but it does."

8. I've observed that most heroin addicts (as well as alcoholics) have childhood histories of traumatic abandonment. Research has shown that separation distress is particularly sensitive to opiates such as heroin and morphine, and high doses of ethanol (alcohol). David Benton and Paul Brain (1988, p. 221) noted that opioids (the body's endogenous opiates) have specific influence on the distress that occurs when the young of a species experiences separation from its attachment.

9. Myron Hofer (1995b, p. 23) addressed the impact of separation on endogenous opiates. A rat pup will put out a distress cry until the mother rat comes and licks it. But if the pup is injected with naloxone, a drug that blocks its opioid receptors, the mother's licking is no longer able to shut down the pup's distress cries, demonstrating that it isn't the licking that calms the pup's distress; it is the opioid produced by the licking that does the job.

   Many heroin addicts are unwittingly self-medicating separation distress (resulting from early childhood losses as well as adult disconnections). Jamie Talan (2002d) reported on buprenorphine, a new drug to treat heroin addiction. She also reported (2002d) that researchers are exploring gene therapies (to increase D-receptors in the nucleus accumbens—found to be depleted in many addicts) to combat addiction.

   Researchers Jaak Panksepp, Eric Nelson, and Marni Bekkedal stated that the main characteristics of narcotic addiction—i.e., dependence, tolerance, and withdrawal—are strikingly similar to the dependence, needing more, and withdrawal of attachment and separation. According to the authors, "No behavior is as powerfully and consistently mediated by opiates as separation distress" (p. 6).

10. Paraphrased from personal dialogues with psychiatrist and author Richard Robertiello.

11. Peter Yelton, A.C.S.W., a friend and colleague, contributed the vivid descriptions of the wounding process.

12. Narcissism as a personality trait and a component of borderline personality disorder has been extensively described. For example, read H. Kohut (1977), Otto Kernberg (1975), and Helen Block Lewis (1971).

13. Explosive rage as a symptom of posttrauma is identified in Bessel Van der Kolk, Alexander McFarlane, Lars Weisaeth (1966, p. 217).

14. The term *involuntary separation* comes from Virginia Colin (1996).

15. The numbing effect associated with grief and mediated by opioids was explored by David Benton and Paul Brain (1988). Judith Herman (1992) discussed trauma's ability to create states of disconnectedness and dissociation. Comprehensive information on dissociative states was also discussed by Bessel Van der Kolk and colleagues (1996, pp. 51–73, 303–33). See also D. Kelly (1986).

Chapter 1: Centering

1. Daniel Goleman (1995) provided a lucid description of the body's alarm system and the cascade of psychological symptoms that are triggered, as did Robert Sapolsky (1994). Also see Jerome Kagan (1994).

2. Mild to severe reality distortions are not uncommon during the early stages of abandonment. Candice Pert (1997) explained the brain circuitry of "mistaken identity" (p. 143).

3. Phraseology and sentiment contributed by Donna Carson, L.C.S.W.

4. Daniel Goleman (1995) described our primal feelings that hearken back to childhood as "wordless blueprints… potent emotional memories dating from the first five years of life." Joseph LeDoux (1996) explained that since memories were laid down before the neocortex and hippocampus (involved in forming explicit memory) were fully developed, "there would be no matching set of articulated thoughts for the vague sensation of reawakened anxieties from childhood."

5. For insight into the gotta-have-it response to drugs and other substances, read Ronald Ruden and Marcia Byalick (1997). The authors noted that the impulses leading to addiction have a high dopamine production in the nucleus accumbens and are associated with low serotonin levels (pp. 5–6). Also read Roy Wise (1988) and William McKinney (1985).

6. The "power of possibility" was contributed by Donna Carson.

7. Donna Carson provided this quote from the inspirational speaker Les Brown.

8. Joseph LeDoux (2002) discussed a shift away from the concept of *limbic system*, a term used by Paul McLean (1990).

9. Read William Smotherman and Scott Robinson (1996). An Associated Press article (*Newsday*, August 15, 2002) reported a study in *Journal of Epidemiology and Community Health* led by David Barker that suggested adult health is set to a significant degree by conditions in the womb. A study led by June Machover Reinisch (2002) demonstrated similar findings—that early environment has lasting impact on cognitive functioning. Reinisch noted that infants who had been breast-fed for up to nine months scored an average of six points higher on I.Q. tests than infants who were nursed for less than one month. Jaak Panksepp, Stephen Siviy, and Lawrence Normansell (1985) reported a doubling of plasma levels of endorphins in lactating women when their infants were suckling. It is believed that casomorphin, an endorphin in breast milk, strengthens the mother-infant bond. For more information, see P. Wolff (1968).

    As a final point of interest, neurobiologist Evan Balaban's research showed that a preference for one's mother's voice is hard-wired into the brain cells and can be transferred surgically from one species into another (reported by Robert Cooke). Also read A. Decasper and W. Fif (1980).

10. Joseph LeDoux (2015) cautions us that the amygdala does not behold emotions per se, but reacts to threat, which other mental capacities interpret as fear.

11. To understand how conditioning works, consult I. V. Pavlov's *Conditioned Reflexes* (1922). Joseph LeDoux (1996) investigated the emotional brain's role in conditioning.

12. Robert Sapolsky (1994) discussed the physiological impact of sustained stress.

13. The amygdala develops before birth, explaining why some of our emotional memories (fear conditioning) were set in prenatally. The hippocampus, responsible for explicit memory, isn't fully developed until several years later, explaining why we cannot recall the contexts in which many of our early emotional memories were created.

14. As a point of interest: Myron Hofer (1995b, p. 211) found that older children, as well as older rats, who had experienced earlier separations responded to signals of impending separation without requiring the actual loss of an object to elicit the response. In other words, they developed anticipatory anxiety to loss, analogous to "insecurity" in humans. Daniel Goleman (1995) called this "lowering the neural setpoint" (p. 203), explaining that if a child had early trauma, the amygdala is primed to find danger later on. The threshold to activating the fight-or-flight response is lowered.

15. Most of these symptoms are part of the fight-or-flight response of the sympathetic branch of our autonomic nervous system. When compiling the mind-body checklist, I drew from many works, including those of Sapolsky, Kagan, Goleman, LeDoux, and Seiver.

16. Robert Sapolsky explained the role of glucocorticoid stress hormones. See also Stephen Suomi (1991a, 1991b).

17. Many abandonment survivors report having memory gaps of significant childhood experiences. Researchers have shown memories to be labile—subject to revision and even deletion, not only at the time the experience is occurring but also at the time of retrieval. Adrenocorticotropic hormone (ACTH)—a stress hormone—is known to interfere in hippocampal memory, explaining why some memories are impossible to retrieve, because they were never recorded in the hippocampus in the first place since stress hormones interfered in the process. It is known that stress causes dendrites (branches on neurons that transport information) to grow in the amygdala and shrink in the hippocampus, explaining why we can have an ongoing emotional response to a triggering event for which we have no explicit memory. See also Eric Kandel (1992) and Kandel, James Schwartz, and Thomas Jessell (1992). Jamie Talan (2002c) reported in studies that show that experiences recalled from childhood are stored in synapses, which change in number and strength depending on the specific memory. Neurons manufacture proteins for memory. Chemicals such as protein kinase M (PKM) are released to strengthen the synaptic connections (thereby facilitating memory). If PKM isn't in good supply within a significant time period after an event, the memory can be weakened or even erased. Alcino Silva pointed to the protein alpha-calmodulin kinase II (alpha-CaMKII) as a factor in "how we establish memories that the brain retains, the ones that become our oldest memories" (reported by Will Boggs, 2001).

    Research on memory is making headway in treatment of memory disorders, as revealed in a lecture by Tim Tully (2001; gratitude to Edith Drucker for providing lucid notes). Psychiatrist, researcher, and author Barry Riesberg (1984) developed the concept *retrogenesis*, which has profound implications for treating Alzheimer's disease.

18. According to Andrew Solomon (2001), "It is clear that stress drives up rates of depression. The biggest stress is humiliation; the second is loss" (p. 63)—covering both conditions of abandonment, for sure.

    Jerome Kagan (1984) discussed the shame associated with prolonged suffering. He noted that attributing suffering to weakness has a long history and quoted Pierre Janet as saying, "Sadness is always a sign of weakness and sometimes of the habit of living weakly." Michael Lewis (1992) explored the psychological impact of shame. See also Helen Block Lewis (1971).

19. John Bowlby throughout his many works, emphasized that the work of grief is to accept the pain of loss. William McKinney (1985) described protest as one of the most commonly observed responses to loss (the other being despair). Protest is an active response characterized by crying and motoric demonstrations of grief; despair is a quiet and withdrawn response to grief. Also see Kenneth Doka (1996; thanks to Helen Dubinsky for this reference).

20. Subject to intensive investigation. Here are a few sources of discussion: Joseph LeDoux (2002) provided neurophysiological and philosophical insight on this subject. Antonio Damasio (1994) discussed the interdependency of emotion and reason. Edward Wilson (1998) addressed the question of mind versus brain, referring to the processing of numerous parallel coding networks and internal mapping of multiple sensory impressions as constituting awareness, rather than a separate entity observing the "who" or "what" of the mind.

21. The health benefits of human connection have been widely researched. When you're in disconnect mode, your body has a background tone of fight or flight. The energy usually deployed to your immune response is diverted to aid your exercise muscles, to decrease your reaction time and to allow you to fight or sprint away from an enemy. The impact of separation stress (versus social bonding) on the immune response is well documented: See Steven Maier, Linda Watkins, and Monika Fleshner (1994); S. J. Schleifer and colleagues (1983); J. Kiecolt-Glaser and colleagues (1987); Christopher Coe and colleagues (1985); J. Eysenck (1987); H. Weiner, M. Hofer, and A. Stunkard (1981); and Esther Sternberg (2001).

22. The advantages to solving problems at the level of the solution (rather than the level of the problem) were emphasized by Paul Watzlaich, John Weakland, and Richard Risch (1974).

23. Visualizing the solution first and then backtracking to determine what obstacles had to be removed is a technique I learned from Richard Belson, family therapist.

24. This quote was contributed by friend and artist Pat Dennis.

Chapter 2: Cleansing

1. *Love map* is a term I borrowed from Tian Dayton (1997).

2. Some drug rehabilitation programs use "shattered defenses" to therapeutic advantage. They promote a therapeutic regression, using provocative techniques to break down the addict's defenses, increasing his reliance on therapeutic principles in hopes that he will internalize a healthier set of behaviors.

3. Tiffany Field (1985) showed how we become attuned to our partners (as seen in the synchrony of pupil dilation, respiration rate, vocal cadences, etc.). Read Virginia Colin (1996) for insight into the psychobiology of forming primary attachments.

4. The chemistries involved in attraction are extensive: Casomorphin, phenylethylamine (PEA), oxytocin, and dehydroepiandrosterone (DHEA), to name a few. Read Helen Fisher (1992).

5. Myron Hofer (1995b) explained that when two people become entwined in a relationship, they meld into a psychobiological unit—a mutual regulatory system involving neurochemicals, hormones, pheromones, and other bodily systems. See also C. M. Parkes, J. Stevenson-Hinde, and P. Marris (1991).

6. For differing views on the subject of arranged relationships and romantic attraction, see Joshua Harris (1997) and Jeremy Clark (2000).

7. For coming up with the alternative term for *abandoholism*—abandonment compulsion—I am indebted to my friend and colleague Peter Yelton.

8. Oxytocin, one of the neurohormones mentioned above, has been called the "interpersonal hormone." Shelly Taylor, Laura Klein, B. P. Lewis, T. L. Gruenewald, R. A. Gurung, and J. A. Updegraff (2000) offered insight about

oxytocin and gender differences involving the stress response. They reported that when oxytocin is released along with stress hormones in women, it helps buffer their fight-or-flight response and encourages them to connect with others. Oxytocin's ability to calm fight-or-flight responses does not occur in men, because testosterone, which men produce in high levels when stressed, is found to reduce the effects of oxytocin, whereas estrogen seems to enhance it. According to the authors of this University of California at Los Angeles study, when women are stressed they tend to befriend; when men are stressed they hole up alone or become aggressive. This article was contributed by Nama Frankel.

   According to researchers John Capitanio, Michael Weissberg, and Martin Reite (1985), oxytocin is involved in milk ejection, uterine contraction, and sperm transport. Antonio Damasio (1994) suggested that oxytocin is released during stimulation of genitals and nipples and orgasm. Oxytocin is believed to disrupt memory of painful childbirth (so that women will continue having children).

9. Robert Sapolsky (1994) offered a possible explanation about why we get caught up in self-defeating patterns. He suggested that organisms will habituate to a stressor if it is applied over and over because it is predictable by them, and it triggers a smaller stress response (p. 214). Joseph LeDoux (2002) noted that once you learn a pattern of avoidance, the amygdala drops out of the circuit because it does not need to involve fear to be aroused (p. 251).

10. Jaak Panksepp, Eric Nelson, and Marni Bekkedal (1997) noted that when we build a close relationship, our brain produces opioids. When we break up, the production of certain opioids decreases, and we go into physical withdrawal similar to heroin withdrawal. In other words, our closest relationships actually are opioid addictions—we become addicted and go into withdrawal from our own internal narcotic drugs.

11. *Abandophobism* (avoiding relationships out of fear of abandonment) is a term invented by Armond Demille during our radio interview in 2000.

12. I learned this paradoxical fact of life from Norman Moore, A.C.S.W., in private consultation.

13. This term is found in the work of Mary Ainsworth (1979). It's important to note that criteria for a "secure attachment" have been examined for possible cultural biases. See Fred Rothbaum and colleagues (2000). For an excellent overview, read Margaret Talbot (1998).

14. Psychologist Melissa Downey enlightened me with the insight into the unstable and labile aspects of young relationships, which contribute to the emotionally provocative social environments of school playgrounds.

15. Incubation of fear is an important finding in Joseph LeDoux's (1996) research on the amygdala.

16. Eric Fromm (1989) suggested that separation anxiety is the root of all emotional distress, disturbance, and dysfunction.

17. Friend and psychotherapist Carole Ann Price, A.C.S.W., contributed this statement.

18. Virginia Colin (1996) provided insight into the primal emotions involved in love, citing similarities between romantic love and infant-to-caregiver attachment. In romance, your mood depends on your perception of whether your beloved is responsive or rejecting, just as the baby's feeling of joy and distress depends on his perceptions of his primary caretaker's availability or responsiveness (p. 297).

19. Lee Alan Dugatkin (2001) provided valuable insight into the acquisition of some of our romantic values and our tendency toward "monkey see, monkey do." He cited an example in which guppy females chose partners based on which other females found the males desirable.

20. Julia Vormbrock (1993) proposed two psychobiological systems involved in human bonds: caregiving and attachment. If a person has difficulty depending on others, she might have an *avoidant attachment* style but be quite comfortable when others are dependent on her (pp. 122–44). A lot of abandonment survivors are most comfortable in a caregiving role and tend to initiate intimacy only when a prospective partner needs their support and is in a nonthreatening position.

Chapter 3: Attending to the Moment

1. I have observed the symptoms of abandonment to match nearly all of the characteristics of posttrauma delineated by Bessel Van der Kolk, Alexander McFarlane, and Lars Weisaeth (1996), pp. 203–59, and Judith Lewis Herman

(1992). For a list of symptoms of posttraumatic stress disorder of abandonment, read my *Journey from Abandonment to Healing* (2000, pp. 41–43).

2. Early emotional memory storage—the domain of the amygdala—is the subject of Joseph LeDoux (1996).

3. Abandonment is a severe enough emotional trauma to create a temporary regression to borderline functioning. Split thinking is highly prevalent in the initial stages of abandonment. The trauma of rejection causes victims to see themselves as all bad—weak and undesirable—and their abandoner as all good—omnipotent and supremely desirable. In clinically deconstructing the self-hatred and panic, I find that always-and-never thinking provides the cognitive fuel. H. Kohut (1977), Otto Kernberg (1975), James Masterson (1978), and others have provided in-depth discussions of borderline regression.

4. Myron Hofer (1995b) pointed out that neural networks are developed in early infancy, causing "separation to be the first innate anxiety state in many animals" (p. 27). Hofer has found that rats, for example, react to their very first experience of separation. This fear reaction is adaptive to ward off the threat of becoming separated from the mother.

5. Jerome Kagan (1994, pp. 51–52) theorized that certain children may have inherited a tendency to produce higher concentrations of norepinephrine (NE) (or may have a higher density of NE receptors in the locus ceruleus), causing them to be "inhibited," suggesting a neurochemical basis for heightened vulnerability and other anxiety-based personality traits.

Michelle Cottle (1999) explored the issue of psychological faddism in identifying "social phobia" as a condition. She offered valuable perspective by suggesting that Americans tend to assume that the norm is to be outgoing—an alien notion to many Chinese and Japanese people. American society tends to glorify celebrities and admires flamboyant personalities and tends to impugn those who fail to stand out in the crowd.

6. Children blame themselves, rather than their parents, in order to preserve their sense of security, adding and not detracting to the sense of their parents' omnipotence. Judith Harris (1998) concurred, pointing out that children remain attached to their abusers (p. 151).

7. Not only do children lack cognitive apparatuses with which to distinguish events that are truly beyond their control but their developing brains are adversely physiologically affected by stressors such as abuse, witnessing violence, and neglect. Allan Schore (1994) presented theories about how the human brain develops corticolimbic circuits as a result of child-to-caretaker experiences.

Psychiatrist Susan Vaughan (1997) noted, "The absence or presence of important others during early childhood may affect the deep brain nuclei directly…which can lead to the development of depressive symptoms later on" (pp. 141–42). Also see Myron Hofer (1995a, pp. 17-38) for discussion about how separations in early childhood lead to conditions in adulthood.

8. The long-term impact of childhood neglect and abandonment has been widely researched. Mary Carlson's study of orphanages revealed that children who were deprived of maternal nurturing exhibit abnormal levels of cortisol, show long-term memory problems, and are slowest in both motor and mental development (reported by Anna Nidecker, 1998). See also note 7.

9. Joseph LeDoux (1996) made a contribution to the above discussion by explaining that fear has a tendency to incubate over time rather than what we expect it to do—to dissipate.

10. The stress created by helplessness has been extensively researched—see, for example, Martin Seligman (1975) and Robert Sapolsky (1994)—and found to lead to posttraumatic behaviors caused by physiological changes (see Sapolsky, 1994, p. 219). To demonstrate the effect of helplessness, Sapolsky cited this experiment: Put two people in adjoining rooms and give a lever to only one. Expose both rooms to loud, noxious noises. Results: The person with the lever has a lower poststress response (even when the lever is not connected to the noise mechanism) than the person without one. In repeated trials of this study, it was found that subjects who have the lever but don't bother to use it do just as well as those who do use it. This shows that even if you don't exercise your control option, just believing you have control is sufficient to reduce stress,

Sapolsky also cited an example from World War II when London was bombed every night on schedule. In the suburbs, the bombing was far less frequent and at random. A study of the postwar impact of these raids found that people in the suburbs who had "fewer stressors but much less predictability" had more poststress symptoms (that is, they developed more ulcers) than did their more heavily bombed London counterparts. Your ability to predict events lessens your sense of helplessness and reduces the traumatic impact.

11.   Joseph LeDoux (1996) explored the neurophysiological basis for the arousal of emotional memories.

12.   The point that witnessing violence constitutes a real trauma was underscored at a Voices Set Free conference at Portland State University in Oregon, directed by Margi McCue and Louise Bouschard. Voices Set Free provided information and services to victims of family violence. Witnesses, a targeted at-risk group, were offered programs such as trauma-reduction therapy. See Louise Bouschard and Mary Kimbrough (1986).

13.   I have received hundreds of personal stories from abandonment survivors who describe childhoods disrupted by family violence and who ask me how this caused them to develop unstable and emotionally abandoning adult relationships. How does the posttrauma set in? According to researcher Bruce McEwen, stress makes dendrites grow in the amygdala (center of the emotional brain) and shrink in the hippocampus (part of the brain involved in memory) (reported by Jamie Talan, 2002a). Prolonged stress—as experienced by children within dysfunctional families—affects brain structure and function. In the same article, Talan reports that Rachel Yehuda, an expert on posttrauma, suggested that there are biochemical markers for long-term abnormal stress reaction (or posttraumatic stress disorder).

14.   See Myron Hofer (1995a, 1995b).

15.   Parent-child relationships help mold the structure of a developing brain. During separation, the bodies of rats and humans alike produce cortisol, a stress hormone known to lower levels of growth hormone, leading to speculation that stress can cause slower growth of important brain connections in a child's developing brain. For example, the vagus nerve, responsible for priming the body for fight or flight, is believed to be affected, setting the brain to a higher level of reactivity and leading to anxiety disorders in adolescence and adulthood. For more information, read Allan Schore (1994) and John Madden (1991). Hara Estroff Marano (1999) provided an excellent overview of how childhood stressors affect brain development. Robert Sapolsky (1994) explained how stress affects learning, including social and academic learning.

16.   When examining the neurobiological level of human experience, many researchers caution against mechanistic thinking and oversimplifying, including Joseph LeDoux (1996 and 2015), Antonio Damasio (1994), Virginia Colin (1996), and E. O. Wilson (1998).

17.   See David Benton and Paul Brain (1998); Jaak Panksepp, Eric Nelson, and Marni Bekkedal (1997); and Roy Wise (1988).

18.   The ability for mother-infant separation to produce depressive disorders in adulthood has been widely studied. Darlene Francis and Michael Meaney (1999) provided insight into environmental stressors and maternal care, showing that early deprivations in licking or handling in rat pups produce illnesses, such as depression in response to fear. For rhesus monkeys, repeated periods of maternal separation increase serotonin and norepinephrine responses to stress later on. "Considering the importance of the ascending noradrenergic and serotonergic systems in depression, these findings suggest a mechanism whereby early life events might predispose an individual to depression in later life" (p. 5).

   There's important research and meta-analysis in regard to the effectiveness of antidepressants, especially selective serotonin reuptake inhibitors (SSRI) such as Prozac, suggesting that placebo is nearly as effective. These studies raise the following question: If placebo can mimic effects of SSRIs, then how can we maximize its potential benefits for health? See John Salamone (2002), Irving Kirsch and Thomas J. Moore (2002), Shankar Vedamtam (2002), and D. Klein (1998).

19.   Ronald Ruden and Marcia Byalick (1997) explored the psychobiological dynamics of the "gotta have it" response.

20.   According to Sol Gordon (1983), the earmark of low self-esteem is the need for immediate gratification.

21.   Bessel Van der Kolk, Alexander McFarlane, and Lars Weisaeth (1996) stated that owing to the deregulation of stress hormones and other factors, trauma victims have difficulty going through a linear process of rational planning and instead tend to go directly from impulse to action (p. 203).

22.   Bessel Van der Kolk, Alexander McFarlane, and Lars Weisaeth (1996, p. 227) explained that even decades after a traumatic event, victims will continue to have an opioid-mediated response to a stimulus. In other words, a

detached emotional state can persist as a result of the neurobiology of trauma. See also D. D. Kelly (1986) for an explanation about stress/trauma leading to numbing to surroundings.

23. An interesting note: According to Jean West (2001), the popular amphetamine Ritalin (used to treat attention deficit disorder with hyperactivity) has a greater potency in the brain than cocaine. It takes Ritalin (pill form) an hour or so to raise dopamine levels in the brain; however, cocaine does so in seconds if smoked or injected—but with less potency.

24. According to grief pioneers John Bowlby (1983) and Elisabeth Kübler-Ross (1969), the primary task of grief work is acceptance—accepting the reality of loss, accepting its pain.

25. Larry Seiver and William Frucht (1997) explained that fear promotes the release of norepinephrine, which functions to turn attention outward (in the service of attending to the whereabouts of predators or potential food sources, etc.). Conversely, when attention turns inward, norepinephrine declines. This explains the hypervigilance we experience toward our ex during abandonment, the attention we place on the details of the breakup, the tendency to be unable to concentrate on anything else, and the tendency to remain jumpy.

26. Joseph LeDoux (1996) explained that adrenaline increases impulse to action, promoting quick life-saving action. This comes in handy during a real life-or-death battle, but the response seems overblown when the battle is the internal kind, like heartbreak.

27. Jamie Talan (2001) reported on a new finding that should be of interest to clinicians treating abandonment trauma. Conventional wisdom suggests that we should feel our grief and talk about our feelings and problems, but George Bonanno's (2002) research at Columbia University showed that people who do not display overt grief over the death of a spouse are not necessarily suppressing grief but demonstrating resiliency. The researchers reviewed methods for debriefing victims of traumas (such as might be used to help victims of the terrorist attacks of 2001) and discovered that asking people to talk about details of the event exposes them to traumatic imagery and can actually impede recovery.

28. A lot of abandonment's pain and anguish is made worse by trying to rail against reality (rather than accepting it). People say they feel relieved when they are finally able to face up to the situation squarely. It allows them to stop the futile outlay of emotional energy in trying to defend against the loss. Only then can they discover their ability to stand on their own two feet, withstand the torrent of emotion, and move forward.

29. "Now is all there ever is"—a broad perspective of the true nature of reality offered by psychologist Roseanne McAward at Bellmore Union Free School District in 1999.

Chapter 4: Separating

1. Psychiatrist and author Irving Yalom (1992) presented the concept of *amor fati*, which is Latin for "love your fate," suggesting the benefits of accepting your reality rather than resisting it, allowing you to move forward and make the best of life.

2. Roy Baumeister and Mark Leary (1995) addressed the need for linkage with others, saying grief creates depression because it is not just a reaction to loss but a reaction to the "loss of a linkage with another person."

3. Read R. Weiss (1973) and Erika Chopich and Margaret Paul (1990).

4. From Virginia Colin (1996).

5. What makes witnessing family violence so stressful is the helplessness it creates. The violence isn't happening to the witness, You can't fight back or cope with the pain for the other person. You have no lever of control.

6. Robert Sapolsky (1994) reviewed research about the stress created when we have no control. See also chapter 3, note 10.

7. Your need for control began during your terrible twos. If your parents allowed you to make some choices for yourself and honored your decisions, you most likely grew up feeling a sense of control over your life. On the other hand, if you were constantly bombarded with unpredictable events, you might have felt that life was happening *to* you or *at* you rather than feeling like an active participant in your life.

8. Here's some advice for parents going through separation or divorce to help their children cope. I learned this

technique from psychotherapist Amy Wapner, who showed me how it helps mitigate separation trauma. It involves creating a family calendar that includes visitation schedules and upcoming family events. Mount it up on the refrigerator or kitchen wall where even the youngest child can reach it. Make sure you've already discussed all of these events and changes with your children before posting them. For very young children, use pictures along with words to allow them to keep track of what's going on in their lives. This calendar is a simple device that helps children emotionally prepare for the comings and goings of their parents, as well as postponements in the visitation schedule. It allows them to look forward to future occasions. Providing children with a predictable environment helps them feel secure and in control, even in the most difficult of times.

9. For comprehensive exploration into bereavement, consult the works of John Bowlby (1983) and Elisabeth Kübler-Ross (1969). To understand the connection between grief and clinical depression, read Sigmund Freud's famous treatise *Mourning and Melancholia* (1917).

10. This phrase came from Pauline Boss (1999).

11. Separation creates prolonged anxiety, traumatic stress, and depression. Read R. Weiss (1973, 1975), Julia Vormbrock (1993), Myron Hofer (1995b), and Virginia Colin (1996).

12. For insight into secure versus insecure attachments, see Mary Ainsworth (1979, 1991).

13. Clinical discussion about the ways in which parents pass their wounds along to their children is found in Alice Miller (1997).

14. The exception to giving your kids better than you had it is when a serious disruption to family functioning is involved, such as alcoholism or grave financial stress.

15. See Jerome Kagan (1984).

16. From Donald Winnecott (1965). Also read Margaret Mahler (1968).

17. Patrick Seely, a friend and health professional.

18. Sophia, friend and colleague.

19. Comments of Peter Yelton, friend and colleague, during an informal consultation.

20. Abandonment creates a tendency toward repetition compulsion—one of the symptoms of posttraumatic stress disorder. I proposed a list of symptoms for abandonment's posttrauma in *The Journey from Abandonment to Healing* (pp. 42–44).

21. Read Harold Kushner (1997).

22. To accept the transience of life, see the following two books: Sogyal Rinpoche (1994) and Pema Chödrön (1997).

23. According to Steven Maier, Linda Watkins, and Monika Fleshner (1994), stress is immunosuppressive. Herbert Weiner (1992) stated that the sympathetic branch of the nervous system (responsible for fight or flight) controls the immune system, encompassing bone marrow, thymus, spleen, gut, and lymph nodes. Myron Hofer (1995b) suggested that social companions offer comfort by stimulating opioid release. See also J. Kiecolt and colleagues (1987); S. Schleifer and colleagues (1983); Christopher Coe (1994); Sandra Weiner, Leon Rosenbert, and Seymour Levine (1985); Hans Selye (1994); and an informative overview by Esther Sternberg (2001).

Chapter 5: Beholding the Importance of Your Existence

1. Sandra Blakeslee (2000) reviewed research that explains how our memories can become embellished, distorted, changed. When an old memory is pulled into consciousness, the brain reconfigures and updates it. Memories are transformed to reflect each person's life experiences, not the memory itself. She quoted Harvard psychology professor and memory expert Daniel Schacter as saying, "It's a mistake to think that once you record a memory, it is forever fixed." Researchers at New York University reported that laboratory rats' memories remain open to manipulation for about six hours. The brain then synthesizes proteins (during a time-limited window) that set memories in place (Karim Nader, Glenn Schafe, and Joseph LeDoux, 2000). The authors reported that by using anisomycin, a protein-synthesis inhibitor, they were able to determine that once your consolidated fear memories are reactivated, they return to a labile state (reported by Jamie Talan, 2002a).

2. See Robert Gossette and Richard O'Brien (1990, 1992).

3. Joseph Ledoux (1996) explored the feedback loop between amygdalal and cortical processes.

4. Elisabeth Kübler-Ross (1969).

5. Ellen Barohn (2002) reported on research that shows that writing helps people assimilate trauma and can also reduce disease severity.

6. Bonding is something we have in common with other members of the animal kingdom, making it possible to investigate the biobehavioral impact of separation and attachment through animal studies. See Myron Hofer (1995a).

7. Relationships are mediated through many neurochemicals, including one that is addictive: endogenous opiate. See Jaak Panksepp, Stephen Siviy, and Lawrence Normansell (1985); David Benton and Paul Brain (1988); Roy Wise (1988); and Ronald Ruden and Marcia Byalick (1997).

8. Bessel Van der Kolk, Alexander McFarlane, and Lars Weisaeth (1996, p. 227) stated that people who experience posttraumatic stress disorder can have an endogenous opioid analgesia in response to a stimulus as long as two decades after the initial trauma.

9. John Bowlby (1958).

10. Joseph LeDoux (1996). Fear's tendency to incubate explains why old traumas can create overwhelming emotional memories many years later—a concomitant to abandonment posttrauma stress.

11. People going through abandonment report masturbatory increase and heightened sexual cravings. This may be due to opioid withdrawal. An interesting piece of this puzzle comes from G. Serra, M. Collu, and G. Gessa (1988): adrenocorticotropic hormone (ACTH) released during an emotional crisis has been found to block endogenous opioids. Opiates like heroin, morphine, and methadone are known to decrease libido, retard ejaculation, and contribute to impotence in males. I conclude that stress hormones (ACTH and others) produced during abandonment, by reducing the endogenous narcotic effect, thereby arouse the potential for heightened sexual response.

12. Candace Pert (1997) said that we have "our own personal pharmacopoeia within our bodies" (p. 271), and it manufactures the drugs needed for health, well-being, sexuality, and love. Science has identified many of the chemicals involved in attachment, separation, and sexuality. Jaak Panksepp, Eric Nelson, and Marni Bekkedal (1997) said that future medication targeting oxytocin receptors (associated with social bonding) will someday help alleviate loneliness (p. 85), just as opiates are effective, but without the addictive side effects. Also see Jaak Panksepp (1996); Myron Hofer (1995b); David Benton and Paul Brain (1988); John Capitanio, Michael Weissberg, and Martin Reite (1986); Theresa Crenshaw (1996); Helen Fisher (1992); William McKinney (1985); and Herbert Weiner (1992).

13. From Candace Pert (1997, p. 143).

14. John Bowlby (1983).

15. Psychologist Lauren Slater (2002) stated that self-esteem programs in schools are based on the notion that self-esteem is at the heart of bad behaviors (including terrorism). Slater said that researchers Nicholas Emler and Roy Baumeister argued that people "with low self-esteem...may in fact do better" in life (p. 45–48). Their research showed that people with "high self-regard" are known to maim and even kill. In their tests, the researchers noted that people with favorable views of themselves were more likely to administer loud blasts of ear-piercing noise to a subject than those who scored lower on self-esteem scales. In another experiment, they found that men with high self-esteem were more willing to put down victims to whom they had administered electric shocks than were those who'd scored lower on self-esteem scales. They put antisocial men through all known self-esteem tests and concluded, "These men are racist and violent because they don't feel bad enough about themselves." Owing to these considerations and the popular misconstruing of the value of self-esteem, I emphasize substantial principles on which to build a sense of self—avoiding the tendency to base your self-esteem on favorably comparing your physical, social, or intellectual attributes to others.

16. The Four Cornerstones of Self, of which "recognizing the importance of your existence" is one, represent a non-narcissistic approach to building your sense of self. For more information, see Anderson (2000, pp. 149–51).

17. Herbert Weiner (1992, p. 76) suggested the need to "reinvest your emotional currency elsewhere."

18. Performing the Big You / Little You exercise helps make unconscious emotional material conscious. This method of separation therapy brings psychoanalytic psychotherapy to a self-help level, allowing *you*, not your analyst, to administer to your primal needs and feelings. To create a closer relationship with yourself and develop a solid inner core, please read Grace Kirsten and Richard Robertiello (1977).

Chapter 6: Accepting the Unchangeable

1. Peter Yelton made the following statement extemporaneously during an informal dialogue: "Abandonment is a severe enough crisis to implant an invisible drain deep within the self. The paradox for abandonment survivors is that no matter how many 'esteemable' things they try to do to build their self-esteem, the invisible wound of abandonment is always working to leech it away."

2. Thanks to the efforts of my research mentor, Robert Gossette, I was able to read an article by Robert Sapolsky that helped me realize that to understand the special nature of abandonment grief, I'd have to investigate the stress hormones and the research on helplessness and lack of control.

3. Insight offered to me by Amy Wapner and Peter Moriarty during a trip to Vermont.

4. Read Roy Baumeister and Mark Leary (1995).

5. Referring again to Lauren Slater (2002), we learn that Freud's concept of "superego" represents the part of the personality that strives to be realistic (rather than narcissistic) and takes a global view in an effort at honesty. Self-appraisal (a role of the superego) makes an effort to "oversee, edit, praise, and prune" (pp. 45–48) the personality in the direction of making disciplined actions.

6. This term was offered by Suzanne Phillips, Ph.D., during psychoanalytic group therapy.

7. An issue affecting women (particularly when going through heartbreak) is the one that equates her romantic value with her physical appearance. If she's fifty pounds overweight, she's likely to assume that her chances of finding a new partner are nil, which adds to feeling hopeless and doomed. Ideally, women would benefit by challenging this emphasis on looks than competing to be thinner and more beautiful. Read Susannah Meadows (2002), Harriet Rubin (1997), and Susan Faludi (1991). The point here is not that men don't have difficult issues to overcome when surviving abandonment, just different emphases. In fact, men struggle with the "boys don't cry" edict of early tribal socialization. Read Terrance Real (1997) for sensitivity to this issue.

8. Read Joseph LeDoux (2002), which explores the neurobiology of sense of self.

9. Jamie Talan (2002b) reported that scientists have targeted the frontal lobe's right hemisphere as the locus of identity. An eighteen-month-old child begins to recognize himself in the mirror, setting in place a sense of self that will continue throughout life, unless there is disruption to the right frontal lobe. A condition called frontotemporal dementia involves a depletion of serotonin in the region. Patients developing this condition experience significant changes in identity. For example, they may appear more comfortable breaking rules than before, or they may go from gourmet or health food tastes to a sudden preference for fast food, from wearing designer apparel to sweat clothes, or from conservative political affiliations to liberal.

10. From Michael Balint (1992, p. 287).

11. See Dan Schacter (2001): one of his "seven sins of memory" is misattribution.

12. Read Michael Lewis (1992) and Helen Block Lewis (1971) regarding shame.

13. Andrew Solomon (2001, p. 65) echoes Freud (1917).

14. One of many life-sustaining slogans from Alcoholics Anonymous.

15. Psychiatrist and author Richard Robertiello said "Everybody needs a mountain to climb" during a private consultation.

Chapter 7: Increasing Your Capacity for Love

1. People who are love challenged rarely recognize their "disability" and may provide examples of what Antonio Damasio (1994, p. 63) called "anosognosia"—the inability to recognize illness, especially "when the denial of illness results from the loss of a particular cognitive function."

2. For a complete list of symptoms for posttraumatic stress disorder of abandonment, see my *Journey from Abandonment to Healing* (pp. 42–44).

3. Betsy O'Shae, friend and business advisor, contributed insight about life's relationships being a series of triangles.

4. Competition for a lover can create jealousy—an issue discussed by Joseph LeDoux (2002). He quotes Donald Hebb

as saying, "Jealousy is readily detected by impartial observers but denied by the jealous person, who may instead characterize his state as indignation or annoyance" (p. 202).

5. *Triangulated* has a different usage in the field of systemic family therapy. If a child is caught in the middle of his parent's marital problems, serves as a pawn in their power struggles, or is expected to keep them distracted from their problems, he is said to be triangulated.

6. Theresa Crenshaw (1996) explored love chemicals.

7. Helen Fisher (1992) discussed one of the key substances involved in attachment—phenylethylamine (PEA)—a natural amphetamine designed to rev up the brain. When our brain is saturated with PEA, we feel infatuated. Monoamine oxidase (MAO) inhibitors block a substance that is known to break down PEA (and other neurochemicals) and can diminish the lovesick craving for a mate.

8. Insecure mating relationships activate your autonomic nervous system, preparing you for the Four Fs of Survival. The problem is that infatuated feelings are transferable. Unless there is substantial caring (deeper love), it is easy to transfer these romantic feelings onto a new partner, leaving the original partner open to abandonment.

9. Helen Fisher (1992) referred to "love blindness," a condition typified by people who believe they've never felt romantic love. In some cases, love blindness is caused by hypopituitarism, a rare disease causing malfunction in the pituitary gland.

10. Read Jaak Panksepp, Stephen Siviy, and Lawrence Normansell (1985); Myron Hofer (1995b); and David Benton and Paul Brain (1988).

11. According to psychotherapist and mentor Norman Moore, A.C.S.W., depression depletes energy, cutting you off from the creative process of love.

12. Marilyn Barker, an artist friend of mine, commented on mistakes women tend to make that keep them isolated: "Taking men too seriously; not showing enough humor; wanting to have heavy conversations all the time; expecting men to resolve the heavy issues of their lives; allowing themselves to get too dependent; not keeping their female friendships active enough; not knowing how to flirt; not being in tune with their own sexuality; not staying in good shape. They don't have to be beautiful, they just have to take care of themselves." She commented on what men aren't embarrassed to do that women tend to be afraid to do: "They show nerve by opening up a conversation—simple as that."

13. To understand positive and negative reinforcements in conditioning, read Ivan Pavlov (1922). To understand the neurobiology of amygdalal conditioning, read Joseph LeDoux (1996).

14. Taking constructive actions to increase your sense of self and well-being involves neurological reward systems within the brain. Jamie Talan (6/11/2002) reported that researchers Barry Richmond and Munetaka Shidara said that reward is most likely centered in the anterior cingulate, a structure that helps keep us on task when we're working on a distant goal, even when we don't like what we are doing. Joseph LeDoux (2002, p. 250) discussed amygdalal mediation of positive incentive in the nucleus accumbens.

15. "Fake it till you make it" is a slogan of Alcoholics Anonymous. Paul Ekman's (1992) research showed that make-believe smiles create patterns of brain waves that differ from real smiles. I draw the conclusion that acting "as-if" can improve your mood but cannot completely eliminate your true response to life.

16. Chapter 5, note 13.

17. Read Michele Kodis, David Moral, and David Berliner (1998) and L. Motni-Bloch and B. Grosser (2001).

18. Myron Hofer (1995b, p. 222) said that the relationship between mother and infant regulates hidden psychological and physiological systems. They come to be stored in the memory as mental representations that later primary relationships are built on and become regulatory in terms of the functioning of the whole system.

19. Myron Hofer (1995b, p. 222) stated that loss creates discomfort because of withdrawal of physical and temporal interactions with the lost object and that the physical and cognitive changes of grief are similar to those seen in sensory deprivation. Each target area—muscles, lungs, heart, skin—is controlled by local physiological mechanisms. Pulling the relationship apart affects all systems. Nathan Fox (1985, p. 401) discussed patterns of attunement between parents and children, involving highly attuned smile responses and heart rate—applicable to adult primary relationships. Tiffany Field (1985, pp. 445–48) added pupil dilation, circadian rhythms, speech patterns, and pheromones to the list of attuned functions.

20. Herbert Weiner (1992, p. 75) pointed out that separation is more difficult for adults if it recapitulates childhood loss (particularly loss of mother before the age of seventeen), placing people at risk for developing major depressive disorders. David Benton and Paul Brain (1988) said that common neural mechanisms include regulation of endogenous opioids. During separation, they induce "crying, irritability, depression, insomnia, and anorexia" (p. 221).

Chapter 8: Letting Go

1. The Serenity Prayer is borrowed from Alcoholics Anonymous.
2. A slogan borrowed from Alcoholics Anonymous.
3. Another slogan borrowed from Alcoholics Anonymous.
4. Read Mavis Hetherington and John Kelly (2002), whose book summarizes three decades of research. Compare the more dire conclusions drawn by Judith S. Wallerstein (2001). For a comprehensive overview, read Malcolm Gladwell (1998).
5. From Pauline Boss (1999).
6. From Paul Watzlawick, John Weakland, and Richard Risch (1974).
7. I've been looking for evidence in neuroscience to explain the effectiveness of creative visualization in promoting healing and growth. Although I have yet to find any authoritative scientific research on the subject, I find myself drawn to Allan Hobson's work on dreaming. Hobson and Jonathan Leonard (2001) purported that psychotic states show a parallel brain-processing pattern to dream states. I've wondered if visualization may possibly represent an intermediate brain state. Researcher Candace Pert (1997, p. 146) made the point that visualization increases blood flow to the body part that is being focused on in a meditation exercise. This, in turn, increases the availability of blood, oxygen, and nutrients to carry away toxins and nourish the cells, but what about when you're visualizing a house?

Chapter 9: Reaching Out

1. Daniel Goleman (1995) provided a lucid overview of the psychobiology of anger. He drew from the work of Dolf Zillman (1992) and Diane Tice and Roy Baumeister (1992).
2. See Daniel Goleman (1995).
3. The tenth step of Alcoholics Anonymous enjoins us to continue to take personal inventory, and when we are wrong, promptly admit it. The ability to take a realistic look at yourself, even to the extent that you admit to your character defects, is an important step in changing deeply entrenched patterns.
4. I gained this insight from friend and mentor Linda Bergman, Ph.D.
5. Feeling critical toward a friend is one of our more vexing (to self and others) Outer Child behaviors. In reacting to heedless behaviors in others, we know full well that this person needs support, compassion, and patience. A way to channel our critical energies—rather than judge people who are enslaved by their impulses—is to understand that there are reasons ranging from biological to psychological for their difficulty exercising restraint. It might help to think of it as a problem going on in the wiring or conditioning of their emotional brains. Their amygdalae may be chronically aroused and prone to hijacking their ability to exercise better judgment (although you may not know, or need to know, the exact reason for this). People who succumb to immediate gratification are evincing low self-esteem. Due to the psychobiological urgencies they feel, they have difficulty giving substantial rewards to themselves. Instead of working toward goals, they grab for quick fixes. No matter how hopelessly out of control we act, all of us are capable of learning how to pick up the reins in our lives and regain self-control. Our higher selves can face the personal lesson in it for ourselves and provide encouragement and compassion to our friends so that we can grow in the direction of our human potential.
6. Outer Child is a vehicle that allows victims of heartbreak (whose abandonments have already created the tendency

to be self-critical and self-blaming) to take a look at their patterns and personal defects without excoriating themselves in the process. When we discover a personal glitch, we can reassure ourselves that we are in good company, as human nature has been widely recognized. Robert Sapolsky (2001) pointed out that, when baboons (our fellow primates) are able to displace their anger on lower-ranking males, they have lower glucocorticoid levels—suggesting the unfortunate conclusion that it's good for one's health to "kick the dog."

An additional piece of unsavory news comes from a study conducted by Robert Feldman at the University of Massachusetts. More than 60 percent of the 121 pairs of study subjects lied an average of two to three times. "Men and women lied about the same—but women lied to make the other person feel better, while men lied to make themselves look better" (see *Newsday* Health and Discovery section, June 25, 2002).

Another example: A controlled study showed that "people hate a winner so much they'll pay handsomely just to damage that person"—demonstrating the role of envy in the motivation of economics (reported by Jack Lucentini, 2002). Outer Child impulses are hardwired in humans and other animals, it would seem.

7. Joseph LeDoux (2002) provided insight into the "automatic" nature of our persistent patterns. He explained that once an emotional habit is learned, the brain simplifies the process, leaving the amygdala out of the loop (since once you learn the behavior, fear no longer needs to be the arousing factor). The accumbens also drops out of the response (since the behavior is already well learned). With a learned behavior (such as patterns of abandoholism), the learning is transferred to another region(s) in the brain, which LeDoux suspected is the cortex; research is ongoing.

8. Taking up physical activity may be a truly restorative way to invest your aggressive energy—and may help your brain cells to grow. Researcher Fred Gage said that immature cells have been identified in the brain and they can be induced to grow, mature, and function: "Exposure to an enriched environment increases neurogenesis" (nerve cell growth in the dentate gyrus), and certain types of physical activity (such as voluntary running in rats) can enhance the number of neurons the brain needs to function; reported by Robert Cooke (2002). Oprah Winfrey's *Make the Connection* is all about making the connection between health and full engagement in life activity (see Bob Greene and Oprah Winfrey, 1999).

9. "100-Item Outer Child Inventory" is excerpted from Susan Anderson (2000, pp. 192–200).

Chapter 10: Integrating and Owning

1. Dominant culture's attempt to separate the human species into separate races is a form of wholesale abandonment intended to exploit an "outside" group. Alan Templeton (2002), professor of biology and genetics at Washington University, stated that whereas one can make a biological case for the existence of subspecies within some other animal populations, when applying the criteria for subspecies to human populations, our species cannot be divided into subspecies or races.

2. Some researchers have suggested that wrapping your arms around yourself is a body signal for keeping people out. At times, the gesture may be defensive, as when we use this self-nurturing gesture to cushion ourselves when feeling unsafe within a social interaction.

3. Traumatic bonding is a widely researched issue. See Howard Hoffman (1994), whose writing created suspense as he made a case for opioid-mediated bonding—the way a mystery writer presents a "whodunit."

4. This came from Judith Harris (1998).

5. From Steve Smale (1980).

6. The startle reflex, caused by unexpected sights, sounds, or touches, is mediated in the brainstem. According to Malaysian societal belief, anyone can be made into a *latah* if startled persistently and afterward will obey commands. Read Ronald Simons (2001).

7. Yvonne Rivers referred me to William Lynch (1999).

8. In Alcoholics Anonymous, step one is admitting you are powerless over alcohol and that your life has become unmanageable.

9. The mother is usually the primary caretaker and, therefore, the one to shoulder the guilt of not being able to

live up to society's expectations of how a mother is "supposed" to parent on a day-to-day basis. She is always on duty, mishaps are constant, and she receives little validation for what she goes through. She conducts her role in isolation, with little to show for her efforts at the end of the day except that the children survived and the house is still standing. It's a relentless and emotionally demanding occupation, but the severity of its emotional toll tends to be minimized by society. Mothers, worn down by the daily grind, sometimes raise their voices (shout, yell, scream, cry, bark, curse, and throw temper tantrums along with their kids). They do so in the privacy of their homes, never imagining that other mothers are succumbing to the same "imperfect" parenting techniques in the privacy of their own homes. Mothers who fail to recognize the universality of these behaviors suffer their guilt in relative secrecy. For all of the joys and blessings of motherhood, it can wreak havoc on a woman's sense of self and can cause her to lose confidence in being able to be competent in an outside job.

10. Forgiveness may have pragmatic benefits. Studies have shown that unforgiving people have higher levels of stress hormones, which elevate their fight-or-flight responses. This is okay on a short-term basis but physiologically harmful on a long-term basis (from Everett Worthington, 2002). Also read Fred Luskin (2002).

Chapter 11: Transcending

1. For further discussion of this issue, see my *Journey from Abandonment to Healing* (pp. 212–36).
2. As if life weren't complicated enough, Andrew Solomon (2001) mentioned "post-joy stress." "Depression," he wrote, "can as easily be the consequence of too much that was joyful as of too much that was horrible" (p. 99).
3. Andrew Solomon (2001, p. 412).
4. Read Sharon Begley (2001) for insight into the variety of spiritual experiences and speculation about brain regions involved in these phenomena.

Chapter 12: Connecting

1. Amy Wapner, movement/dance therapist, psychotherapist, and friend, taught me about nonverbal cues, wordless defenses, and movement signatures, revealing to me a whole new level of clinical and personal observation and uncovering a wealth of emotional meaning in human behavior.

Appendix A

1. Losing a primary bond leads to an increase in glucocorticoid stress hormones, interfering in group dominance themes (see Robert Sapolsky, 1995).
2. Bassel Van der Kolk, Alexander McFarlane, and Lars Weisaeth (1996) addressed the impact of adrenaline.
3. Behavior among competing alpha baboons holds insight for human dynamics. See Robert Sapolsky's article.

Appendix C

1. From Michael Gershon (1998).
2. This expression was contributed by psychotherapist Carole Ann Price, A.C.S.W., during an informal discussion.

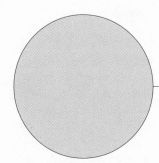

Bibliography

Ainsworth, Mary D. S. "Attachments and Other Affectional Bonds Across the Life Cycle." In *Attachments Across the Life Cycle*. New York, NY: Routledge, 1991.

———. "Infant-Mother Attachment." *American Psychologist* 43 (1979).

Anderson, Susan. *Black Swan: The Twelve Lessons of Abandonment Recovery*. New York, NY: Rock Foundations, 1999.

———. *The Journey from Abandonment to Healing*. New York, NY: Berkley, 2000.

———. "A Peer Model of Group Dynamics and Adult Education." In *Enhancing Creativity in Adult and Continuing Education*. Eds. Paul Edelson and Patricia L. Malone. San Francisco, CA: Jossey-Bass, 1999.

———. *Taming Your Outer Child*. Novato, CA: New World Library, 2015.

Balint, Michael. *The Basic Fault: Therapeutic Aspects of Regression*. Evanston, IL: Northwestern University Press, 1992.

Barohn, Ellen. "Journaling. When the Pen Really Can Be Mightier." *Newsday*, March 19, 2002, p. D5.

Baumeister, Roy F., and Mark R. Leary. "The Need to Belong. Desire for Interpersonal Attachments as a Fundamental Human Motivation." *Psychological Bulletin* (1995).

Beck, Aaron. *Anxiety Disorders and Phobias*. New York, NY: Basic Books, 1990.

Begely, Sharon, "Religion and the Brain." *Newsweek*, May 14, 2001.

Benton, David, and Paul F. Brain, "The Role of Opioid Mechanisms in Social Interaction and Attachment." In *Behavioral Processes*. Eds. R. J. Rodgers and S. J. Cooper. New York, NY: Wiley, 1988.

Blakeslee, Sandra. "Brain-Updating Machinery May Explain False Memory." *New York Times*, October 19, 2000.

———. "Placebo Proves So Powerful Even Experts Are Surprised." *New York Times*, October 13, 1998.

Boggs, Will. "Mystery of Permanent Memory Revealed." *Reuters*, May 16, 2001.

Bonanno, George. "Not All Grievers Need Therapy." *Newsday*, May 7, 2002, p. D2.

Boss, Pauline. *Ambiguous Loss: Learning to Live with Unresolved Grief*. Cambridge, MA: Harvard University Press, 1999.

Bouschard, Louise, and Mary Kimbrough. *Voices Set Free: Battered Women Speak from Prison*. St. Louis, MO: Women's Self-Help Center, 1986.

Bowen, Murry. *Family Therapy*. New York, NY: Aronson, 1978.

Bowlby, John. "Loss, Sadness and Depression." In *Attachment and Loss III*. New York, NY: Basic, 1983.

———. "The Nature of the Child's Tie to His Mother." *International Journal of Psychoanalysis* 39 (1958).

Bretherton, Inge, and Kristine A. Munholland. "Internal Working Models of Attachment Relationships: A Construct Revisited." In *Handbook of Attachment*. Eds. Jude Cassidy and Phillip R. Shaver. New York, NY: The Guilford Press, 1999.

Capitanio, John, Michael Weissberg, and Martin Reite. "Biology of Maternal Behavior." In *Psychobiology of Attachment and Separation*. Eds. Martin Reite and Tiffany Field. San Diego, CA: Academic Press, 1985.

Chödrön, Pema. *When Things Fall Apart.* Boston, MA: Shambhala, 1997.

Chopich, Erika J., and Margaret Paul. *Healing Your Aloneness: Finding Love and Wholeness Through Your Inner Child.* San Francisco, CA: Harper, 1990.

Clark, Jeremy. *I Gave Dating a Chance.* Colorado Springs, CO: Waterbrook Press, 2000.

Cloninger, Robert. "A Unified Biosocial Theory of Personality and Its Role in Personality States." *Psychiatric Development* 4, no. 3 (1986): 167–226.

Coe, Christopher, Sandra Wiener, Leon Rosenbert, and Seymour Levine. "Endocrine and Immune Response to Separation and Maternal Loss in Nonhuman Primates." In *The Psychobiology of Attachment and Separation.* Eds. Martin Reite and Tiffany Field. San Diego, CA: Academic Press, 1985.

Colin, Virginia A. *Human Attachment.* Philadelphia, PA: Temple University Press, 1996.

Cooke, Robert. "Hatching a New Theory: Chick Experiment Sheds Light on Newborn Perception." *Newsday* (2002), p. A3.

———. "Mice over Matter: New Studies Counter Long-Held Beliefs about Brain Cell Growth." *Newsday,* February 26, 2002, pp. D3–11.

Coopersmith, Stanley. *The Antecedents of Self-Esteem.* San Francisco, CA: Freeman, 1967.

Cottle, Michelle. "Selling Shyness: How Doctors and Drug Companies Created the 'Social Phobia' Epidemic." *The New Republic,* August 2, 1999, pp. 24–29.

Crenshaw, Theresa. *The Alchemy of Love and Lust.* New York, NY: Putnam, 1996.

Damasio, Antonio. *Descartes' Error: Emotion, Reason, and the Human Brain.* New York, NY: Grosset/Putnam, 1994.

Dayton, Tian. *Heartwounds: The Impact of Unresolved Trauma and Grief on Relationships.* Deerfield Beach, CA: Health Communications, 1997.

Decasper, A. J., and W. P. Fif. "Of Human Bonding: Newborns Prefer Their Mother's Voices." *Science* 208, no. 4448 (1980).

Doka, Kenneth, ed. *Living with Grief after Sudden Loss: Suicide, Homicide, Accident, Heart Attack, Stroke.* Bristol, PA: Taylor & Francis, 1996.

Dugatkin, Lee Alan. *The Imitation Factor: Evolution Beyond the Gene.* New York, NY: Free Press, 2001.

Ekman, Paul. "Facial Expressions of Emotion: New Findings, New Questions." *Psychological Science* 3, no. 1 (1992): 34–38.

Eysenck, J. J. "Anxiety, Learned Helplessness and Cancer." *Journal of Anxiety Disorders* 1 (1987): 87–104.

Faludi, Susan. *Backlash: The Undeclared War against American Women.* New York, NY: Crown, 1991.

Field, Tiffany. "Attachment as Psychobiological Attunement: Being on the Same Wavelength." In *The Psychobiology of Attachment and Separation.* Eds. Martin Reite and Tiffany Field. San Diego, CA: Academic Press, 1985.

Fisher, Helen. *Anatomy of Love.* New York, NY: Faucet Columbine, 1992.

Fox, Nathan A. "Behavioral Antecedents of Attachment in High-Risk Infants." In *The Psychobiology of Attachment and Separation.* Eds. Martin Reite and Tiffany Field. San Diego, CA: Academic Press, 1985.

Francis, Darlene D., and Michael J. Meaney. "Maternal Care and the Development of Stress Response." *Current Opinion in Neurobiology* 9 (1999): 128–34.

Freud, Sigmund. *Mourning and Melancholia.* 1917.

Fromm, Eric. *The Art of Loving.* New York, NY. HarperCollins, 1989.

Gershon, Michael D. *The Second Brain.* New York, NY: HarperCollins 1998.

Gladwell, Malcolm. "Do Parents Matter?" *New Yorker,* August 17, 1998, pp. 54–64.

Goleman, Daniel. *Emotional Intelligence.* New York, NY: Bantam, 1995.

Gordon, Sol. *When Living Hurts.* New York, NY: Dell, 1983.

Gossette, Robert L., and Richard M. O'Brien. "The Efficacy of Rational Emotive Therapy in Adults: Clinical Fact or Psychometric Artifact?" *Journal of Behavior Therapy and Experimental Psychiatry* 23, no. 1 (1992): 9–24.

———. "Irrational Beliefs and Maladjustment: When Are Psychometric Effects Clinically Meaningful?" Paper presented at the 1990 Convention of the American Psychological Association, Boston, August 11, 1990.

Greene, Bob, and Oprah Winfrey. *Make the Connection: Ten Steps to a Better Body and Mind.* New York, NY: Hyperion, 1999.

Harris, Joshua. *I Kissed Dating Goodbye.* Sisters, OR: Multnomah Publishers Inc., 1997.

Harris, Judith. *The Nurture Assumption: Why Children Turn Out the Way They Do*. New York, NY: Free Press, 1998.

Hazon, Cindy, and Debra Zelfman. "Pair Bonds as Attachments: Evaluating the Evidence." In *Handbook of Attachment*. Eds. Jude Cassidy and Phillip R. Shaver. New York, NY: The Guilford Press, 1999.

Herman, Judith Lewis. *Trauma and Recovery*. New York, NY: Basic, 1992.

Hetherington, Mavis, and John Kelly. *For Better or for Worse: Divorce Reconsidered*. New York, NY: Norton, 2002.

Hobson, J. Allan. *The Dreaming Brain*. New York, NY: Basic, 1988.

Hobson, J. Allan, and Jonathan A. Leonard. *Out of Its Mind, Psychiatry in Crisis: A Call for Reform*. Cambridge, MA: Perseus, 2001.

Hofer, Myron. "An Evolutionary Perspective on Anxiety." In *Anxiety as Symptom and Signal*. Eds. S. Roose and R. Glick. Hillsdale, NJ: Analytic Press, 1995a.

———. "Hidden Regulators, Implications for a New Understanding of Attachment, Separation, and Loss." In *Attachment Theory: Social, Developmental and Clinical Perspectives*. Eds. S. Goldberg, R. Muir, and J. Kerr. Hillsdale, NJ: Analytic Press, 1995b.

Hoffman, Howard S. *Amorous Turkeys and Addicted Ducklings: A Search for the Causes of Social Attachment*. Sarasota, FL: Authors Cooperative Inc., 1994.

Holzel, Britta, E. Hoge, D. Greve, T. Gard, D. Creswell, et al. "Neural Mechanisms of Symptom Improvements in Generalized Anxiety Disorder Following Mindfulness Training." *Neuroimage: Clinical* 2 (2013): 448–58.

Horney, Karen. *Our Inner Conflicts: A Constructive Theory of Neurosis*. New York, NY: Norton, 1993.

Iacoboni, Marco. *Mirroring People*. New York, NY: Farrar, Straus and Giroux, 2008.

Kagan, Jerome. *Galen's Prophecy*. New York, NY: Basic, 1994.

———. *The Nature of a Child*. New York, NY: Basic, 1984.

Kandel, Eric R., James H. Schwartz, and Thomas M. Jessel. *Essentials of Neural Science and Behavior*. Norwalk, CT: Appleton & Lange, 1992.

———, eds. *Principals of Neural Science and Behavior*. Norwalk, CT: Appleton & Lange, 1992.

Kelly, D. D. "Stress-Induced Analgesia." *Annals of the New York Academy of Sciences* (1986).

Kernberg, Otto F. *Borderline Conditions and Pathological Narcissism*. Northvale, NJ: Aronson, 1975.

Kiecolt-Glaser, J. K., L. D. Fisher, P. Ogrocki, J. C. Stout, C. E. Speicher, and R. Glaser. "Marital Quality, Marital Disruption, and Immune Function." *Psychosomatic Medicine* 49, no. 1, (1987).

Kirsch, Irving, and Thomas J. Moore. "The Emperor's New Drugs: An Analysis of Antidepressant Medication Data Submitted to the U.S. Food and Drug Administration." *Prevention and Treatment* 5 (2002).

Kirsten, Grace Elish, and Richard Robertiello. *Big You Little You: Separation Therapy*. New York, NY: Dial Press, 1977.

Klein, D. F. "Listening to Meta-Analysis but Hearing Bias." *Prevention and Treatment* (1998).

Klein, Donald. "Anxiety Reconceptualized." In *Anxiety: New Research and Changing Concepts*. Eds. Donald Klein and Judith Rabkin. Philadelphia, PA: Raven Press, 1981.

Klein, Melanie. *Love, Guilt, and Reparation and Other Works 1921–1945*. New York, NY: Free Press, 1984.

———. "On the Theory of Anxiety and Guilt." In *Envy and Gratitude and Other Works 1946–1963*. New York, NY: Delacorte Press, 1975.

Kodis, Michele, David T. Moral, and David Berliner. *Love Scents: How Your Pheromones Influence Your Relationships, Your Moods, and Who You Love*. New York, NY: Dutton, 1998.

Kohut, H. *The Restoration of the Self*. Madison, WI: International Universities Press, 1977.

Kübler-Ross, Elisabeth. *On Death and Dying*. New York, NY: Simon & Schuster, 1969.

Kushner, Harold. *When Bad Things Happen to Good People*. New York, NY: Avon, 1997.

LeDoux, Joseph, *Anxious*. New York, NY: Viking, 2015.

———. "Emotion, Memory and the Brain." *Scientific American*, June 1994.

———. *Emotional Brain*. New York, NY: Simon & Schuster, 1996.

———. *The Synaptic Self*. New York, NY: Viking, 2002.

Lewis, Helen Block. *Shame and Guilt in Neurosis*. Madison, WI: International Universities Press, 1971.

Lewis, Michael. *Altering Fate: Why the Past Does Not Predict the Future*. New York, NY. Guilford, 1998.

———. *Shame: The Exposed Self*. New York, NY: Free Press, 1992.

Lucentini, Jack. "A Game of Cash and Carry a Grudge." *Newsday*, July 9, 2002, pp. D1–3.

Luskin, Fred. *Forgive for Good*. San Francisco, CA: Harper, 2002.

Lynch, William. *The Willie Lynch Letter and The Making of a Slave*. Chicago, IL: Lushena, 1999.

Madden, John, ed. *Neurobiology of Learning, Emotion and Affect*. New York, NY: Raven Press, 1991.

Mahler, Margaret. "On Human Symbiosis and the Vicissitudes of Individuation." In *Infantile Psychosis*. Madison, WI: International Universities Press, 1968.

Maier, Steven F., Linda R. Watkins, and Monika R. Fleshner. "Psychoneuroimmunology: The Interface Between Behavior, Brain and Immunity." *American Psychologist* 49 (1994): 1004–17.

Masterson, James F., ed. *New Perspectives of Psychotherapy of the Borderline Adult*. New York, NY: Brunner Mazel, 1978.

McKinney, William T. "Separation and Depression: Biological Markers." In *The Psychobiology of Attachment and Separation*. Eds. Martin Reite and Tiffany Field. San Diego, CA: Academic Press, 1985.

McLean, Paul. *The Triune Brain in Evolution*. New York, NY: Plenum Press, 1990.

Meadows, Susannah, "Meet the Gamma Girls." *Newsweek*, June 3, 2002.

Meaney, M. J., D. H. Aitken, and S. R. Bodnoff. "The Effects of Postnatal Handling on the Development of the Glucocorticoid Receptor Systems and Stress Recovery in the Rat." *Neuropsychopharmocology* 9, nos. 5–6: 731–34.

Miller, Alice. *The Drama of the Gifted Child*. New York, NY: Basic, 1997.

Millman, Marcia. *The Seven Stories of Love: How to Choose Your Happy Ending*. New York, NY: William Morrow, 2001.

Monti-Bloch, L., and B. I. Grosser. "Effect of Putative Pheromones on the Electrical Activity of the Human Vomeronasal Organ and Olfactory Epithelium." *Journal of Steroid Biochemistry and Molecular Biology* 39, no. 48 (2001): 537–82.

Morano, Hara Estroff. "Depression: Beyond Serotonin." *Psychology Today*, April 1999, pp. 30–76.

Murphy, Joseph. *The Power of Your Subconscious Mind*. New York, NY: Bantam, 2000.

Nader, Karim, Glenn E. Schafe, and Joseph E. LeDoux. "Fear Memories Require Protein Synthesis in the Amygdala for Reconsolidation after Retrieval." *Nature* 406 (2000): 722–26.

Nhat Hahn, Thich. *The Miracle of Mindfulness: A Manual on Meditation*. Boston, MA: Beacon Press, 1987.

Nidecker, Anna. "Maternal Deprivation Reduces Cortisol Levels." *Pediatric News* 32, no. 1 (1998): 10.

Panksepp, Jaak. *Advances in Biological Psychiatry*. Vol. 1. Greenwich, CT: JAI Press, 1996.

———. "The Emotional Brain and Biological Psychiatry." In *Advances in Biological Psychiatry* (269–86). Greenwich, CT. JAI Press, 1996.

Panksepp, Jaak, Eric Nelson, and Marni Bekkedal. "Brain Systems for the Mediation of Separation Distress and Social Reward." *Annals of the New York Academy of Sciences* 807 (1997): 78–100.

Panksepp, Jaak, Stephen M. Siviy, and Lawrence A. Normansell. "Brain Opioids and Social Emotions." In *The Psychobiology of Attachment and Separation*, Eds. Martin Reite and Tiffany Field. San Diego: Academic Press, 1985.

Parkes, C. M., and J. Stevenson-Hinde. *The Place of Attachment in Human Behavior*. New York, NY: Basic, 1982.

Parkes, C. M., J. Stevenson-Hinde, and P. Marris. *Attachments across the Life Cycle*. New York, NY: Routledge, 1991.

Pavlov, I. V. *Conditioned Reflexes*. Mineola, NY: Dover, 1922.

Pert, Candace B. *Molecules of Emotion*. New York, NY: Scribner, 1997.

Real, Terrance. *I Don't Want to Talk about It*. New York, NY: Scribner, 1997.

Riesberg, Barry. *Guide to Alzheimer's Disease*. New York, NY. Free Press, 1984.

Rinpoche, Sogyal. *The Tibetan Book of Living and Dying*. San Francisco, CA: Harper, 1994.

Robertiello, Richard. *Hold Them Very Close, Then Let Them Go*. New York, NY: Dial, 1975.

Robertiello, Richard, and Hollace M. Beer. "Bulimia as a Failure in Separation." *Journal of Contemporary Psychotherapy* 23, no. 1 (1993):41–45.

Robertiello, Richard, and Terril T. Gagnier. "Sado-Masochism as a Defense against Merging: Six Case Studies." *Journal of Contemporary Psychotherapy* 23, no. 3 (1993): 183–92.

Rothbaum, Fred, John Weisz, Martha Pott, Kazuo Miyake, and Gilda Morelli. "Attachment and Culture." *American Psychologist* 55, no. 10 (2000): pp. 1093–1104.

Rubin, Harriet. *The Princessa: Machiavelli for Women*. New York, NY: Doubleday, 1997.

Ruden, Ronald A., and Marcia Byalick. *The Craving Brain: The Biobalance Approach to Controlling Addiction*. New York, NY. HarperCollins, 1997.

Salamone, John D. "Antidepressants and Placebos: Conceptual Problems and Research Strategies." *Prevention and Treatment* 5 (2002).

Sapolsky, Robert M. *A Primate's Memoir: A Neuroscientist's Unconventional Life among Baboons.* New York, NY: Scribner, 2001.

———. "Social Subordinance as a Marker of Hypercortisolism." In *Social Subordinance: Annals of the New York Academy of Sciences* (626–38). New York, NY: Routledge, 1995.

———. *Why Zebras Don't Get Ulcers.* New York, NY: Freeman, 1994.

Schacter, Daniel. *The Seven Sins of Memory.* Boston, MA: Houghton Mifflin, 2001.

Schleifer, S. J., S. E. Keller, M. Camerino, J. C. Thornton, and M. Stein. "Suppression of Lymphocyte Stimulation Following Bereavement." *Journal of the American Medical Association* 250, no. 3 (1983): 374–77.

Schore, Allan. *Affect Regulation and Origin of Self: The Neurobiology of Emotional Development.* Mahwah, NJ: Erlbaum, 1994.

Seiver, Larry J., and William Frucht. *The New View of Self: How Genes and Neurotransmitters Shape Your Mind, Your Personality and Your Mental Health.* New York, NY: Macmillan, 1997.

Seligman, Martin. *Helplessness: On Depression, Development and Death.* San Francisco, CA: Freeman, 1975.

Selye, Hans. In *Advances in Psychoneuroimmunology.* Eds. Istvan Berczi and Judith Szelenyi. New York, NY: Plenum Press, 1994.

Serra, G., M. Collu, and G. L. Gessa. "Endorphins and Sexual Behavior." In *Endorphins, Opiates and Behavioral Processes.* New York, NY: Wiley, 1988.

Simao, Paul. "Study Contradicts Theory Suicide Is 'Contagious.'" *Reuters,* July 13, 2001.

Simons, Ronald. *Boo! Culture, Experience and the Startle Reflex.* New York, NY: Oxford University Press, 1996.

Slater, Lauren. "The Trouble with Self-Esteem." *New York Times Magazine,* February 3, 2002, pp. 45–48.

Smale, Steve. "The Prisoner's Dilemma and Dynamical Systems Associated to Noncooperative Games." *Econometrica* 48 (1980): 1617–34.

Smotherman, William P., and Scott R. Robinson. "The Development of Behavior before Birth." *Developmental Psychology* 32 (1996): 425–34.

Solomon, Andrew. *Noonday Demon: An Atlas of Depression.* New York, NY: Scribner, 2001.

Stanford, S. C., and P. Salmon. *Stress: From Synapse to Syndrome.* San Diego, CA; Academic Press, 1993.

Sternberg, Esther. *The Balance Within: The Science Connecting Health and Emotions.* New York, NY: Freeman, 2001.

Suomi, Stephen. "Early Stress and Adult Emotional Reactivity in Rhesus Monkeys." In *The Childhood Environment and Adult Disease.* New York, NY: Wiley, 1991.

Suomi, Stephen J. "Primate Separation Models of Affective Disorders." In *Neurobiology of Learning, Emotion and Affect.* Vol. 4. Ed. John Madden. Philadelphia, PA: Raven Press, 1991b.

Talan, Jamie. "Doubts on Debriefing." *Newsday,* October 2, 2001, pp. C3–6.

———. "A Neuron Link to Motivation, Reward." *Newsday,* June 11, 2002e.

———. "New Drug Treats Heroin Addiction." *Newsday,* May 22, 2002d, p. A22.

———. "Special Protein Linked to Less Forgetful Fruit Flies." *Newsday,* April 2, 2002c, p. D5.

———. "Targeting the Structure of Horrific Memories." *Newsday,* January 29, 2002a, pp. D5–7.

———. "Technique Offers Hope to Addicts." *Newsday,* 2002f, p. A35.

———. "Where in the Brain Is Our Identity?" *Newsday,* January 29, 2002b.

Talbot, Margaret. "Attachment Theory: The Ultimate Experiment." *New York Times Magazine,* May 24, 1998, pp. 24–54.

Tavris, Carol. *Anger: The Misunderstood Emotion.* New York, NY: Touchstone, 1989.

Taylor, Shelly, L. C. Klein, B. P. Lewis, T. L. Gruenewald, R. A. Gurung, and J. A. Updegraff. "Female Responses to Stress: Tend and Befriend, Not Fight or Flight." *Psychological Review* 107, no. 3 (2000): 41.

Templeton, Alan R. "The Genetic and Evolutionary Significance of Human Races." In *Race and Intelligence: Separating Science from Myth.* Ed. Jefferson M. Fish. Mahwah, NJ: Erlbaum, 2002.

Tice, Diane, and Roy Baumeister. "Self-Induced Emotion Change." In *Handbook of Mental Control.* Eds. Daniel M. Wegner and James W. Pennebaker. Paramus, NJ: Prentice Hall, 1992.

Tully, Tim. "Fruit Flies, Mind, You." Lecture presented at the Cold Spring Harbor Laboratory, Cold Spring Harbor, NY, November 6, 2001.

Van der Kolk, Bessel A., Alexander C. McFarlane, and Lars Weisaeth. *Traumatic Stress: The Effects of Overwhelming Experience on Mind, Body, and Society.* New York, NY: Guilford Press, 1996.

Vaughan, Susan. *The Talking Cure. The Science Behind Psychotherapy.* New York, NY: Grosset/Putnam, 1997.

Vedamtam, Shankar. "Against Depression, a Sugar Pill Is Hard to Beat: Placebos Improve Mood, Change Brain Chemistry in Majority of Trials of Antidepressants." *Washington Post*, May 7, 2002.

Vormbrock, Julia K. "Attachment Theory as Applied to Wartime and Job-Related Marital Separation." *Psychological Bulletin* 114 (1993): 122–44.

Wallerstein, Judith S. *The Unexpected Legacy of Divorce: A 25-Year Landmark Study.* New York, NY: Hyperion, 2001.

Wapner, S., R. Ciottone, G. Hornstein, O. McNeil, and A. M. Pacheco. "An Examination of Studies of Critical Transitions throughout the Life Cycle." In *Toward a Holistic Developmental Psychology* (111–32). Eds. S. Wapner and B. Kaplan. Mahwah, NJ: Erlbaum, 1983.

Watzlawick, Paul, John Weakland, and Richard Risch. *Change: Principles of Problem Formation and Problem Resolution.* New York, NY: Norton, 1974.

Weiner, H., M. A. Hofer, and A. J. Stunkard. *Brain, Behavior and Bodily Disease.* New York, NY: Raven Press, 1981.

Weiner, Herbert. *Perturbing the Organism: The Biology of Stressful Experience.* Chicago, IL: University of Chicago Press, 1992.

Weiss, Jay M. "Stress-Induced Depression: Critical Neurochemical and Electrophysiological Changes." In *Neurobiology of Learning, Emotion and Affect.* Ed. John Madden. New York, NY: Raven Press, 1991.

Weiss, R. S. *Loneliness: The Experience of Emotional and Social Isolation.* Cambridge, MA: MIT Press, 1973.

———. *Marital Separation: Coping with the End of a Marriage and the Transition to Being Single Again.* New York, NY: Basic Books, 1975.

West, Jean. "Children's Drug Is More Potent Than Cocaine." *The Observer*, September 9, 2001.

Wilson, E. O. *Consilience: The Unity of Knowledge.* New York, NY: Knopf, 1998.

Winnecott, Donald W. "The Capacity to Be Alone." In *The Maturational Processes and the Facilitating Environment: Studies in the Theory of Emotional Development.* Madison, WI: International Universities Press, 1965.

Wise, Roy A. "The Neurobiology of Craving: Implications for the Understanding and Treatment of Addiction." *Journal of Abnormal Psychology* 97, no. 2 (1988): 118–32.

Wolff, P. H. "The Serial Organization of Sucking in the Young Infant." *Pediatrics* 42 (1968): 943–56.

Worthington, Everett. *Five Steps to Forgiveness: The Art and Science of Forgiving.* New York, NY: Crown, 2002.

Yalom, Irvin. *When Nietzsche Wept.* New York, NY: Basic, 1992.

Zillman, Doll. "Mental Control of Angry Aggression." In *Handbook of Mental Control.* Eds. C. M. Wegner and J. W. Pennebaker. Paramus, NJ: Prentice Hall, 1992.

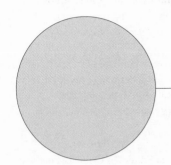

Index

About the Author

Susan Anderson is a psychotherapist who has specialized in heartbreak, loss, and abandonment for more than thirty years. The author of *The Journey from Abandonment to Healing, Taming Your Outer Child*, and *Black Swan: 12 Lessons of Abandonment Recovery*, she founded the abandonment recovery movement, offering a program of abandonment support groups and new techniques. She leads workshops across the country and reaches out through her website (www.abandonment.net) to bring her message of healing to abandonment survivors as well as clinicians.

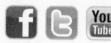
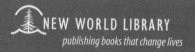